Rethinking Artful Politics: Bodies of Difference Remaking Body Worlds

Rethinking Artful Politics: Bodies of Difference Remaking Body Worlds

Editors

Nadine Changfoot
Carla Rice
Eliza Chandler

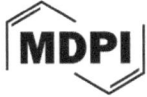

Basel • Beijing • Wuhan • Barcelona • Belgrade • Novi Sad • Cluj • Manchester

Editors
Nadine Changfoot
Trent University
Peterborough, ON
Canada

Carla Rice
University of Guelph
Guelph, ON
Canada

Eliza Chandler
Toronto Metropolitan University
Toronto, ON
Canada

Editorial Office
MDPI AG
Grosspeteranlage 5
4052 Basel, Switzerland

This is a reprint of articles from the Special Issue published online in the open access journal *Social Sciences* (ISSN 2076-0760) (available at: https://www.mdpi.com/journal/socsci/special_issues/Artful_Politics).

For citation purposes, cite each article independently as indicated on the article page online and as indicated below:

Lastname, Firstname, Firstname Lastname, and Firstname Lastname. Article Title. *Journal Name* **Year**, *Volume Number*, Page Range.

ISBN 978-3-7258-2109-9 (Hbk)
ISBN 978-3-7258-2110-5 (PDF)
doi.org/10.3390/books978-3-7258-2110-5

Cover image courtesy of Aimée Anctil and Nadine Changfoot.
This image evokes amplification, amplification of diverse disability arts-based knowledge within these articles.

© 2024 by the authors. Articles in this book are Open Access and distributed under the Creative Commons Attribution (CC BY) license. The book as a whole is distributed by MDPI under the terms and conditions of the Creative Commons Attribution-NonCommercial-NoDerivs (CC BY-NC-ND) license.

Contents

About the Editors vii

Preface ix

Nadine Changfoot, Carla Rice and Eliza Chandler
Introduction to the Special Issue "Rethinking Artful Politics: Bodies of Difference Remaking Body Worlds"
Reprinted from: *Soc. Sci.* **2024**, *13*, 304, doi:10.3390/socsci13060304 1

Evadne Kelly, Carla Rice and Mona Stonefish
Towards Decolonial Choreographies of Co-Resistance
Reprinted from: *Soc. Sci.* **2023**, *12*, 204, doi:10.3390/socsci12040204 7

Jenelle Rouse, Amelia Palmer and Amy Parsons
Reconstruct(ing) a Hidden History: Black Deaf Canadian Relat(ing) Identity
Reprinted from: *Soc. Sci.* **2023**, *12*, 305, doi:10.3390/socsci12050305 22

Chelsea Temple Jones, Joanne Weber, Abneet Atwal and Helen Pridmore
Dinner Table Experience in the Flyover Provinces: A Bricolage of Rural Deaf and Disabled Artistry in Saskatchewan
Reprinted from: *Soc. Sci.* **2023**, *12*, 125, doi:10.3390/socsci12030125 40

May Chazan
Crip Time and Radical Care in/as Artful Politics
Reprinted from: *Soc. Sci.* **2023**, *12*, 99, doi:10.3390/socsci12020099 59

Luis R. Alvarez-Hernandez and Maureen Flint
Epistemological Weaving: Writing and Sense Making in Qualitative Research with Gloria Anzaldúa
Reprinted from: *Soc. Sci.* **2023**, *12*, 408, doi:10.3390/socsci12070408 76

Ben Barry, Philippa Nesbitt, Alexis De Villa, Kristina McMullin and Jonathan Dumitra
Re-Making Clothing, Re-Making Worlds: On Crip Fashion Hacking
Reprinted from: *Soc. Sci.* **2023**, *12*, 500, doi:10.3390/socsci12090500 90

Allison Taylor, Allyson Mitchell and Carla Rice
Performing Fat Liberation: Pretty Porky and Pissed Off's Affective Politics and Archive
Reprinted from: *Soc. Sci.* **2023**, *12*, 270, doi:10.3390/socsci12050270 113

Meredith Bessey, K. Aly Bailey, Kayla Besse, Carla Rice, Salima Punjani and Tara-Leigh F. McHugh
Revisioning Fitness through a Relational Community of Practice: Conditions of Possibility for Access Intimacies and Body-Becoming Pedagogies through Art Making
Reprinted from: *Soc. Sci.* **2023**, *12*, 584, doi:10.3390/socsci12100584 128

Rosa Lea McBee
"It Really Put a Change on Me": Visualizing (Dis)connections within a Photovoice Project in Peterborough/ Nogojiwanong, Ontario
Reprinted from: *Soc. Sci.* **2023**, *12*, 488, doi:10.3390/socsci12090488 144

An Kosurko and Melisa Stevanovic
Beyond Utterances: Embodied Creativity and Compliance in Dance and Dementia
Reprinted from: *Soc. Sci.* **2023**, *12*, 304, doi:10.3390/socsci12050304 161

Andrea LaMarre, Siobhán Healy-Cullen, Jessica Tappin and Maree Burns
Honouring Differences in Recovery: Methodological Explorations in Creative Eating Disorder Recovery Research
Reprinted from: *Soc. Sci.* **2023**, *12*, 251, doi:10.3390/socsci12040251 . . . . **182**

About the Editors

Nadine Changfoot

Nadine Changfoot is a Full Professor in Political Studies at Trent University, Peterborough/ Nogojiwanong (Canada, part of Turtle Island), which is on the traditional territories of the Michi Saagig Anishinaabeg covered by the Williams Treaties (1818). She serves as Acting Director of the Trent Centre for Aging & Society and as Board Member of EC3, the City of Peterborough's Arts Council. She is a Senior Research Associate with Re•Vision: The Centre for Art and Social Justice (University of Guelph). With Re•Vision and as the Trent Lead of the SSHRC funded partnership project *Bodies in Translation: Activist Art, Technology and Access to Life*, she leads projects partnering with Anishinaabekwe e/Elders and settler, Black, racialized, queer, disabled, older adults, and youth to bring new and prideful cultural representations and embodied movement of Anishinaabe knowledge, aging, and disability into the world. She has published widely in journals that focus on aging, the arts, community development, community-engaged research, philosophy, political science, and sociology.

Carla Rice

Dr. Carla Rice is a Tier I Canada Research Chair in Feminist Studies and Social Practice at the University of Guelph. She is an internationally known scholar who specializes in non-normative embodiments, feminist/intersectionality studies, and arts-based research methods. At the University of Guelph, Rice founded the Re•Vision Centre for Art and Social Justice, a cutting-edge research creation centre and state-of-the-art traveling media lab, which explores how communities can use story and arts-informed research methods to advance social inclusion, well-being, and justice. She has published five books with three more under contract, 110 refereed papers (published/in press/submitted to the world's highest-ranking feminist and critical theory/methods journals), over 40 refereed book chapters, 32 invited papers/articles, and 17 reports/ manuals; mentored 50+ students in scholarships and research; produced an archive of close to 1000 films; and delivered hundreds of training workshops, consultations, and presentations, including over 290 refereed paper presentations and 200+ non-refereed talks and workshops. Her co-edited book (with Marg Hobbs) *Gender and Women's Studies: Critical Terrain* is now in its second edition. Achieving the rank of full professor, she has received five awards for advocacy, research, mentorship, and teaching and was inducted into the Royal Society of Canada, College of New Scholars, Artists and Scientists, in 2017. She currently directs 10 research programs and co-investigates nine initiatives, representing close to CAD 10 million, 180+ researchers, and 40 Canadian and 7 international universities.

Eliza Chandler

Dr. Eliza Chandler is the Executive Director of the Office of Social Innovation and an Associate Professor in the School of Disability Studies at Toronto Metropolitan University. In these roles she leads a research program that animates disability arts and its connections to disability rights and justice. This research interest came into focus when, from 2014 to 2016, she was the inaugural artistic director of Tangled Art + Disability, an organization based in Toronto dedicated to showcasing disability arts and advancing accessible curatorial practice. Dr. Chandler teaches in the areas of disability arts, critical access studies, social movements, and crip technoscience and participates in a number of research projects in these areas, including co-directing the SSHRC-funded partnership project *Bodies in Translation*: *Activist Art*, *Technology*, and *Access to Life*. Chandler regularly gives lectures on disability arts, accessible curatorial practices, and disability politics in Canada, and she is a member of the Royal Society of Canada's College of New Scholars.

Preface

"Rethinking Artful Politics: Bodies of Difference Remaking Body Worlds" was imagined and proposed as the COVID-19 pandemic was becoming less severe and less deadly in the mainstream. Yet, there are body–minds constituted and positioned by power relations in ways that are exclusionary and deny the quality of life of those whose struggles prior to and after COVID-19 were/are ignored and continue to be. Under "return-to-normal" conditions that deny the continuation of a pandemic for vulnerable groups, lower income, poor, disabled, racialized, older, queer, and Indigenous peoples continue to be impacted by multiple intersecting crises related to the pandemic in addition to issues concerning high inflation, housing, food, income, healthcare, long term care, and climate change. Still, we know from our own research contexts that artist–researchers continue to act in response to the pandemic and its aftermath, and in spite of this, pursue meaningful and transformative change in the daily and future life/lives of themselves and communities proudly non-normatively identified.

We designed our call for proposals as an intervention to shine a light on the work done by arts-based research to provide much-needed space for examining the agency and vitality of difference while creating and transforming new/old agential possibilities as new worlds affirming differences come into view. We cast as wide a creative net as possible, welcoming all arts and arts-based research and bodies of difference as they are located and engaged in the wide-ranging and diversely located political work of disrupting and re-engaging power to create worlds where difference can find a home, understanding that "home" is iterative and an ongoing political project. We know that non-normative difference is active in the world, intent on remaking worlds for bodies of difference. This volume brings together research that represents diverse communities (Indigenous, aging, Black, disabled, Deaf, fat, low income, racialized, queer, urban, and rural communities) and serves as a collective exemplar of the political possibilities of art by and for the proudly non-normative.

The eleven chapters in this reprint exceed our expectations in both scope and depth, and we express our deep gratitude to our contributors. For those interested and engaged in arts-based methodology as generative, non-normative worldmaking, this collection provides an impressive array of arts-based research that includes autoethnography, archival review, artful community-based research, choreography as political movement, communities of practice, dance, Deaf jams, digital storytelling, epistemological weaving, ethnomethodology, fashion hacking, and photovoice. Another layer of generative complexity of the collection is that the arts-based methodologies explored herein are located within critical bodies of knowledge that orient toward new world makings, including aging studies, Black studies, critical disability studies, critical race studies, Deaf studies, disability studies, fat studies, feminist studies, Indigenous studies, posthumanism, and queer studies.

This volume is intentionally interdisciplinary, attracting interdisciplinary advocates, activists, artists, students, and researchers from different social locations and positionalities. Reading this volume will enlighten readers of the pathways made possible by and for bodies of difference and worldmaking that come into view and can be effectively experienced. We feel energized and hopeful for all of the ongoing artistic and artful labour and crip time that the chapters convey even while we understand that this labour is undertaken at odds and within dominant normative contexts and timescapes to create possibilities otherwise.

We are profoundly grateful to and deeply respect each of our fine contributors: Luis Alvarez-Hernandez, Abneet Atwal, Aly Bailey, Ben Barry, Kayla Besse, Meredith Bessey, Maree Burns, May Chazan, Alexis De Villa, Jonathan Dumitra, Maureen Flint, Siobhán Healy-Cullen, Chelsea Temple Jones, Evadne Kelly, An Kosurko, Andrea LaMarre, Rosa McBee, Tara-Leigh McHugh, Kristina

McMullin, Allyson Mitchell, Philippa Nesbitt, Amelia Palmer, Amy Parsons, Helen Pridmore, Salima Punjani, Jenelle Rouse, Melisa Stevanovic, Mona Stonefish, Jessica Tappin, Allison Taylor, Joanne Weber. It has been a joy and generative experience working with you. We also thank Aimée-Marie Anctil, Emmaleigh Dew, Megan Johnson, and Isabelle Row for their much appreciated research assistance.

Our gratitude also extends to the always positive and supportive Yvaine Sun of *Social Sciences* and the Multidisciplinary Digital Publishing Institute (MDPI). Yvaine and her editorial team have been with us every step of the way in the process of bringing this collection together and understanding our crip timescapes informed by and in resistance to Covid and neoliberal, normative systems.

Nadine Changfoot, Carla Rice, and Eliza Chandler
Editors

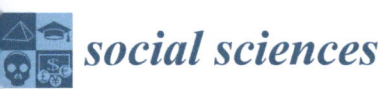

Editorial

Introduction to the Special Issue "Rethinking Artful Politics: Bodies of Difference Remaking Body Worlds"

Nadine Changfoot [1,*], Carla Rice [2] and Eliza Chandler [3]

1. Department of Political Studies and Trent Centre for Aging & Society, Trent University, Peterborough, ON K9L 0G2, Canada
2. Re•Vision: The Centre for Art and Social Justice, University of Guelph, Guelph, ON N1G 2W1, Canada; carlar@uoguelph.ca
3. School of Disability Studies, Toronto Metropolitan University, Toronto, ON M5B 2K3, Canada; eliza.chandler@torontomu.ca
* Correspondence: nadinechangfoot@trentu.ca

"Rethinking Artful Politics: Bodies of Difference Remaking Body Worlds" is a robust Special Issue comprising 11 scholarly articles on the nexus of art and politics. Together, the collection aims to demonstrate how critical scholarship/artistic praxis, which affirms difference within difference-attuned contexts, can carve out change-making pathways and build new worlds wherein non-normativity itself materializes differently—as political, as artful, and as vital. Such work is critically important as imagining worlds desirous of difference provides members of justice movements with multiple and potent directions for transformational change. Attentive to this desire, we begin with a question posed by one of us (Carla Rice) prior to the start of this project: "How do we create a world where difference is not merely tolerated, but anticipated and welcomed as basic to life and as critical to the story of humanity itself"? As we developed our Call for Proposals (CFP) and began working directly with contributing authors, we realized anew how an important part of the answer to this question lies in the worldmaking potential of art. As such, the collection of manuscripts that make up "Rethinking Artful Politics" animates worlds made by those living with difference via art, art-based research, and research creation methods. We conducted what we refer to as 'friendly reviews' of all articles prior to kickstarting the official peer review process. We also worked with each of the authors and their manuscripts until we agreed (found consensus among us) that the pieces were ready for anonymous review. All articles were reviewed by at least two peer reviewers. Where there was discrepancy between reviewers and authors, we provided authors with the opportunity to respond to the reviewers' comments and sent the revised articles to reviewers for re-review. A compelling collection was compiled through this multiple review process.

Art, as a method for prefiguring and imagining worlds, is a political intervention (Haritaworn et al. 2018). Art orients to (re)worlding in affective, cultural, imaginative, and justice-attuned (re)ordering ways (Chandler 2018; Cachia 2022; Fatona 2014; Kuppers 2022; Rice et al. 2024; Weber 2024). In so doing, art (re)visions, activates, produces, and propels cultural and political transformations with ripple effects through assemblages (the coming together of art with human bodies, technologies, relationalities, physical spaces, audience meanings and affects, cultural and social institutions, economies, etc.) at multiple scales—local, regional, national, and transnational. Art that leads with, centres, and desires difference prefigures and materializes an infinite array of lived experiences into new aesthetics and possibilities for worldmaking (Rice and Mündel 2018). Art practices, performances, exhibitions, curatorial framings, and documentary artifacts become spaces for artists, critical theorists, and creative methodologists to engage directly in cultural expression and resistance, imagining and enacting social justice as praxis, and offering rich spaces for political possibilities for difference. Art expresses and ciphers diverse and divergent materialities and futurities. Therefore, accessing art is necessary for accessing

---

Citation: Changfoot, Nadine, Carla Rice, and Eliza Chandler. 2024. Introduction to the Special Issue Rethinking Artful Politics: Bodies of Difference Remaking Body Worlds". *Social Sciences* 13: 304. https://doi.org/10.3390/socsci13060304

Received: 3 April 2024
Accepted: 4 April 2024
Published: 5 June 2024

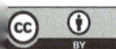

Copyright: © 2024 by the authors. Licensee MDPI, Basel, Switzerland. This article is an open access article distributed under the terms and conditions of the Creative Commons Attribution (CC BY) license (https://creativecommons.org/licenses/by/4.0/).

life. This issue understands art broadly and expansively, as including the creation of new aesthetics; methodologies/artful methods of inquiry; and new futurities, politics, and political possibilities. Moreover, activist art also enables us to open up performance, installation, curation, and audience reception practices. Similarly, we understand "politics" broadly and expansively, as in opposition, resistance, redistribution, movement(s), intervention(s), or assemblages within relations of power visible and invisible for equity and/or world-(re)making.

This Special Issue is inspired by "Bodies in Translation: Activist Art, Technology and Access to Life", a research project based in Canada at the University of Guelph with projects at Toronto Metropolitan University and Trent University, among many other universities and arts organizations in and beyond the northern part of Turtle Island. Research within "Bodies in Translation" is animated by two guiding propositions: First, we incite and catalyse generative collaborations among artists and academics across disciplinary, sectorial, cultural, and other divides. Second, we centralize diverse artist practitioners culturally, cognitively, affectively, and physically as members of communities whose perspectives, agency, and self-representations have been marginalized from mainstream social discourses, cultural landscapes, and art institutions across the land now called Canada (the northern part of Turtle Island) (Bobier and Ignagni 2021; Bodies in Translation n.d.; Changfoot 2016; Gold 2021; Mohr-Blakeney and Changfoot 2018; Swain 2019). The perspectives and communities within these articles proudly include the following: Anishinaabeg, Black, d/Deaf, people of colour, disabled, fat/thicc, low income, mad, neurodivergent, queer, persons living with dementia, and persons living with mental differences and distresses.

We solicited and welcomed proposals that address the methodology and process, including inter- and transdisciplinary approaches to art as a methodology and to methodology as an art. The impact of the work included is felt broadly and at diverse scales. For example, the manuscripts have impacts for artists/art generators themselves, communities and audiences, and curators and curational approaches, including collaborations, partnerships, and policies. We especially welcomed articles that include and/or incorporate perspectives and voices of non-academic partners because we understand that partnerships are often at the centre of art generation, curation, and production.

Common to all the articles in "Rethinking Artful Politics" is the diverse worldmaking well underway from diverse localities of difference. Worldmaking emerges from the realization that complex relationalities propelled by uneven power relations (including both power to and power over) shape spaces, places, notions of time, humans, cultures, and human responses to/interactions with the more-than-human world (technology, the built environment, living environments, land, animals, and plants). Through putting these and other human/more-than-human relationalities under question, critical scholars and artists create microworlds for difference to become and to flourish—in research processes and ideas generated, in the relationalities enacted and extended, and in the artistic works created (Simpson 2017; Piepzna-Samarasinha 2022; Rice et al. 2022). For bell hooks, this entails "imagining possible futures, a place where life could be lived differently" (Hooks 1994, p. 61). Worldmaking encompasses many imagined possibilities.

Decolonizing and indigenizing worlds led by Indigenous persons is crucial (Lavallee 2020; Stonefish et al. 2019). This is especially the case for us writing from the Anglo-Franco settler colonial context of Canada where Indigenous peoples and settler allies continue to make political strides to hold Canadian governments accountable to the 94 Calls to Action recommended by our national Truth and Reconciliation Commission of Canada (2015). This world building can be achieved artfully and collaboratively. As Evadne Kelly, Carla Rice, and Mona Stonefish (Bear Clan) demonstrate, rethinking movement by a "coalition of co-resisters" (2023, p. 1) is itself a critical methodology that reveals at once the eugenics entwined with settler movement practices *and* the decolonizing interventions that reclaim/enact the Anishinaabe understanding of the inseparability of our bodies and worlds—or the connectedness of the human with land, water, and sky that affirms our "mutual difference." They do this with and alongside their co-curation of the award-winning exhibit "Into the Light" (Stonefish et al. 2019; Kelly et al. 2021), which examines how eugenics thinking continues to influence education, healthcare, culture, and politics. With their movement practice, they demonstrate that meaningful decolonizing/reclaiming/enacting of Anishinaabe knowledge cannot be achieved without attention to eugenics in the ongoing legacy of settler colonialism in quotidian life. This is a powerful example of an artistic and artful rethinking and enacting of politics.

All the articles in "Rethinking Artful Politics" employ art-based methodologies and research creation methods informed by a range of critical theories and activist research practices, including critical disability and access studies, critical race theory, fashion studies, fat studies, posthumanism, feminism, participatory action research, human-centred design, and auto and ethnomethodology, etc. These theoretical and methodological approaches not only become sites from which to imagine possible futures, but these ways of thinking and doing also *materialize* them—that is, bring futures just out of reach into the thick present through co-created, collective efforts (Rice et al. 2024). Part of this imagining comes from identifying possibilities in diverse places and everyday life anew. This can be, for example, at a d/Deaf-centred jam session dinner table where improvisation brings into being a desired, cripped collective assemblage (Jones et al. 2023). Possibilities can also emerge through a social media call that brings together Black Deaf persons who then collectively and inaugurally materialize Black Deaf Canadian identities using community-based research to (re)discover and affirm "relating" Black Deaf persons in Canada (Rouse et al. 2023). When neoliberal timescapes become crushing, crip agency enacts crip time and possibilities that bring together work, care, and community to create workable and caring spaces (Chazan 2023).

From the articles in "Rethinking Artful Politics", spaces of difference and otherwise worlds can also include fashion hacking workshops as well as online dance classes with persons living with dementia and in community-created neighbourhood spaces. For example, fashion researchers create a series of fashion hacking workshops inviting disabled, D/deaf, and mad-identified men and masculine non-binary people to explore how they might recreate existing wardrobe items "to support their physical, emotional and spiritual needs" (Barry et al. 2023). In an online dance class, persons with dementia and co-present facilitators use improvisation and reciprocal interaction-expanded and -transformed understandings of co-creation itself (Kosurko and Stevanovic 2023). Further. through the NeighbourPLAN photovoice project in Peterborough/Nogojiwanong, downtown residents at the intersections of disability and low-income come together using photovoice to understand renewed connections with places meaningful to them and with one another (McBee 2023).

These articles artfully demonstrate how researchers use arts-based methodologies to refuse dominant understandings of normativity (norms premised upon mythical ableist, ageist, white, cisgender, heteronormative standards that become normalizing) associated with a range of norms that govern our lives: notions of what it means to "recover" from eating and body-related distresses, from contemporary ideals of fitness, from fat hate, and from the difficult intellectual-affective work of producing decolonial knowledge inside colonial institutions. Art making becomes a series of refusals to remain contained within the given lines through unpredictable expressive acts that seek to proliferate possibilities for care and repair. Artful recoveries move away from universalizing and standardized responses for recovery from mental health distresses that systemically pressure persons labelled with them in healthcare structures (LaMarre et al. 2023). A Fitness Community of Practice (CoP) comprised of gender diverse disabled, queer, fat, thicc, and racialized persons is thickened, cripped, and made queer when these bodies come together to co-create, celebrate, and welcome rest in a fitness world replete with micro-activist affordances (Bessey et al. 2023). Auto/ethnographic explorations into the archive (consisting of performance videos, posters, emails, administrivia, etc.) of the queer feminist fat performance collective *Pretty, Porky, and Pissed Off* show the "liberatory, life-affirming, and life-giving potential" of fat embodiment and activism (Taylor et al. 2023). Even relational spaces thought more traditional, such as professor-doctoral student relationships, transform when students and professors centre difference, demonstrating that writing can become a creative conversation between supervisor, student, and guiding theorist, in this case, Gloria Anzaldúa, that opens onto new thresholds of Anzaldúa-inspired and informed queer Chicana knowledge (Alvarez-Hernandez and Flint 2023).

These places each have a vitality made intelligible by the authors and their research partners. How they are brought into the present and explored also demonstrates the extraordinary care with which the makers create their work, and the vulnerability and agency associated with their co-creation. Without collapsing difference within the worlds collectively prefigured across the articles, strong affective and reciprocal relations clearly come across in the research relationship evoked by each of them. Affect and reciprocity are entwined through the interactions of research partners/participants as well as research and art creation to materialize multidimensional affects and effects of joy, identity-creation and identity-validation, connection, community, alternative herstories/theirstories, and liveable lives. This represents life-giving and life-sustaining politics through art in the refusal and resistance to power "over" relations that control, extract, manipulate, and deny life (e.g., colonialism, racism, ableism, fat hatred, normative recovery). These articles do not claim that art in its political intent and activism is the only pathway to justice that is truly welcoming and sustaining of difference. While not directly policy-oriented, each article offers difference-attuned inspiration (Rice et al. 2021) for policy that is equity-focused rather than based on narrow, normative standards of neoliberal individualism. Such standards often assume and endorse mythical self-sufficiency, able-bodiedness and enmindedness, cisheteronormativity, successful aging, and being well resourced. The research specific to each article and the worlds brought to light are given a provisional "ending" that occurs within the framing of the genre of the "scholarly article". Yet, there is important natality to them that researchers identify for continued research for worldmaking. Additionally, readers will wonder, hope, and support their continued flourishment and growth that is iterative for possibilities to carry and continue to enact these new worlds into the future. In doing so, we are excited for the continued and generative centring of difference with art-based methodologies in service of bodies of difference and the worlds they prefigure and create.

Funding: We acknowledge and thank "Bodies in Translation: Activist Art, Technology, and Access to Life", a research project funded by the Social Sciences and Humanities Research Council of Canada (#895-2016-1024) that supports our collective work.

Acknowledgments: We are also indebted to the artists and scholars featured in this Special Issue for creating and theorizing work that pushes our thinking and provokes us to consider anew the centrality of art in the making of difference-attuned worlds. We thank Aimée-Marie Anctil, Emmaleigh Dew, and Megan Johnson for their much-appreciated research assistance in support of this Special Issue.

Conflicts of Interest: The authors declare no conflicts of interest.

List of Contributions:

1. Alvarez-Hernandez, Luis R., and Maureen Flint. 2023. "Epistemological Weaving: Writing and Sense Making in Qualitative Research with Gloria Anzaldúa". *Social Sciences* 12: 408. https://doi.org/10.3390/socsci12070408.
2. Bessey, Meredith, K. Aly Bailey, Kayla Besse, Carla Rice, Salima Punjani, and Tara-Leigh F McHugh. 2023. "Revisioning Fitness through a Relational Community of Practice: Conditions of Possibility for Access Intimacies and Body-Becoming Pedagogies through Art Making". *Social Sciences* 12: 584. https://doi.org/10.3390/socsci12100584.
3. Barry, Ben, Philippa Nesbitt, Alexis De Villa, Kristina McMullin, and Jonathan Dumitra. 2023 "Re-Making Clothing, Re-Making Worlds: On Crip Fashion Hacking". *Social Sciences* 12: 500 https://doi.org/10.3390/socsci12090500.
4. Chazan, May. 2023. "Crip Time and Radical Care in/as Artful Politics". *Social Sciences* 12: 99 https://doi.org/10.3390/socsci12020099.

5. Jones, Chelsea Temple, Joanne Weber, Abneet Atwal, and Helen Pridmore. 2023. "Dinner Table Experience in the Flyover Provinces: A Bricolage of Rural Deaf and Disabled Artistry in Saskatchewan". *Social Sciences* 12: 125. https://doi.org/10.3390/socsci12030125.
6. Kelly, Evadne, Carla Rice, and Mona Stonefish. 2023. "Towards Decolonial Choreographies of Co-Resistance". *Social Sciences* 12: 204. https://doi.org/10.3390/socsci12040204.
7. Kosurko, An, and Melisa Stevanovic. 2023. "Beyond Utterances: Embodied Creativity and Compliance in Dance and Dementia". *Social Sciences* 12: 304. https://doi.org/10.3390/socsci12050304.
8. LaMarre, Andrea, Siobhán Healy-Cullen, Jessica Tappin, and Maree Burns. 2023. "Honouring Differences in Recovery: Methodological Explorations in Creative Eating Disorder Recovery Research". *Social Sciences* 12: 251. https://doi.org/10.3390/socsci12040251.
9. McBee, Rosa Lea. 2023. "It Really Put a Change on Me: Visualizing (Dis)connections within a Photovoice Project in Peterborough/Nogojiwanong, Ontario". *Social Sciences* 12: 488. https://doi.org/10.3390/socsci12090488.
10. Rouse, Jenelle, Amelia Palmer, and Amy Parsons. 2023. "Reconstruct(ing) a Hidden History: Black Deaf Canadian Relat(ing) Identity". *Social Sciences* 12: 305. https://doi.org/10.3390/socsci12050305.
11. Taylor, Allison, Allyson Mitchell, and Carla Rice. 2023. "Performing Fat Liberation: Pretty Porky and Pissed Off's Affective Politics and Archive". *Social Sciences* 12: 270. https://doi.org/10.3390/socsci12050270.

References

Bobier, David, and Esther Ignagni. 2021. Interview with David Bobier (Dispatch). *Studies in Social Justice* 15: 282–87. [CrossRef]
Bodies in Translation: Activist Art, Technology, and Access to Life. n.d. Projects. Available online: https://bodiesintranslation.ca/projects/ (accessed on 2 April 2024).
Cachia, Amanda. 2022. Introduction: Committed to Change—Ten Years of Creative Access. In *Curating Access: Disability Art Activism and Creative Accommodation*. Edited by Amanda Cachia. New York: Routledge, pp. 1–14.
Chandler, Eliza. 2018. Disability Art and Re-Worlding Possibilities. *A/b: Auto/Biography Studies* 33: 458–63. [CrossRef]
Changfoot, Nadine. 2016. Creative socialist-feminist space: Creating moments of agency and emancipation by storytelling outlawed experiences and relational aesthetic. *Socialist Studies/Études Socialistes* 11: 62–82. [CrossRef]
Fatona, Andrea. 2014. The State of Blackness: From Production to Presentation. Available online: https://thestateofblackness.format.com/ (accessed on 2 April 2024).
Gold, Becky. 2021. Neurodivergency and interdependent creation: Breaking into Canadian disability arts. *Studies in Social Justice* 15: 209–29. [CrossRef]
Haritaworn, Jin, Ghaida Moussa, and Syrus Marcus Ware, eds. 2018. *Queering Urban Justice: Queer of Colour Formations in Toronto*. Toronto: University of Toronto Press.
Hooks, Bell. 1994. *Teaching to Transgress: Education as the Practice to Freedom*. New York: Routledge.
Kelly, Evadne, Dolleen Tisawii'ashii Manning, Seika Boye, Carla Rice, Dawn Owen, Sky Stonefish, and Mona Stonefish. 2021. Elements of a counter-exhibition: Excavating and countering a Canadian history and legacy of eugenics. *Journal for the History of Behavioural Sciences* 57: 12–33. [CrossRef] [PubMed]
Kuppers, Petra. 2022. *Eco Soma: Pain and Joy in Speculative Performance Encounters*. Minneapolis: University of Minnesota Press.
Lavallee, Lynn. 2020. Is Decolonization Possible in the Academy? In *Decolonizing and Indigenizing Education in Canada*. Edited by Sheila Cote-Meek and Taima Moeke-Pickering. Toronto: Canadian Scholars, pp. 117–35.
Mohr-Blakeney, Victoria, and Nadine Changfoot. 2018. Phantom, stills & vibrations: An interview with Lara Kramer. *Dance Current: Canada's National Dance Magazine*. March. Available online: https://thedancecurrent.com/article/phantom-stills-vibrations/ (accessed on 30 March 2024).
Piepzna-Samarasinha, Leah Lakshmi. 2022. *The Future Is Disabled: Prophecies, Love Notes and Mourning Songs*. Vancouver: Arsenal Pulp Press.
Rice, Carla, and Ingrid Mündel. 2018. Story-making as methodology: Disrupting dominant stories through multimedia storytelling. *Canadian Review of Sociology/Revue Canadienne de Sociologie* 55: 211–31. [CrossRef] [PubMed]
Rice, Carla, Chelsea Temple Jones, Ingrid Mündel, Patty Douglas, Hannah Fowlie, May Friedman, Elisabeth Harrison, Devan Hunter, Evadne Kelly, Madeleine Kruth, and et al. 2022. Stretching Our Stories (SOS): Digital worldmaking in troubled times. *Public* 33: 154–77. [CrossRef]
Rice, Carla, Eliza Chandler, Fady Shanouda, Chelsea Temple Jones, and Ingrid Mündel. 2024. Misfits meet art and technology: Cripping transmethodologies. *Cultural Studies <=> Critical Methodologies*. ahead of print. [CrossRef]
Rice, Carla, Katie Cook, and K. Alysse Bailey. 2021. Difference-attuned witnessing: Risks and potentialities of arts-based research. *Feminism & Psychology* 31: 345–65. [CrossRef]
Simpson, Leanne Betasamosake. 2017. *As We Have Always Done: Indigenous Freedom through Radical Resistance*. Minneapolis: University of Minnesota Press.

Stonefish, Mona, Peter Park, Dolleen Tisawii'ashii Manning, Evadne Kelly, Seika Boye, and Sky Stonefish. 2019. *Into the Light: Living Histories of Oppression and Eugenics in Southern Ontario*. Museum Exhibition, Guelph Civic Museum. Guelph: Guelph Museums and Re•Vision: The Centre for Art and Social Justice. Available online: https://guelphmuseums.ca/event/into-the-light-eugenics-and-education-in-southern-ontario/#:~:text=Into%20the%20Light%20examines%20local,white,%20able-bodied%20settlers (accessed on 2 April 2024).

Swain, Gloria. 2019. The healing power of art in intergenerational trauma: Race, sex, age and disability. *Canadian Journal of Disability Studies* 8: 15–31. [CrossRef]

Truth and Reconciliation Commission of Canada. 2015. *Honouring the Truth, Reconciling for the Future: Summary of the Final Report of the Truth and Reconciliation Commission of Canada*; Ottawa: Government of Canada.

Weber, Joanne. 2024. Making Multiple Deaf Worlds Intelligible: A Posthumanist Arts-based Cartography of Apple Time. *Studies in Social Justice* 18: 16–34. [CrossRef]

Disclaimer/Publisher's Note: The statements, opinions and data contained in all publications are solely those of the individual author(s) and contributor(s) and not of MDPI and/or the editor(s). MDPI and/or the editor(s) disclaim responsibility for any injury to people or property resulting from any ideas, methods, instructions or products referred to in the content.

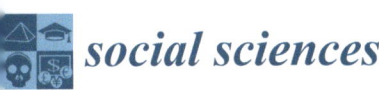

Article

Towards Decolonial Choreographies of Co-Resistance

Evadne Kelly *, Carla Rice and Mona Stonefish

Re•Vision: The Centre for Art and Social Justice, College of Social and Applied Human Sciences, University of Guelph, Guelph, ON N1G 2W1, Canada; carlar@uoguelph.ca (C.R.)
* Correspondence: evadne@uoguelph.ca

Abstract: This article engages movement as a methodology for understanding the creative coalition work that we carried out for a project series called *Into the Light* (ITL) that used research from university archives to mount a museum exhibition and then develop an interactive public education site that counters histories and ongoing realities of colonial eugenics and their exclusionary ideas of what it means to be human in Canada's educational institutions. We address different movement practices, both those initiated by ableist-colonial forces to destroy difference and by our coalition of co-resistors to affirm difference. We apply a decolonizing and Anishinaabe philosophical lens alongside a feminist disability-informed neomaterialist and dance studies one to theorize examples of ITL's "choreographies of co-resistance". Anishinaabe knowledge practices refuse and thus interfere with colonial-eugenic practices of erasure while enacting an ethic of self-determination and mutual respect for difference. The ripple effect of this decolonizing and difference-affirming interference reverberates through our words and moves at varying tempos through our bodies—traveling through flesh, holding up at bones, and passing through watery, stretchy connective tissue pathways. These are our choreographies of co-resistance as actions of mattering and world-building.

Keywords: co-creation; decolonization; difference; disability justice; art; choreography; eugenics; Original Peoples; Anishinaabe; neomaterialism

Citation: Kelly, Evadne, Carla Rice, and Mona Stonefish. 2023. Towards Decolonial Choreographies of Co-Resistance. *Social Sciences* 12: 204. https://doi.org/10.3390/socsci12040204

Academic Editor: Nigel Parton

Received: 14 December 2022
Revised: 23 March 2023
Accepted: 24 March 2023
Published: 30 March 2023

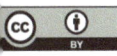

Copyright: © 2023 by the authors. Licensee MDPI, Basel, Switzerland. This article is an open access article distributed under the terms and conditions of the Creative Commons Attribution (CC BY) license (https://creativecommons.org/licenses/by/4.0/).

This article engages movement as a methodology for understanding the creative coalition work that we carried out for a project series called *Into the Light* (ITL) that works in solidarity across our differences to counter histories and ongoing realities of colonial eugenics and its exclusionary ideas of what it means to be human in Canada's educational institutions. We situate our work in relation to the Anishinaabeg of the Three Fires Confederacy among the Ojibwe, Odawa, and Potawatomi upon whose ancestral lands our work takes place, and we honor, respect, and prioritize Original Peoples (First Nations) of this hemisphere and their worldviews as co-authors of ITL. The authors of this article are Mona Stonefish, Ogichidaakwe of the Anishinaabeg Three Fires Confederacy (Bkejwanong Territory), Doctor of Traditional Medicine, international activist for peace, women's and disability rights, and Grandmother Water Walker who was recently honoured by Chief Charles Sampson and Council of Bkejwanong First Nation for her thriving and determination as a residential school survivor, whose wisdom has guided ITL from the start, and who is receiving an Honorary Doctorate of Laws (16 June 2023) from the University of Guelph for her dedication to the pursuit of truth through centralizing the preservation of Anishinaabe language, culture, and tradition, advocacy for human rights, restorative justice, and decolonial education; Carla Rice, a crip-queer white settler critical embodiment scholar, who supervised Kelly's research and collaborated on ITL; and Evadne Kelly, a white settler dance-artist and scholar and project lead of ITL, whose curvy spine and large body regularly challenge normative constructions of the body upheld by western theatrical dance conventions. As justice-seeking artists, scholars, and activists who are invested in the power of the body and its movements to bring new possibilities for non-normative life into the world, we understand movement as encompassing the sensory, perceptual, affective, emotive, communicative, cognitive, physical, psychic, spiritual, and all other actual and potential doings of bodies that ripple out into the world to have formative and transformative effects (Rice 2015, 2018; Rice et al. 2021b, 2022). The following draws on both Anishinaabe (or Nishnaabe to use Stonefish's and Michi Saagiig Nishnaabeg scholar-artist Leanne Betasamosake Simpson's spelling and pronunciation preference) and feminist disability-informed understandings to explore movement as a decolonial crip methodology for creative coalition work that resists collapsing difference and counters Canadian histories and ongoing realities of colonial eugenics. We call our movements together "choreographies of co-resistance" to foreground the agentic desires of bodies to live relationships marked by non-interference and respect for difference through mapping how these relations might materialize if we attend closely to process, place, time, and moving bodies (Foster 2011).

Into the Light aims to uncover histories of southern Ontario educational institutions producing and disseminating colonial "race betterment" (including eugenics) to trace those histories to present-day oppressions, and to counter them directly in our process and outcome. Southern Ontario is an important site for this work as it is often wrongfully assumed by many white, non-disabled middle-class settler Ontarians that race betterment belongs to another time and place, with Nazi Germany often thought of as the epitome of such violence. Instead, as central to the Canadian nation-state-in-formation's land occupation, southern Ontario has been an epicenter of white supremacist race betterment through strategic state interventions in families through forced and coerced sterilization and the forced placement of individuals from groups targeted for elimination in socially engineered residential environments including Indian Residential Schools, the so-called 60s Scoop, training schools, and reformatories. With knowledge of this history, the first author Kelly conducted research into university archives, organized a call for curators, and co-mounted an award-winning exhibition titled *Into the Light: Eugenics and Education in Southern Ontario* at the Guelph Civic Museum (Ontario Heritage Trust 2020). In addition to Kelly, exhibition co-curators included Stonefish, Peter Park (survivor of Oxford Regional Centre, co-founder of Respecting Rights, a project at ARCH Disability Law Centre, and founder of People First), Dolleen Tisawii'ashii Manning (Anishinaabe contemporary artist, philosopher, and Assistant Professor at Queen's University), Seika Boye (scholar, educator, dancer, and Assistant Professor Teaching Stream at the Centre for Drama, Theatre and Performance Studies, University of Toronto), and Sky Stonefish (Anishinaabe jingle dress dancer, photographer, and activist). Key collaborators and partners supporting and co-sponsoring the project included Rice (PI, Bodies in Translation), Sue Hutton (coordinator of Respecting Rights, a project led by people labeled with intellectual disability), and Dawn Owen (curator of Guelph Museums). *Into the Light*'s co-curatorial exhibition team made a conscious choice to prioritize stories of survivor-activists who have lived experiences of surviving and fighting eugenics. Stories they chose to share publicly are intimate and simultaneously protect their individual privacy. Since the knowledge of survivor-activists often becomes silenced and diminished, we asked visitors to engage with the stories as primary sources of expert knowledge of lived experience as well as the testimonies embedded in the stories that illuminate the histories and ongoing realities of systemic violence that comes from colonialism and eugenics. The exhibition incorporated artistic, sensory, and material expressions of memory in addition to archival artifacts as evidence of the role of education in accelerating and bolstering eugenics in Ontario.

Building on the exhibition's success, between May 2021 and August 2022, Kelly assembled another team to extend the reach of the knowledge generated through the survivor-activist testimony, her own ongoing archival research, and her learnings from audience engagement with the exhibition itself to create a new online learning platform entitled *Into the Light: Living Histories of Oppression and Education in Ontario*. To guide the development of this accessible, interactive, and multi-media platform full of artistic expressions of lived experience, we held 12 team meetings over eight months with Nishnaabeg, Métis, Black, racialized, white, disabled, labeled-as-disabled, verbal, non-verbal, and non-disabled contributors. Music, visual art, and creative movement guided the development of our learning platform and our relational work together. At least half of our meetings featured guided movement activities led by Stonefish and Kelly as accessible, life-affirming, and decolonizing creation activities.

Our methodology of "choreographing co-resistance" works from the belief that socio-material realities engage and influence our embodied actions, which positions embodied action as a potent site for reproducing and/or intervening in the existing social order (Schneider 2015). Southern Ontario, as an early, sustained, and strategic site of colonial eugenics within which our embodied actions occur is imbued with sociopolitical and ecological significance for Anishinaabeg (Tuck and McKenzie 2015) and disabled peoples and thus is deeply relevant to our work. The term "co-resistance" centers the experiential wisdom of both Nishnaabeg and disabled survivor-activists who decentre the human-centric, unidirectional, and hierarchical ideas that agents of colonial eugenics have attempted to impose onto bodies and minds of difference. For us, choreographing co-resistance affirmed and altered our modes of embodiment without assimilating differences or imposing a normative standard during our ethically precarious creative processes of decolonial counter-eugenic political engagement.

Through the findings and makings that our methodology affords, we argue that choreographies of co-resistance using shared decision-making processes of self-determination and non-assimilation can create conditions of possibility through the collective generation of desires and practices for decolonization and accessibility. We believe that our coalitional experiences of collaborative research on ITL are emblematic of the complexly overlaid relationships that occur between bodies enacting settler and those enacting Anishinaabe worldviews, and between ableist-colonial and disability-affirmative decolonial orientations that unevenly center on and impact our moving bodies. By celebrating difference, the choreographies we co-create challenge ableist-colonial practices that aim to fold different embodiments into sameness and rank them against ableist-colonial aesthetic standards for bodily appearance and movement (Rice et al. 2021c). The choreographies that we surface in our learning platform push against the colonial-eugenic compulsion still evident in many university programs that involve the study of movement, including dance programs (Mitra 2021), kinesiology and physical education (Bailey et al. forthcoming a, forthcoming b; Bessey et al. forthcoming), public and preventative health care (Rice et al. forthcoming, 2015; Viscardis et al. 2019), and rehabilitation (Gibson et al. 2020).

In what follows, we offer three examples that demonstrate these choreographies of co-resistance that flow from different lived experiences of surviving and resisting colonial eugenics: the first focuses on the centrality of movement practices to the ITL exhibition and in the creation process of our learning platform. For our second example, we resurface selected passages of an 1844 debate that took place on Walpole Island (located in Bkejwanong Territory known today as southwestern Ontario) between Anishinaabe leaders who defended their sovereignty against Jesuit Missionary encroachment as local context to Anishinaabe understandings of difference. The debate shows how difference is welcomed from this Anishinaabe philosophical perspective because spirit is integral to everything in the universe, organic and non-organic. Spirit is not isolated to a transcendent god-figure that rules over and above humans and who imposes a hierarchy of life onto the material world. We bring this debate into dialogue with Stonefish's expressions of sovereignty during ITL to acknowledge and foreground the Anishinaabeg traditions of honoring the body, its movements, and its relationship to the universe (land, water, and sky or ecosystem). Revisiting this debate also allows us to attend to the force of Anishinaabeg ideas in countering Christian colonial language that seeks to diminish Anishinaabe knowledge and political orders, especially those regarding body–mind difference. Our third example builds on the two prior examples to show how Stonefish drew from her lived knowledge of Anishinaabe language, culture, and tradition and activated this knowledge in her approach to guiding us toward transformative understanding and action. Leading an ITL co-design session with a guided movement activity called "Touching the Universe with Love" Stonefish encouraged participant-contributors to centralize our place-specific bodies, knowledge, traditions, and movements as unique sources of creativity within a communal process that rippled knowledge differently into being. The intention in reporting on our building of the learning platform in this way is not only to provide people with information about the locally specific operations/effects of colonial eugenics but also to provide some insight about the epistemologically and ethically charged processes of bringing to light the lived impacts of such life-destroying knowledge. This we worked to accomplish by creating a difference-affirming space that could foster and support a deeply felt-sensed engagement with ITL through responsiveness, connection, and accountability. To explore and theorize the three examples of ITL's "choreographies of co-resistance", we draw on research team discussions, personal correspondences between Stonefish, Rice, and Kelly, and we apply a decolonizing (Jimmy and Andreotti 2019) and Anishinaabe philosophical (Simpson 2011, 2017) lens alongside a feminist disability-informed neomaterialist (Barad 2006; Rice et al 2021a, 2021b, 2022), and dance and performance studies one that disrupts a focus on conventional western theatrical notions of dance and performance (Foster 2011; Perazzo Domm 2019; Schneider 2015; Larasati 2013; Kelly 2019). Ultimately, our methodology prioritizes lived experience in our moving together as kinetics or doings that generate transformative and decolonizing learning within an ethic of non-assimilation that affirms differences and why they matter.

Choreographies of Co-Resistance in Motion
Example 1: Into the Light Exhibit as a Choreography of Co-Resistance

Into the Light focuses on exposing and resisting eugenics, a so-called "race betterment" theory and practice that sought and still seeks to control the future of humanity as part of a broader Euro-western intellectual and religious-imperial drive to control the direction of all earthly life (Kelly and Rice forthcoming). Over the 20th century, agents of race betterment, who included white settler researchers, politicians, doctors, social workers, educators, nurses, and other status figures prominent across social spheres, have embedded race betterment ideas and practices across institutions and institutional practices. These eugenic agents aimed to accelerate the cultivation of an ideal norm or "fit" "Canadian race", understood as white, Christian, non-disabled, hetero-patriarchal, and propertied, through two main strategies: providing those deemed as "fit" with incentives to reproduce, have families, and excel in life and work; and targeting those deemed "unfit", namely First Nations and racialized, poor, disabled, and labeled-as-disabled settler groups for dehumanization, diminishment, erasure, and elimination (Kelly et al. 2021a, 2021b; McLaren 1990; Stonefish et al. 2019). They created a hierarchy of mind over body to undermine embodied and experiential knowledge of groups that were largely excluded from the ranks of those deemed as knowers, leaders, and experts in institutions. For example, residential institutions (including Indian Residential Schools, training schools, poor houses, and asylums), organized and run by white religious and professional actors, took shape as immobilizing places of confinement and control that carried out ableist-racist aims of removal, incarceration, and ultimately, elimination of First Nations, racialized settlers, and settlers with body–mind differences, disabilities, and labeled-as-disabled (Ben-Moshe et al. 2014; Diverlus et al. 2020; McLaren 1990).

Despite ongoing resistance and the massive scientific and political discrediting of eugenics from the 1940s onwards due to the unprovability of its theories and the culpability of these in the atrocities of the Holocaust, eugenic praxis continues now, albeit in more stealthy, indirect, and insidious forms (Kelly and Rice forthcoming). Today, eugenic desires for race betterment continue to take the form of carceral logics, or practices of surveillance, regulation, discipline, and punishment embedded in and enacted by state systems (social welfare, healthcare, education, immigration), as abolitionists (Davis et al. 2022) and disability and transformative justice scholars point out (Ben-Moshe et al. 2014). Child welfare agencies continue to systematically take First Nations and Black children from their families and communities to be placed in white settler homes (Ontario Human Rights Commission 2018) and medical practitioners continue to control human reproduction through, for example, forced and coerced sterilizations (Ataullahjan et al. 2021). Canadian colonial eugenics does not limit itself to control over human life: taking and controlling land and non-human life for settler benefit and profit comprises another eugenic impulse with disastrous ecological effects (Kelly and Rice forthcoming). These unjust and destructive betterment ideas and practices were woven into the building blocks of the Canadian nation-state, and, as such, continue to target bodies and lives (human and non-human) for dehumanization and elimination (Burch 2021).

The title of our work together, *Into the Light*, carries activist understandings of movement and emergent life that flow from difference-affirming and generating perspectives. From a Nishnaabeg perspective, Simpson understands dance, kinetics, or acts of doing, as "the crucial intellectual mode for generating knowledge", and as a methodology that enacts Nishnaabeg "embedded practices and processes" (Simpson 2017, p. 20) to animate knowledge that sustains diverse life. Referring to embedded practices of Nishnaabe-kwe that recuperate and revitalize knowledge specifically, Stonefish explains, "When we walk for the water, it reminds us of the sacredness of water and our responsibility to water. . . . We are the winds of change . . . traditions, language, and culture connect us to our land, water, and sky, *our* ecosystem, and that is what will truly sustain us" (Stonefish, pers. comm. with Kelly, 7 July 2021). Acknowledging the immobilizing and ecologically devastating effects of Canadian colonial eugenics, Stonefish uplifts the power of moving together to protect and care for earthly life. Thus, in their Nishnaabeg praxis, Simpson and Stonefish show how dancing and moving interactions and relations are world-making in the effects they generate, but in their respective projects, each reveals how these relations are also ethically complex networks or constellations of co-resistance that interfere in white settler colonial ideas/practices. Nishnaabeg knowledge systems generate knowledge through movement that encodes and animates that knowledge; and here Simpson and Stonefish turn to Nishnaabeg relations with land, water, and sky to activate the knowledge that is expressed and expanded through living relationships. These relations sustain balance and support the thriving of all life.

Neomaterialist theory also orients to how the physical world is constantly moving and, thus, aligns with Anishinaabe philosophy in understanding reality as ever-shifting and as continuously materializing differently in service of life's vitality (Rice 2014; Rice et al. 2021b, 2022). We draw on feminist settler physicist Karen Barad's understanding of reality as agentic based on her theoretical physics-informed understanding of diffraction or interference as a force that secures life's ongoing nature through its capacity to create difference. In physics, diffraction or interference comprises the idea that the energies that constitute the world do so through diffracting and interfering with each other (e.g., think about light, sound, and water waves bouncing off and changing the trajectories of each other) to re-produce existing or create new patterns and realities (Barad 2006; Rice et al. 2021b, 2022). Barad views diffraction not only as a metaphor but more so as the material practice of "making a difference in the world . . . taking responsibility for the fact that our practices matter; the world is materialized differently through different practices" (Barad 2006, p. 89). She understands knowledge, methodology, and ethics as entangled in how knowledge, and the research apparatus used to make it, changes reality, and, as she writes, "practices of knowing are specific material engagements that participate in (re)configuring the world". (Barad 2006, p. 91). This ethically entangled process of making knowledge and reality requires that we think with theories and design studies that have the potential to open space for difference to presence and to thrive (Rice et al. 2021b). Whilst materialist and Nishnaabeg thinkers orient to reality as processual, neomaterialists fail to acknowledge the centrality of relationality with the land to knowledge and worldmaking, or to ground their ethical frames in protecting and sustaining the vitalities and animacies of a place (Tuck and McKenzie 2015; Rice et al. 2021c). In response, Stonefish guided the ITL team to consider the significance of land- and place-based knowledge and experience. Knowledge made through creative movement relies upon the specifics of land and place to proliferate diverse life, or difference, as opposed to producing sameness. During our online gatherings, disability activist-survivors Marie Slark and Antoinette Charlebois also shared movement and art practices that signified and generated hope, resistance, creativity, and self-determination in the face of physical confinement and carceral treatment in a residential institution for disabled and labeled-as-disabled children, youth, and adults called the Huronia Regional Centre. Through song, knitting, and needlework, they oriented to what research and creative practice might do for those of us who misfit with normative constructions of the human to generate culture, liberation, and change, and give greater access to life.

Both Anishinaabe and disability-informed neomaterialist approaches foreground movement as significant to knowing and worldmaking, as a methodology for interacting with and altering the world. We hold these differing theoretical traditions as complementary but not the same. Since the movements integral to each system have radically different roots and aims or desires—one in an Anishinaabe philosophical worldview concerned with the wellbeing of land and the universe, and the other in quantum physics interested in unlocking the nature of energy and matter—we work with them contiguously, in ways akin to Cree artist Elwood Jimmy's and settler scholar Vanessa Andreotti's braiding approach (Jimmy and Andreotti 2019). Mobilizing a braiding approach allows us to maintain the distinctions between, and integrity of, each knowledge system whilst materializing the differences in Nishnaabeg and crip experiences of colonial eugenics and in our sense-making of those experiences. We have used the term "interference" intentionally, for example, to not collapse differences in meaning, or appropriate or absorb different knowledge systems and worldviews into a singular framework as colonial systems have tried to do. We mobilize the term interference when we discuss the ableist-colonial drive to interfere with life to erase and eliminate difference. However, we also use the term in a different way. Rice et al (2022) extend Barad's diffractive theory of the dynamism of reality to draw attention to the ways eugenic colonial logics have produced disability as a "lesser than" embodiment, and how biomedicine continues to interfere with the bodies and lives of those who misfit with its mythical norms in ways that still see difference as deficiency (Viscardis et al. 2019). The authors purposely mobilize the word interference rather than diffraction to jolt readers into awareness of the extreme violence done to misfitting body/minds within normative (health, education) systems and how those body/minds resist and re-orient to difference through disability cultures and activisms (Chandler et al. 2023; Rice et al. 2022). In addition to tracking such interferences put in motion by our motions, our methodology complicates neomaterialist notions of interference by foregrounding the Nishnaabeg ethic of noninterference, respect for self-determination, and difference as introduced by Stonefish and Simpson. We carefully hold the Nishnaabeg ethic of noninterference contiguous with the neomaterialist ethic that sees knowledge and ethics as always already entangled to think through our methodology—to think through how different knowledge systems might productively influence without interfering with or assimilating each other.

Importantly, respecting differences at an epistemic level does not mean we remain untouched and unchanged by each other (Rice et al. 2021a); rather, throughout the process of coming together to create ITL projects, we found ourselves opening to being touched and even changed by each other in non-directive and non-prescriptive ways through the movement practices we enacted to affirm Anishinaabe, crip, and other life and (even if fleetingly) (re)configure the world. Referring to our creative coalition or solidarity work together, we use the umbrella concept of "non-assimilation" to signal the ethic of respect for radical difference that emerges across our worldviews. We access and express that solidarity through the feelings and experiences that emerge from our creating together (Gaztambide-Fernández 2012; Rice et al. 2021a; Rice and Mündel 2018). We forefront the ethics that inform our methodological and actual dance together: the conscious, careful, and creative modes of knowledge generation and exchange that center mutual respect and non-assimilation in our decolonizing and accessible creation processes. We recognize that our encounters and configurations within this moving reality carry complex intersectional asymmetries, risk, and ethical precarity (Rice and Mündel 2019). ITL's movement activities, as "choreographies of co-resistance", begin to articulate and map the complex interrelations between the physical and social worlds of ITL contributors and, in that articulation and mapping, ethically engage with land and place-specific socio-political and ecological realities that we, knowingly and unknowingly, reproduce (and disrupt) through our embodied actions.

Our individual understandings of what it means to move "Into the Light" are multifarious and reflect the ways in which difference has always been centered in our collaborative approach. For example, during the ITL museum exhibition, bodies moving through space created patterns of light and shadow. Light sources including focused overhead track lighting, projectors, backlighting, and lamps illuminated eugenic and counter-eugenic ideas. As visitors moved in and out of exhibition lights, their bodies interfered with light waves, and the light waves interfered with their bodies. Through movement, a person's body could block a eugenic idea from being projected into the space, but that also meant the eugenic idea appeared on their body. Bodies interfered with the light cast by projectors, and, in turn, bodies became sources of shadow and light, (potentially) prompting people to query how bodies and movements resist, interfere with, and become implicated in and impacted by the larger story being told (for detailed discussion, see Kelly et al. 2021a, 2021b). Entering the space, visitors moved with and through the rhythms and sound waves of Stonefish's voice delivering a traditional opening thanksgiving in Anishinaabemowin on a looped recording. The co-curatorial team configured her voice recording alongside a looped recording of a song by disability survivor-activist Peter Park. Together, their voices created a rhythm for visitors to move through the space with soundings celebrating difference. Through their vocal and rhythmic presence, Stonefish's and Park's bodies rippled out into the world to have formative and transformative effects on exhibition visitors.

In building our learning platform, we layered land- and place-based knowledge of water waves onto our work with light and sound waves as another source for understanding the movement interferences necessary for transformative decoloniality and disability justice. For example, the "Home" page of the ITL learning platform (go to: intothelight.ca) shows intersecting rivers at the site of our exhibition in Guelph, Ontario. Created by digital designers Jasmine Plumb, Shital Desai, and Ian Garrett in dialogue with the full team, the map of the Speed River joining with the Eramosa River creates three visual pathways in relation to eugenics taught at the Macdonald Institute and Ontario Agricultural College. The pathways center the lives of Stonefish (who survived the Mohawk Institute), Park (who survived Oxford Regional Centre), and Slark and Charlebois (who survived Huronia Regional Centre). The moving rivers show the intersections of colonial eugenics and resistance to it without folding lived experiences and journeys into one.

Through the energetic and sensory modes of learning offered by waves of light, sound, and water, Nishnaabeg living practices not only encode but also generate knowledge by "combining potential energy and kinetic energy as a creative force" (Simpson 2017, p. 183). Simpson's explanation of a "Stone's Throw" into water exemplifies the effects of doing/knowing/creating as acts of resistance with the potential to transform worlds:

[A]cts of resistance are like throwing a stone into water . . . There is the original splash the act of resistance makes, and the stone (or the act) sinks to the bottom, resting in place and time. However, there are also more subtle waves of disruption that ripple or echo out from where the stone impacted the water . . . . Their path of influence covers a much larger area than the initial splash, radiating outward for a much longer period of time. (Simpson 2011, p. 145)

While Stonefish reminds us that "resistance comes at a very high price" (Stonefish, pers. comm. with Kelly, 29 March 2023), for Stonefish and Simpson, moving together to know-access-alter the world aims to affirm and embrace diverse life and to reject drives to determine and control the future as colonial eugenicists did. Such non-determining influence "matters in a dance towards decoloniality" (Mackinlay 2016, p. 220).

From a neomaterialist approach to knowledge making, visitors' movements in the Guelph gallery generated waves of energies that traveled, overlapped, interacted, and changed as they experienced the exhibition, itself produced within the walls of a museum structure born as the Loretto Convent and residential academy. An inaccessible staircase adjacent to the source of Stonefish's voice served as a reminder that the place has been inflected, ordered, and oriented by the tensions that exist within a community impacted by and implicated in Christian colonial-eugenic histories and legacies. Counter to the rigid, exclusionary, and controlling normative ideas of bodies put in motion by the building's very structure, visitors from across and beyond Ontario moved in non-linear ways through the ITL exhibition to the rhythms set by Stonefish and Park in ways that made them more comfortable: some chose to sit directly on the floor, some leaned against walls, some sat on chairs provided by exhibition vignettes (thus implicating themselves in museum scenes), some relied on their mobility devices. The embodied and emplaced experiences and movements of visitors challenged the erasure of difference and put new patterns of thinking and feeling into motion—embodied actions that affirmed difference within local experiences. Bodies in motion were thus central to emergent knowledge. These examples show how we attended to the difference that a research practice makes in the world, using a methodological approach that "maps where the effects of difference appear" (Donna Haraway quoted in Mackinlay 2016, p. 213). These different perspectives regarding the movements of the physical world afford a non-hierarchical understanding of doing-knowing-creating through interaction, encounter, and interference. They invited a proliferation of stories and not a reduction of ideas; they activated visitors in ways we hoped would result from our work together; and they activated ripples that have traveled across and through bodies, which emerged as and with a new aliveness, as new entities unique to the encounters.

Example 2: Moving with a Nishnaabeg Ethics of Difference

The ethical and political complexities of undertaking coalitional research across embodied and embedded differences have reverberated throughout ITL. An ethical space of engagement is, as Cree scholar Willie Ermine writes, "formed when two societies with disparate worldviews, are poised to engage each other" (Ermine 2007, p. 193). For the ITL team, moving together is densely layered and entangled with ethical complexity and uneven power. For example, both scholars and survivor-activist team members embody lived experiences of settler colonial and eugenic interferences, resistance to such genocidal interference, as well as their own ethics of difference. Within this context, our work together across differences could be described as an "Im/possible Choreography" enmeshed within the paradoxical convergence of the possible with the impossible (Perazzo Domm 2019, p. 8). To unmake histories and legacies of oppressive and unethical contact, we needed to enter into relations or make contact through different tools and mechanisms on difference-centered terms (Mitra 2021). These have included a Nishnaabeg ethics of non-interference that upholds mutual respect, self-determination, and sovereignty (Simpson 2011, 2017) and a disability justice ethic that leads with disability to disrupt ableist practices and embrace difference-led decision-making and artistic approaches to research (Rice et al. 2018).

As our process unfolded, Stonefish brought forward her lived wisdom and the wisdom of her Anishinaabe ancestors on Walpole Island to deepen our collective understanding of Nishnaabeg ethics of non-interference and respect for difference and to consider what this understanding might mean for further decolonizing co-resistance. Prioritizing ancestral wisdom also centralizes Anishinaabe governance of the unceded territory, Anishinaabe presence and relations to the universe, and Anishinaabe efforts to challenge persistent settler notions of ownership over the land, water, and sky. Almost 200 years ago, the Anishinaabeg expressed resistance to western encroachment during a formal debate that took place in 1844 on Walpole Island between Ojibwe leaders and Jesuit Missionaries. The debate between Ojibwe leaders Chief Petrokeshig and 83-year-old warrior Oshawana representing thirty Elders present and Father Chazelle occurred within a context of increasing Christian colonial efforts to squeeze Original Peoples off their land and undermine their worldviews, and assimilate or eliminate them (Delâge and Tanner 1994; Krasowski 1999). In rejecting the establishment of a Christian mission on Walpole Island, Chief Petrokeshig spoke for the Ojibwe leaders to refuse Chazelle's assertion of a single truth disconnected from the lived experience of difference, orating that

...the Great Spirit who made all things that exist made them with an infinite variety [...]. The trees are of many different species, and the plants are even more diverse. [...] *It is certainly the Great Spirit who put these innumerable differences in all that he created; consequently, his plan was not that we all have one and the same way of seeking the light.* I have a special way of seeking the light that he gave to me, you have yours that he also gave to you, and it is the same for all nations (quoted in Delâge and Tanner 1994, p. 311, emphasis ours).

Against Chief Petrokeshig's description of spiritual, epistemological, and material movements towards seeking difference, Chazelle argued that there was only one pathway to enlightenment, imposing a monotheist belief in a supreme all-knowing being that reflected the white man's image only and that denied the existence of other spiritual forces and pathways to truth:

Once [the people of my island] accepted prayer they came to know the Great Spirit much better than you do, and since then they know that there is but one way to seek the light. [...] When anyone has Prayer, it is Jesus, the son of the Great Spirit made man himself, who teaches us wisdom by making himself known, by revealing himself. Yes, he reveals himself, not to the eyes of the body, but to the eyes of the spirit. [... .] I need several feet of land, for my dwelling and the House of Prayer. The English to whom this island belongs, give them to me. (Quoted in Delâge and Tanner 1994, pp. 315–17)

By infusing spirit and truth in a singular supreme being that reflected only his image, Chazelle diminished embodied and lived experience as sites for knowledge generation and spiritual practice and refused the spirit, knowledge, and agency that the Anishinaabe understood as integral to everything in the universe. Further, his complete disregard for the Ojibwe leaders' assertion of their own intellectual and spiritual orders also justified the Jesuit's violent colonial interference with Anishinaabe sovereignty and governance. Yet Oshawana's final words reiterated the Ojibwe leaders' unwavering refusal of western encroachment and their demand for mutual respect for different worldviews and forms of worship.

My brother, you have come to teach us that there is only one way, for all people, to know the Great Spirit and deserve his favors? [...] Except our way is different from that of White men. It must be that way, *because we see differences in all things*, according to the will of the Great Spirit. [...] Listen to what I have to say in conclusion. Stop building the cabin you have begun [...]. (Quoted in Delâge and Tanner 1994, pp. 319–20, emphasis ours).

To accelerate white settler supremacy, from the mid-19th to the mid-20th century, the Canadian state-in-formation increasingly used race betterment to form Indian Affairs Policy and the building blocks of the Indian Residential School system, striving to eliminate, assimilate, and suppress difference and dissent in its drive to become a white settler colonial society (Bednasek and Godlewska 2017). Despite ongoing resistance, the effects of Christian colonial interferences on the lives of Original Peoples have been and continue to be egregious. This was recently acknowledged by Pope Francis himself who, during his 2022 visit to Turtle Island to apologize for the church's role in Canada's IRS system, used the term genocide to describe its devastating effects on First Nations (Ka'nhehsí:io 2022). Condemning and eliminating First Nations language, culture, and traditions is, in the Pope's own words, a genocidal tool of colonization, or, in the words of Audra Simpson, a "sovereign death dance" (Simpson 2017, p. 115).

The Anishinaabe evidence their sustained resistance to colonialization in the documentation of the debate and in the way they have intergenerationally transferred the resistance and self-determination encoded in their language, culture, and knowledge (Krasowski 1999). For Simpson, the everyday embodiment comprises "a mechanism for ancient beginnings" that creates "flight paths out of colonialism and into magnificent unfolding" of locally specific resurgences of First Nations sovereignty (Simpson 2017, p. 193). As demonstrated by Stonefish, ancestral knowledge regarding self-determination, consent, and respect for difference on Walpole Island continues to be unwavering in the oratorical teachings, worldviews, and traditions that have been carefully, strategically, and lovingly passed down and inherited. Engagement with these traditions continues within the wider political circumstances of ongoing settler-colonial eugenics. Stonefish explains: "Being human does not rely upon western modes of understanding. We need to counter such thinking and prioritize our language and culture in order to re-learn obligations of mutual care and to move forward together in a good way". By bringing forward the importance of the 1844 debate, Stonefish anchors her movements within a multigenerational choreography that remembers its traditions and refuses assimilation and genocide.[1] Beyond self-determination, bringing forth an understanding of embodied movement as inherent in learning and world-making within an ethic of non-assimilation and respect for difference, quoting Stonefish from our 25 August 2021 team meeting, "also connects us to our land, water, and sky (our ecosystem), which is what will truly sustain us into the future".

Example 3: "Touching the Universe with Love"

Aware of the violent effects of actions, or interferences, that impose singular and immobilizing truths, incorporating movement-based methods of interacting that prioritize difference requires a sensitivity to the relationships between movement and interference. We see decolonizing and difference-centered interferences across worldviews as generative—even and perhaps especially when they are generative refusals. As Simpson notes, centering generative refusal when building a movement that "pivots on (re)connecting with the land and with practices that sustain life and land" has "world-making effects" (Simpson 2017, p. 178). Such refusals include any one or a combination of movements as expressions of agency and self-determination, those that offer ways of resisting colonial eugenics, and those enacted as "deliberate and strategic resurgence", amongst others (Simpson 2017, p. 197).[2] Following Black feminist scholar Jennifer Nash, generative refusals of the status quo also include movements toward another (Nash 2019). This is because a break with the "what is" might facilitate a movement toward others with an openness to transformative change and to be transformed and changed by another (Nash 2019). As Stonefish guides us movements toward another move in relation to the universe, which includes land, water, sky, and all human and non-human beings.

Building on the rippling of lived experience as acts of resistance, we turn towards Stonefish's guided movement creation activity, "Touching the Universe with Love" that emerged during the development of our learning platform. We present this example as a powerful source of creation for us because it offers critically important insights into ableist-colonial interference in Anishinaabe political orders and the generative refusal of Nishnaabeg as expressed through their embodied actions and philosophies of difference. Through her guided movements, Stonefish's living experiences emerged as a powerful source of transformative learning within a Nishnaabeg ethic of noninterference that generated mutual respect and a space of collaborative and sustainable world-making.

The following transcript of a movement activity led and guided by Stonefish during our 18 January 2022, team meeting articulates the power and creative potential of moving within a mixed ethical space to activate non-assimilative ways of creating together to interfere in colonial eugenic logics and shift our experiences of and relations to local ecosystems.

Well, before white settlers came here, this continent was one of love, one of understanding. When we extend our hands when we give our thanksgiving, we always touch the earth, and we touch the water. We do not necessarily just extend our hand to the front, but we always extend our hands to the back as well because there might be little children or people who are like myself that cannot walk real fast. You still let them know that we are of some worth, and everybody is of worth here. Since we are here at this time, and we share this planet together.

So, when we bring our hands together to touch the earth, we also go down to the floor, to the earth.

Since movement is so important, especially throughout your whole life, you should be able to be mobile, you should be able to move around. Even for my granddaughter. I want to tell a story about her because when she was in high school, they have a thing called IEP—an individual education plan—but they had her sitting in a wheelchair facing the wall. So, I would go to the school. I volunteered, so I could help all the children who needed that extra help, to lift their hands, to move all their little fingers and all their bones—just move them around, because we all need that. We all need to feel that safe touching. We need to feel our mother, the earth. We were not meant to just forget about one another, but to come together in a circle as we look at our mother, the earth. So, if you could stand up, and you bring your hands up like this to your own body yourself, and then you go to the floor. You ball yourself up like the earth too, like how she does. You lower your head. Put your head far down on the ground.

Then you touch your toes, massage your toes, because your feet are the ones that carry the whole weight of your body. Our mother the earth carries all of our weight and carries everything, all the unnecessary things that are happening to her right now. She is in a lot of pain.

You come up to your hands. You move every little bone in your hands. You go to your left. You make the motion like in a circle. You go far back as you can behind you, and you make this circle with your hands–every finger spread out. This keeps you in balance.

Now you turn to the other side, and you do it the same way. You reach your hands out in the back. In doing so, we say that we are going to leave this planet the way we found it, or better than we found it, for the sake of the next generations to come. So, when we give our thanksgiving, we give thanksgiving for our ancestors and for those who are not yet born, and we keep our hands rolling in front of us again—almost in a swimming motion.

Then we un-cocoon ourselves, and we reach up into the sky world, the stars, and to the moon, and all those other things that are there that we may not know about. Yet, they are what sustains us here.

Then you put your hands, not together, but you intertwine your fingers like this. You put your fingers out. You bring them into your abdomen. You breathe in. You make some sounds of a rushing lake, always keeping your hands by your abdomen because when we have challenges in our life, that is where it affects us—in our abdomen and then our lower backs.

So now we cross our hands over to our shoulders. We feel the weight of our mother, the earth, because we held a lot of things that we should not be holding. We bring that out to our fingertips, and we shoo it out for the universe to take, to re-energize ourselves again always in a circular motion.

We put our hands over our faces, making sure that they are both on the left and right cortex of our brains and the front and back of our brains as well. We touch our ears so that we can hear the birds singing, so that we can hear the cries of the needy, so that we can hear the joyful laughter of those who are happy. Then we take two fingers and put them in front of our ears, like in our high cheekbone area, then we bring them over into our eyes. Whether we can see or not, feel the eye sockets that we all bestow.

Then you touch your nose, touch your nostrils. Then you bring your fingers down and you touch your mouth. You touch your chin. You say to the strongest muscle in your body, the tongue, that I watch my tongue and what I say, because I may hurt somebody. That is the strongest muscle in our body, and that is the one that is most hurtful.

That is why, there are some to remind us, to give us the patience, the love, and the understanding for those who cannot speak words, who are nonverbal. Then we go to our voice box and say not to waste our voice box with anger, not to say things that are going to hurt other people, because we are all a part of creation.

Now we lift our hands up high. Then we put another circle and touch our bosom, and for those of us who are life givers, like our mother, the earth, we were given breasts so that we could nourish our children. We have to give thanksgiving for that. We touch our abdomen again. Then we go to our navel. Where we have carried life, and if we have not carried life, you are an auntie to many, many children of the world, and always remember that and see the beauty in yourself and the beauty that Mother Earth, the moon, and we as co-creators of the universe still bestow today.

With that, I'm going to caress my hair again. Since this is what they tried to take away from me. Yet I still have it.

Again, I put my hands out like I have the world in my hands, and we do have the world in our hands, and we must be mindful of that. The decisions that we make today are the decisions that are going to either harm or be helpful for future generations to come.

Okay now we have spoken, and now we can relax our bodies, carry on with our business, and take a break. I thank you for taking this time to touch the earth.

Stonefish's guided movement activity was embedded with the knowledge of bodies moving towards connection to the universe, and how our actions matter. Stonefish reminded us of how settler colonial structures and processes interfered with Anishinaabe practices of touching the universe with love—an ongoing violence that continues to the present day. In placing and leaving Stonefish's granddaughter (Sky) in a wheelchair facing the wall, settler education enacts erasure by refusing mutual respect and self-determination and by preventing her from doing-knowing-creating relationally and communally. Stonefish contrasts this with the embodied practices that she and Sky mutually engage in including how she lovingly moves Sky's hands, fingers, and bones to help Sky activate her body-world of experience and relationship. Stonefish's loving touch and Sky's loving acceptance and response to/return of that touch, they together enact a doing-knowing-creating that generates life-affirming ethical effects. As a creative, non-assimilative, and life-affirming methodology of resistance to colonial eugenics in education, Stonefish guided the team in creating a safe, inclusive space where we could "combin[e] potential energy and kinetic energy as a creative force" (Simpson 2017, p. 183). Through her touch and her movements, she was accessing the entire universe through her practice. Her lived wisdom guided our movements towards affirming the vitality of our unique embodiments while also opening our embodiments towards new understandings of the ways our non-assimilated bodies are central to direct decolonial and counter-eugenic engagement and change.

Through our entangled movements towards decolonization, accessibility, and justice, the world of our digital co-created space "materialized differently through different practices" (Barad 2006, p. 89). As we moved together toward the universe with love, our bodies also opened to being transformed by each other through solidarity that celebrates difference Opening towards Stonefish's guided movement activity created felt-sensed interferences in the ways we each experience our bodies differently and drew greater awareness to the lived experience of thriving despite the violence of colonial eugenics. The ripple effect of Stonefish's lived wisdom and resulting decolonizing interferences reverberates into this writing and continues to move at varying tempos through our bodies—traveling through flesh, holding up at bones, and passing through watery, stretchy connective tissue pathways.

Conclusions

In this paper and our larger *ITL* project, we aim to model ethics of listening, feeling, sensing, and moving differently, to learn about obligations of mutual care and respect, and how to collectively hold dissenting views in generative ways for more just and sustainable futures on Nishnaabeg and crip survivor-activists' terms. Our process for interacting creatively is informed by Stonefish's and other survivor-activists' lived knowledge of Canadian colonial eugenic interference as well as resistance to it. Simultaneously, their lived experiences as decolonizing anti-eugenic interferences have had life-affirming and transformative effects on our creation process. They continue to inform our doing-knowing-creating in ways that bring bodies into proximity without folding into sameness. Guided by the lived wisdom of survivor-activists, our movements together have developed into a particularly potent and meaningful methodology for interfering with colonial eugenic ideas and practices while also maintaining an ethic of non-assimilative mutual respect for difference. Throughout ITL, lived fleshy interferences of survivor-activists have reverberated between us. Moving, feeling, sensing, and opening toward one interference, then another and another. This is our choreography of co-resistance and our rhythm-relation into the writing of this work as actions of mattering and world-building centered on and across differences. As Stonefish has reminded us, "we do have the world in our hands, and we must be mindful of that. The decisions that we make today are the decisions that are going to either harm or be helpful for the future generations to come".

Author Contributions: Conceptualization, E.K., C.R. and M.S.; Methodology, E.K., C.R. and M.S.; Formal analysis, E.K., C.R. and M.S.; Investigation, E.K., C.R. and M.S.; Writing—original draft, E.K.; Writing—review & editing, E.K., C.R. and M.S.; Supervision, C.R.; Project administration, E.K.; Funding acquisition, E.K. and C.R. All authors have read and agreed to the published version of the manuscript.

Funding: eCampusOntario: GUEL—564; University of Guelph: Learning Enhancement Fund; Social Sciences and Humanities Research Council's Partnership fund #895-2016-1024.

Institutional Review Board Statement: This article describes a co-created knowledge creation and dissemination project series. The participants, including the authors of this article, collectively created methods of working together and the projects' outcomes.

Data Availability Statement: Not applicable.

Conflicts of Interest: The authors declare no conflict of interest.

Notes

[1] Tsimshian Art History scholar Mique'l Dangeli uses the term "dancing sovereignty" to describe song and dance performances that activate protocols "in ways that affirm hereditary privileges [. . .] and territorial rights to land and waterways" (Dangeli 2016, p. 75).

[2] Examples include forcing First Nations onto reservations and then creating a pass system (between 1885 and 1945) that made it illegal to move outside of ones reserve without a pass (Cram 2016), forced relocation of First Nations children to residential schools, and banning traditional and ceremonial dancing. The so-called potlatch ban, for example, could result in six months of jail time for those found guilty of participating in dances and festivals (Anderson 2018). Yet, First Nations continue to remember and embody power in their language, culture, and tradition, including their dances and movements (Anderson 2018).

References

Anderson, Charnel. 2018. The Resurgence of Powwows in Ontario | TVO Today. July 31. Available online: https://www.tvo.org/article/the-resurgence-of-powwows-in-ontario (accessed on 18 September 2022).

Ataullahjan, Salma, Wanda Elaine Thomas Bernard, and Nancy J. Hartline. 2021. *Forced and Coerced Sterilization of Persons in Canada*. Ottawa: Standing Senate Committee on Human Rights.

Bailey, Alysse, Kayla Besse, Meredith Bessey, Bonji Dube, Evadne Kelly, Tara McHugh, Seeley Quest, Carla Rice, Skylar Sookpaiboon, and Salima Punjani. Forthcoming a. Working Along the Contours of Interdisciplinary Research: Vulnerabilities and Possibilities of ReVisioning Fitness. In *Contemporary Vulnerabilities: Reflections on Social Justice Methodologies*. Edited by Claire Carter, Chelsea Jones and Caitlin Janzen. Edmonton: University of Alberta Press.

Bailey, Alysse, Meredith Bessey, Carla Rice, Evadne Kelly, Tara McHugh, Salima Punjani, Seeley Quest, Bonji Dube, Paul Tshuma, Kayla Besse, and et al. Forthcoming b. In the Wake of Canada's Violent Eugenic Legacies: An Urgency to ReVision Fitness. *Leisure/Loisir Journal*.

Barad, Karen. 2006. *Meeting the Universe Halfway: Quantum Physics and the Entanglement of Matter and Meaning*. Durham: Duke University Press.

Bednasek, C. Drew, and Anne M. C. Godlewska. 2017. The Influence of Betterment Discourses on Canadian Aboriginal Peoples in the Late Nineteenth and Early Twentieth Centuries. *The Canadian Geographer/Le Géographe Canadien* 53: 444–61. [CrossRef]

Ben-Moshe, Liat, Chris Chapman, and Allison C. Carey, eds. 2014. *Disability Incarcerated*. New York: Palgrave Macmillan US. [CrossRef]

Bessey, Meredith, Alysse Bailey, Kayla Besse, Carla Rice, Salima Punjani, and Tara McHugh. Forthcoming. ReVisioning Fitness as a Community of Practice: Conditions of Possibility for Access Intimacies and Body-Becoming Pedagogies. *Social Sciences*.

Burch, Susan. 2021. *Committed: Remembering Native Kinship in and beyond Institutions*. Chapel Hill: University of North Carolina Press.

Chandler, Eliza, Carla Rice, Sean Lee, and Max Ferguson. 2023. Curating Together: A Tangled, Intergenerational, Interdependent Community of Practice. In *Curating Access: Disability Art Activism and Creative Accommodation*. Edited by Amanda Cachia. New York: Routledge, pp. 206–18.

Cram, Stephanie. 2016. Dark History of Canada's Pass System Uncovered in New Documentary | CBC News. *News. CBC.* February 19. Available online: https://www.cbc.ca/news/indigenous/dark-history-canada-s-pass-system-1.3454022 (accessed on 18 September 2022).

Dangeli, Mique'l. 2016. Dancing Chiax, Dancing Sovereignty: Performing Protocol in Unceded Territories. *Dance Research Journal* 48: 74–90. [CrossRef]
Davis, Angela, Gina Dent, Erica Meiners, and Beth Richie. 2022. *Abolition. Feminism. Now*. Va Vergne: Haymarket Books.
Delâge, Denys, and Helen Hornbeck Tanner. 1994. The Ojibwa-Jesuit Debate at Walpole Isb. *Ethnohistory* 41: 295–321.
Diverlus, Rodney, Sandy Hudson, and Syrus Marcus Ware, eds. 2020. *Until We Are Free: Reflections on Black Lives Matter in Canada*. Regina: University of Regina Press.
Ermine, Willie. 2007. The Ethical Space of Engagement. *Indigenous Law Journal* 6: 193–203.
Foster, Susan Leigh. 2011. *Choreographing Empathy: Kinesthesia in Performance*. London and New York: Routledge.
Gaztambide-Fernández, Rubén A. 2012. Decolonization and the Pedagogy of Solidarity. *Decolonization: Indigeneity, Education & Society* 1: 41–67.
Gibson, Barbara, Gareth Terry, Jenny Setchell, Felicity Bright, Christine Cummins, and Nicola Kayes. 2020. The Micro-Politics of Caring: Tinkering with Person-Centered Rehabilitation. *Disability and Rehabilitation* 42: 1529–38. [CrossRef]
Jimmy, Elwood, and Vanessa Andreotti. 2019. *Towards Braiding*. Gesturing towards Decolonial Futures. Available online: https://decolonialfutures.net/towardsbraiding/ (accessed on 18 September 2022).
Ka'nhehsí:io, Deer. 2022. Pope Says Genocide Took Place at Canada's Residential Schools I CBC News. July 30. Available online: https://www.cbc.ca/news/indigenous/pope-francis-residential-schools-genocide-1.6537203 (accessed on 18 September 2022).
Kelly, Evadne. 2019. *Dancing Spirit, Love, and War: Performing the Translocal Realities of Contemporary Fiji*. Madison: University of Wisconsin Press.
Kelly, Evadne, and Carla Rice. Forthcoming. Eugenics and Epistemologies of Ignorance in Ontario. In *Psychiatric and Disability Institutions after Deinstitutionalisation: Memory, Sites of Conscience, and Social Justice*. Edited by Elisabeth Punzi and Linda Steele. Vancouver: UBC Press.
Kelly, Evadne, Dolleen Tisawii'ashii Manning, Seika Boye, Carla Rice, Dawn Owen, Sky Stonefish, and Mona Stonefish. 2021a. Elements of a Counter-exhibition: Excavating and Countering a Canadian History and Legacy of Eugenics. *Journal of the History of the Behavioral Sciences* 57: 12–33. [CrossRef]
Kelly, Evadne, Seika Boye, and Carla Rice. 2021b. Projecting Eugenics and Performing Knowledges. In *Narrative Art and the Politics of Health*. Edited by Sara Blanchette and Brooks Neil. New York: Anthem Press, pp. 37–62.
Krasowski, Sheldon. 1999. *A Numiany (The Prayer People) and the Pagans of Walpole Island First Nation Resistance to the Anglican Church, 1845–1885*. M.A. Canadian Heritage and Development Studies. Peterborough: Trent University.
Larasati, Rachmi Diyah. 2013. *The Dance That Makes You Vanish: Cultural Reconstruction in Post-Genocide Indonesia*. Minneapolis: University of Minnesota Press.
Mackinlay, Elizabeth. 2016. A Diffractive Narrative About Dancing Towards Decoloniality in an Indigenous Australian Studies Performance Classroom. In *Engaging First Peoples in Arts-Based Service Learning*. Edited by Brydie-Leigh Bartleet, Dawn Bennett, Anne Power and Naomi Sunderland. Landscapes: The Arts, Aesthetics, and Education. Cham: Springer Publishing, pp. 213–26. [CrossRef]
McLaren, A. 1990. *Our Own Master Race: Eugenics in Canada, 1885–1945*. Toronto: McClelland & Stewart.
Mitra, Royona. 2021. Unmaking Contact: Choreographic Touch at the Intersections of Race, Caste, and Gender. *Dance Research Journal* 53: 6–24. [CrossRef]
Nash, Jennifer. 2019. *Black Feminism Reimagined: After Intersectionality*. Durham: Duke University Press.
Ontario Heritage Trust. 2020. 2019 Lieutenant Governor's Ontario Heritage Awards Recognize Heritage Excellence in Ontario. Ontario Heritage Trust. February 21. Available online: https://www.heritagetrust.on.ca/en/media-releases/2019-lieutenant-governors-ontario-heritage-awards-recognize-heritage-excellence-in-ontario-1 (accessed on 18 September 2022).
Ontario Human Rights Commission. 2018. *Interrupted Childhoods: Over-Representation of Indigenous and Black Children in Ontario Child Welfare*. Toronto: Ontario Human Rights Commission. Available online: http://www.ohrc.on.ca/en/interrupted-childhoods (accessed on 18 September 2022).
Perazzo Domm, Daniela. 2019. Im/possible Choreographies: Diffractive Processes and Ethical Entanglements in Current British Dance Practices. *Dance Research Journal* 51: 66–83. [CrossRef]
Rice, Carla. 2014. *Becoming Women*. Toronto: UT Press.
Rice, Carla. 2015. Rethinking Fat: From Bio-to Body-Becoming Pedagogies. *Cultural Studies <=> Critical Methodologies* 15: 387–97.
Rice, Carla. 2018. The Spectacle of the Child Woman. *Feminist Studies* 44: 535–66.
Rice, Carla, Alysse Bailey, and Katie Cook. 2022. Mobilizing Interference as Methodology and Metaphor in Disability Arts Inquiry. *Qualitative Inquiry* 28: 287–99. [CrossRef]
Rice, Carla, and Ingrid Mündel. 2018. Story-making as Methodology: Disrupting Dominant Stories through Multimedia Storytelling. *Canadian Review of Sociology/Revue Canadienne de Sociologie* 55: 211–31. [CrossRef] [PubMed]
Rice, Carla, and Ingrid Mündel. 2019. Multimedia Storytelling Methodology: Notes on Access and Inclusion in Neoliberal Times. *Canadian Journal of Disability Studies* 8: 118–48. [CrossRef]
Rice, Carla, Andrea LaMarre, and Roxanne Mykitiuk. 2018. Cripping the Ethics of Disability Arts Research. In *The Palgrave Handbook of Ethics in Critical Research*. Edited by Catriona Ida Macleod, Jacqueline Marx, Phindezwa Mnyaka and Gareth J. Treharne. Cham: Springer International Publishing, pp. 257–72. [CrossRef]

Rice, Carla, Eliza Chandler, Elisabeth Harrison, Kirsty Liddiard, and Manuela Ferrari. 2015. Project Re•Vision: Disability at the Edges of Representation. *Disability & Society* 30: 513–27.

Rice, Carla, Katie Cook, and Alysse Bailey. 2021a. Difference-attuned Witnessing: Risks and Potentialities of Arts-based Research. *Feminism & Psychology* 31: 345–65. [CrossRef]

Rice, Carla, Meredith Bessey, Andrea Kirkham, and Kaley Roosen. Forthcoming. Transgressing Professional Boundaries through Fat and Disabled Embodiments. *Canadian Woman Studies*.

Rice, Carla, Sarah Riley, Andrea LaMarre, and Alysse Bailey. 2021b. What a Body Can Do: Rethinking Body Functionality through a Feminist Materialist Disability Lens. *Body Image* 38: 95–105. [CrossRef]

Rice, Carla, Susan Dion, and Eliza Chandler. 2021c. Decolonizing Disability and Activist Arts. *Disability Studies Quarterly* 41. [CrossRef]

Schneider, Rebecca. 2015. New Materialisms and Performance Studies. *TDR: The Drama Review* 59: 7–17. [CrossRef]

Simpson, Leanne B. 2011. *Dancing on Our Turtle's Back: Stories of Nishnaabeg Re-Creation, Resurgence and a New Emergence*. Winnipeg: Arbeiter Ring Publishing.

Simpson, Leanne B. 2017. *As We Have Always Done: Indigenous Freedom Through Radical Resistance*. Minneapolis: University of Minnesota Press.

Stonefish, Mona, Peter Park, Dolleen Tisawii'ashii Manning, Evadne Kelly, Seika Boye, and Sky Stonefish. 2019. *Into the Light: Eugenics and Education in Southern Ontario*. Museum Exhibition, Guelph Civic Museum. Guelph: Guelph Museums and Re•Vision: The Centre for Art and Social Justice.

Tuck, Eve, and Marcia McKenzie. 2015. *Place in Research: Theory, Methodology, and Methods*. Routledge Advances in Research Methods 9. New York: Routledge.

Viscardis, Katharine, Carla Rice, Victoria Pileggi, Angela Underhill, Eliza Chandler, Nadine Changfoot, Phyllis Montgomery, and Roxanne Mykitiuk. 2019. Difference Within and Without. *Qualitative Health Research* 29: 1287–98. [CrossRef] [PubMed]

Disclaimer/Publisher's Note: The statements, opinions and data contained in all publications are solely those of the individual author(s) and contributor(s) and not of MDPI and/or the editor(s). MDPI and/or the editor(s) disclaim responsibility for any injury to people or property resulting from any ideas, methods, instructions or products referred to in the content.

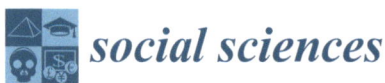

Article

Reconstruct(ing) a Hidden History: Black Deaf Canadian Relat(ing) Identity

Jenelle Rouse [1,2,*], Amelia Palmer [3] and Amy Parsons [4]

1. Faculty of Education, Western University, London, ON N6A 3K7, Canada
2. Centre for Community Services and Early Childhood, George Brown College, Toronto, ON M5R 1M3, Canada
3. Center for Black Deaf Studies, Gallaudet University, Washington, DC 20002, USA
4. Gallaudet Interpreting Service, Gallaudet University, Washington, DC 20002, USA
* Correspondence: research.blackdeafcanada@gmail.com

Abstract: Black Deaf Canadians are under-represented in every facet of life. Black Deaf Canadian excellence, history, culture, and language are under-documented and under-reported. *Where are we in history? Where are we now? Why are we not being documented?* Black Deaf Canada was established to address these long-standing issues and went on to create an independent research team that led a project called "Black Deaf History in Canada". This article provides an early account of how the community-based research team conducted a relationship-building practice prior to and during a three-week research trip. Black Deaf Canadians' relat(ing) experience in history has inspired us to fight for inclusivity.

Keywords: Black Deaf Canadian; identity; relationship-building; sign language; reworlding

Citation: Rouse, Jenelle, Amelia Palmer, and Amy Parsons. 2023. Reconstruct(ing) a Hidden History: Black Deaf Canadian Relat(ing) Identity. *Social Sciences* 12: 305. https://doi.org/10.3390/socsci12050305

Academic Editors: Nadine Changfoot, Eliza Chandler and Carla Rice

Received: 9 December 2022
Revised: 29 April 2023
Accepted: 8 May 2023
Published: 17 May 2023

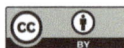

Copyright: © 2023 by the authors. Licensee MDPI, Basel, Switzerland. This article is an open access article distributed under the terms and conditions of the Creative Commons Attribution (CC BY) license (https://creativecommons.org/licenses/by/4.0/).

1. Introduction

The year 2020 is when everything in our lives shifted: the global pandemic; lockdown; social and physical distancing; job loss. Lives were senselessly lost—specifically, the life of George Floyd. A series of losses and chaos provoked many Black Deaf Canadians to reach out for a safe space to obtain comfort, support, and resilience. Natasha "Courage" Bacchus, a Black Deaf Canadian athlete turned performer, decided to reach out and host a private group talk to reflect on the idea of a Deaf Black Lives Matter (Deaf BLM) movement. Through social networking and online communication, Bacchus invited Black Deaf Canadian leaders of different professions—such as teachers, artists, athletes, and business owners—to come together for regular online sessions over several months to share individual experiences. During these sessions, our upbringings, identities, languages, cultures, and education were shared amongst the group.

There was a sense of understanding and belonging within the group. Black Deaf Canadians live in predominantly white Deaf communities, separated by long distances within a large country, making it quite challenging to find each other. While we live in various provinces and territories, we have a shared experience of isolation in the face of abnormal circumstances. Despite each member of the group identifying as Black and Deaf (what we term "Black Deaf"[1]), our understanding of, and access to, Black Deaf Canadian scholarship is challenged by audist attitudes and practices around Sign Language and the Deaf community. Audism describes audiocentric, audiosupremacist assumptions and attitudes around hearing, speaking, and behaving (Humphries 1977). Several questions emerged from the Canadian Deaf Black Lives Matter (BLM) group: Where are we in history? Where are we now? Why are we not being documented? These questions led to the formation of the research project "Black Deaf History in Canada". This research project explores these questions through a theoretical framework that brings together the concepts of Black Deaf Gain (Moges 2020) and DisCrit: Disability Studies and Critical Race Theory (Annamma et al. 2016).

Rezenet Tsegay Moges' (2020) seminal work on Black Deaf identity theorizes Black Deaf Gain as an unintended consequence of segregation and the use of Sign Language as a vehicle towards positive identity formation among Black Deaf individuals in educational contexts (From White Deaf People's Adversity to Black Deaf Gain, pp. 81–84). Moges' work is a critical counternarrative response to Bauman and Murray's (2009, 2014) coining of the initial assent term "Deaf Gain" that counters the deficit frame of terms such as "hearing loss". "Deaf Gain" refers to "unique cognitive, creative, and cultural gains manifested through deaf ways of being in the world" (Bauman and Murray 2014, pp. xv, 15). Moges (2020) built on Bauman and Murray's (2009, 2014) work to further reframe ontological notions of Deaf identity—for example, regaining a Sign Language that was historically excluded as well as studying "new" linguistic growth in Sign Languages at different ages, geographic spaces, and/or stages of cognitive development. Moges (2020) proposed that Black Deaf Gain, overlooked by Bauman and Murray (2009, 2014), needs to be acknowledged. Additionally, Moges (2020) focused on the social and historical experiences of Black Deaf people and Black Sign Language as being worthy of celebration and preservation.

In the United States, Black American Sign Language (in this case, Black ASL) has since been preserved. According to McCaskill et al. (2011), Black ASL is perceived as distinct from the use of American Sign Language (ASL) by white individuals. This is because the vernacular of African American English (AAE) is derived from middle-class white English people. Social and historical experiences of Black Deaf people are featured in Dr. Carolyn McCaskill et al.'s (2011) sociolinguistic research, as observed in historic literature on racial segregation and Civil War America, including racial desegregation in the South (after cases such as Brown vs. the Board of Education).[2] McCaskill et al. recognized, identified, and understood the differences between Black Deaf individuals and the social conditions that impact the emergence of various Sign Languages. Other than the differences between Black and white use of their respective Sign Languages, there are some identified varieties with the Black Deaf community, such as locations, ages, segregated deaf schools, integrated deaf schools, mouth movements, and education. McCaskill and her research team (McCaskill et al. 2011, 2022; McCaskill and Hill 2016) confirmed that signing while Black is evidenced in natural, traditional Sign Languages with distinct phonological, syntax, and grammatical structures and cultural, regional, and linguistic features, as found in policies and reports, some dictionaries, and ASL teaching classes.

Although the author and contributing writers ("authors" going forward) of this article appreciate these facts, a Canadian perspective is needed to determine whether Black Deaf Canadians who prefer Sign Language similarly benefit from history shaping their "language, culture, and identities" (Moges 2020, p. 73). Although the authors of this article concur with McCaskill et al.'s (2011) point that there are several geographic and social factors involved in the formation of language varieties (from a sociolinguistic perspective), the benefits and historical preservation of Black ASL within communities are different between Canada and the United States. Black ASL is influenced differently by, for example, Plains Indian Sign Languages (lingua franca), Caribbean Creole Languages, African Languages, French, and English. As proposed by McCaskill et al. (2011), the changes within Canadian Black Sign Languages are affected by upbringing, language contact, and social interactions and norms that, in turn, influence the understanding of identifying as a Black Deaf Canadian who uses Sign Language.

While adopting Moges' (2020) Black Deaf Gain theory with an embedded Canadian perspective, the authors observed Annamma et al.'s (2016) combined theories of Disability Studies and Critical Race (or DisCrit). DisCrit has seven foundational tenets, wherein it (1) observes the ways ableism, racism, (and audism) demonstrate interdependence and behavior that upholds a standard of "normalcy"; (2) celebrates intersectional or multi-dimensional identities and rejects either/or notions of identity, such as race, dis/ability, class, gender, and sexuality; (3) recognizes Western cultural norms of labeling social constructions of race and ability; (4) unveils invisible narratives of marginalized populations that are not traditionally acknowledged within research; (5) thinks about how legal and historical information (e.g., policies) un/intentionally deny rights to some citizens based on dis/ability and race; (6) notices a variety of superficial relations that racialized people with disabilities have to endure; and (7) requires activism and supports all forms of resistance (Annamma et al. 2016). Ultimately, each tenet serves to strengthen a theoretical framework for a radically intersectional approach to the topic of race and disability in institutional and community contexts. The authors of this article focus on tenets three through six as they are most relevant to this study.

The combined theories of Black Deaf Gain and DisCrit with lived Canadian perspective deliver continuous growth in societal, artistic, and academic areas to "branch out, build, and increase our understanding by considering different sides and exploring various perspectives to find deeper insights or greater truths than presently exist" (Moges 2020, p. 94). As such, "Black Deaf History in Canada" is a significant contribution to a growing body of narratives that were previously neglected. Furthermore, the present research— along with historical information and lived experiences of Black Deaf Canadians—will inspire a paradigm shift in multidisciplinary academic-, professional-, and community-based fields, such as Black Deaf Studies, Black Disability, Black History, Black Arts, Deaf Education studies, and so on. This practice of genuine community-building relationships will encourage us to rethink how we, as Black individuals, relate to our identity. It will lead to a more precise identity (re)definition with full transparency and communication and easier partnerships and community building.

This article provides an account of how establishing our organization enabled the authors, as community-based researchers, to build their individual and collective personal and professional relationships and conduct a research project. This article also shares the authors' commitment to restore and (re)construct histories of Black Deaf Canadians and outlines their research methods at various research sites (archives and museums). New insights that emerged at the early stage of data collection are presented next. This is followed by the concluding considerations of how vital community-building engagement is for incidental or direct learning to ensure that narratives of Black Deaf Canadians are identifiable, tangible, and relatable.

Throughout this article, the authors argue that Black Deaf/Black disabled Canadians are excluded from Canadian history as a result of layered oppression. Black Deaf Canadian narratives are identified as under-documented/under-represented. The processes of relationship-building and decision-making emerging from the research project and (re)constructing history with the Black community lead to the redefinition of Black Deaf Canadian relatable identity/ies.

2. Under-Documentation and Under-Representation of Black Deaf Canadians[3]

Our literature review into the work of scholars focusing on Black disabilities primarily revolves around three major themes: (a) the theory and praxis of critical race and/or critical disabilities within education (McCaskill et al. 2011; Stapleton 2015); (b) the acquired disability experience of Black Americans in later life (Harder et al. 2019); and (c) contrasting the Black disabled experience with the white disabled experience—through a white lens (Moges 2020; Renken et al. 2021). Lived experiences of cultural identities are often overlooked in various traditional research paradigms and bodies of literature. It remains imperative that Deaf researchers from their aligned cultural groups have the opportunity and access to explore, identify, and name how and in what ways our respective Black communities embrace and accept us as Deaf beings.

Deaf identities within the dominant "hearing society" face oppression, as evidenced by white American author Tom Humphries (1977), who identified its root cause of audism.[4] For him, audism means that "one is superior based on one's ability to hear or behave in the manner of one who hears. It is being understood as the bias and prejudice of hearing people against deaf people" (Humphries 1977, pp. 12–13). Over time, the term has gained more nuanced and complex meanings relevant to the authors' experiences These definitions range across multiple contexts, such as individual—an assumption that

Deaf people cannot live independently (Gertz 2008; Humphries 1977; Lane [1992] 1999); institutional—making authoritative decisions about Deaf people's lives without their engagement (Bauman 2004; Lane [1992] 1999); metaphysical—attitudinal prioritization of speaking over signing (Bauman 2004); and finally, an incorporated critical race perspective regarding laissez-faire prejudices—recognizing and dismissing the existence of Deaf people with intersectional identities (Eckert 2010).

Cho et al. (2013, p. 786) discussed the meaning of external and internal layered and intersectional oppression within audiocentric Black communities, defining "the multiple ways that race and gender interact with class in the labor market" and "interrogating the ways that states constitute regulatory regimes of identity, reproduction, and family formation" to determine "whether the subject is statically situated in terms of identity, geography, or temporality". Oppression is intersectional given the instances where race and gender are noticeably discussed, yet the experiences of race, gender, and disability are often excluded.

One example of this occurs when discussing the experience of Viola Desmond—a Black Canadian woman—who was arrested for sitting in a whites-only section at a theatre in the middle of the 20th century. She had to negotiate for her preferred seating and consequently became a civil rights activist: "... I told [the movie theatre manager] that I never sit upstairs because I can't see very well from that distance" (Backhouse 2017, p. 103). The significance of this reasoning is often not included in contemporary analyses of her story. If the previously mentioned statement is closely and carefully considered, it would reveal the possibility that Desmond had a disability (i.e., low vision). While she experienced racial discrimination, her accessibility needs as a person with a disability were also denied. At that time, fundamental human rights and disability rights were apparently not Canada's top priority when individuals with disabilities put forth their experiences of such barriers. It is our observation that Black disability/critical disability academic research is largely reserved for chronic, noncongenital medical conditions such as heart disease, diabetes, obesity, and so on. Based on this observation, Black Canadians are often considered to be Black or not Black when discussing the experiences of oppression and/or barriers.

In another example, a discussion of how race has become a more insidious aspect of the African Canadian experience in Carl James et al.'s (2010) Race and Well-Being: The Lives, Hopes and Activism of African Canadians, there is scant mention of disability or Deaf ways of being in the entire, otherwise essential, text. Black Deaf Canadian identity is clearly under-represented in academic research and in Canadian contexts; being Deaf or disabled becomes buried and invisible under layers of oppression.

When considering the identities held by Black Deaf Canadians, especially those who prefer Sign Language, the experience of audism is conflated with racism. For example, while Eckert (2010) acknowledged racism and audism within Deaf identity studies, the study was largely conducted through a white lens. This can also be seen in Eckert and Rowley (2013), Humphries (1977), and Ladd's (2003) seminal Deafhood work. These works serve as a critical praxis for understanding how white (audio-centric) supremacy is designed to prevent and/or eradicate nonwhite Deaf ways of being within educational, societal, and medical contexts; the latest frameworks serve as the de facto ways of interpreting the Deaf experience, the majority of them operating within a white lens.

Deaf academic research is overwhelmingly white. Research participants are also overwhelmingly white. Participants either have ties to Deaf schools or multigenerational Deaf families where there were no barriers to the language of access—Sign Language. Deaf scholarship, as a burgeoning field, lies mainly in the hands of Deaf elites—those with higher levels of education, from the middle class, and/or from strong Deaf ecosystem networks. The parallel discussions, research, and analysis of Deaf and Black identities are often born from an either/or approach: Black or Deaf. It was not until very recently that discussions of the Black Deaf experience emerged in academic work, such as Chapple (2019), McCaskill and Hill (2016), McCaskill et al. (2011), and Stapleton (2015). Respectively, these works discuss the Black Deaf female experience, Black Sign Language, the experience of Black

Deaf learners, and the process of working with Black Deaf participants. Black Deaf Canada is interested in the Black Deaf Canadian experience as a holistic and encompassing area of research.

It is crucial to make an explicit distinction between audism and ableism—the former focuses on the Deaf experience of moving about in a world that is audiocentric. In contrast, the latter focuses on the experience of the disabled as enforced by the abled society. Scholarship focusing on ableism in Black hearing contexts is scarce, adopting a deficit rather than celebratory mindset. Chapple (2019) reinforced this point by positing a Black Deaf feminist framework that is inclusive of disability analysis; however, her work is rooted in the feminist and female experience, whereas we are more interested in a broader systematic analysis of the Black Deaf Canadian experience. The literature captures systemic oppression that has continued to work against Black individuals and communities to create an "othering" of the Black Deaf experience (McCaskill and Hill 2016; McCaskill et al. 2011; Stapleton 2015). Harder et al. (2019) discussed ableism in communities where they found that implicit (indirect) prejudice against people with disabilities was strongest among Black and male participants. This type of prejudice has increased in older segments of the community (see Harder et al. 2019; see also Gillborn 2015).

Language shaming is another example of prejudice affected by ableism and audism when Black Deaf history is not accounted for in Canadian studies. Language shaming, the enactment of language subordination, is further defined at an institutional/governmental level with respect to Sign Language (Haualand and Holmstrom 2019; Piller 2017). Language shaming is a definite, tangible experience for Black Deaf Sign Language users, of whom there are few. Although Sign Language has been identified as a language in its own right for decades (see Stokoe 1960), it is very much an othered experience within Black communities. Piller (2017, n.p.) argued that "like other forms of stigma, language shame may have deleterious effects on the groups and individuals concerned and may result in low self-esteem, a lack of self-worth, and social alienation".

The research team recognizes that the terms "Deaf" and/or "Black Deaf" are being excluded from Black audiocentric communities. For example, a survey conducted during a Juneteenth event hosted by the DC Area Black Deaf Advocates revealed that 42 percent of respondents—all of whom were Black Deaf—concurred strongly with the phrase, *"My experience with ASL in the Black hearing community has been somewhat negative"*.[5] In reference to the experience of language shaming, a research team member shared their recollection of the range of public visceral reactions when signing in American Sign Language (ASL) with peers:

> Black Deaf friends and colleagues and I often remark on the uncomfortable experience of communicating and using ASL in Black hearing-dominant spaces. We are often infantilized, dismissed, and/or blessed by our elders. On the streets among our youth, we are on the receiving end of knee-jerk responses for the possibility of using gang signs; dismissed once it becomes evident that our language is just that—language. (Parsons 2022a)

By identifying and exploring the intersectional experiences of Black Canadians with congenital and noncongenital disabilities, specifically Black Sign Language users, we hope to name, spotlight, discuss, and ultimately contribute to an expanded body of work around the lives of Black Deaf Canadians. Racist and ableist stigmatizing attitudes and practices around Sign Language extend beyond the team's own individuality and even beyond their Black Deaf community.

With that in mind, contributions of and to all facets of the lives of Black Canadians have been explored, discussed, and defended since the beginning of the 19th century (e.g., Clifford [1999] 2006; Thomas 2021; Walker 2019). However, as we have outlined, Black Deaf Canadians and those with a disability are rarely discussed in conversations or publications. In response to this absence, two Black Canadian individuals—one Deaf artist, Tamkya Bullen, and one hearing activist[6]—connected and began to advocate together for social justice, creating a club that eventually became our organization, currently known as Black Deaf

Canada. This enabled alternative incidental learning about identities—in particular, history, culture, and language that emerged during the community-based implementation process.

In terms of the implementation process, there are a handful of scholarly sources on Deaf research team building or experiences, including Deaf and hearing team partnerships. In this instance, Renken et al. (2021) conducted a case study on the identity development of three Black Deaf secondary students during their summer course of Science, Technology, Engineering, and Math (STEM). From photographic observations, the researchers learned that students' individual identities were being defined and shaped by social and academic engagements. Peer mentorship—a form of relationship building—reveals sensitive yet complicated interactions in which students experience a sense of racial under-representation that impacts their identity development and decision-making. Student identity development often comes from self-analysis, leading to decisions on whether they identify with the term Black Deaf individual. Renken et al. (2021, p. 1109) referred to Schmitt and Leigh's (2015) literature-related observation that Deaf culture is "based upon white Deaf culture and that Black Deaf individuals may perceive themselves as doubly marginalized, from Deaf culture because of their race, and from Black culture because of their deafness".

Wolsey et al. (2017) explored the importance of clear communication within a partnership between Deaf and hearing professionals. According to the authors, vulnerability occurs through the practice of reflecting on one's power/powerless position concerning their audiological status and Sign Language awareness. The Deaf–hearing relationship takes a transformative form that offers the team guidance in comprehending and enriching their knowledge/skills. The authors add that, in spite of their similar academic statuses, the vulnerability of the power imbalance heightens the level of sensitivity in their relationship building by acknowledging their strengths and areas of need.

These examples reveal that many internalized perceptions impact our identity development. We have observed and discussed ableism, audism, racism, and language shaming. With these forces in mind, lived experiences of Black Deaf Canadians who use Sign Language are typically under-documented and under-represented. In the following section, we look at how Bullen's club, the "Black Deaf Club of Canada", initiated and transformed into Black Deaf Canada.

3. From the Black Deaf Club of Canada to Black Deaf Canada

On the nuances of Deaf identity, Leigh et al. (Leigh et al. [1992] 2020, p. 155) collaboratively wrote

> When we ask [Deaf] individuals to describe themselves, they may accept or not accept calling themselves deaf or Deaf, depending on their situation or experience. This can change over time. Those who identify themselves as culturally Deaf are individuals who use . . . signed language . . . , feel strongly that being Deaf is just fine or a gain, socialize with and get support from other culturally Deaf persons, and live a 'Deaf' way of life. They feel at home with each other.

Being "at home with each other" could describe the feeling at the core of Bullen's club that was formed in 2016. It began when Bullen met the activist (who prefers to remain anonymous) at a community activity. They shared the concern that Black Deaf and Black Deaf individuals with disabilities in Canada were often not being fully included in areas such as mental health resources, mindfulness workshops, and accessibility. The activist and Bullen observed that a Deaf-led club should be formed. Bullen and the activist developed a mission statement and publicly posted the statement on a Facebook page. The name of the club, "Black Deaf Club of Canada" was created.

The Facebook page, "Black Deaf Club of Canada", attracted the attention of Abigail Danquah, a then Canadian college student living in the United States. When Danquah saw the club's statement encouraging Black Deaf Canadians to exchange knowledge, experience, and support, she immediately contacted Bullen to request a meeting. Bullen and Danquah bonded through a series of discussions, which led them to create a safe space in which more individuals could participate.

Bullen and Danquah started small by inviting two Black Deaf Canadians, Bacchus and Andrea Zackary (business owner) to a familiar meeting place at a university. At the campus, Bacchus, Bullen, Danquah, and Zackary met to discuss ideas of how to get Bullen's club recognized on a public scale. After a few gatherings, Danquah and Zackary volunteered to help Bullen to lead the club. They debated how the club could be best established or structured in order to get financial support to afford the resources that Bullen dreamed of. However, Bullen, Danquah, and Zackary had different visions that have yet to be realized cohesively. They eventually chose to keep the club as is, without financial support.

The club operated for two years in a safe space with a few activities (e.g., workshops, social events, and drop-in gatherings). Bullen and Danquah reconnected online in August 2020 to discuss ways to continue the club. They then reached out to a Deaf BLM online group with a request for support in moving the club's initiatives forward. Three individuals answered the call, and the group worked on reviewing the club's mission to ensure that it was clear and achievable. As a result, the "Black Deaf Club of Canada" turned into the community-based project "Black Deaf Canada". Since then, Black Deaf Canada has become primarily a social network space where individuals of all ages can find each other online. The name may be subject to change in the future after a series of research and community-based consultations.

4. Research Team: Relationship-Building and Decision-Making Process

Black Deaf Canada empowers Black Deaf Canadian individuals by engaging, networking, collaborating, and forming community-building practices while resisting ableism, audism, and subtle racism. Black Deaf Canada has the skills and ability to influence changes in social and material circumstances, a practice which takes time. Team building occurs through a shared interest in a project that acknowledges members' human experiences and socioeconomic realities. All members of the research team share some similar experiences, as observed through trust, relationship, and identity development. For example, while our upbringings, practices, and behaviors toward Black Deaf, Black hearing, and non-Black individuals are different, we chose to engage in a series of much needed dialogues together that led us to eventually appreciate who and what we are.

To ensure the effectiveness of this project, relationships with scholars, educators, artists, and the Sign Language community are maintained while also recruiting highly driven Black Deaf Canadian individuals who want to pursue independent studies of Black Deaf Canadian history. At least three research team members were naturally recruited because of their interest in sharing their preliminary findings with the public. Team member/author biographies follow as a means to better elaborate on individual team members' respective and shared motivation in coming together to do this work. These short biographical accounts demonstrate some of our decision-making processes that helped us arrive to the point of adopting critical, transformative race theory as our methodology.

Abigail Danquah:

I was the one who saw the original founder's club posted online and became a co-founder. I identified as a Black person and later identified as Black Deaf. I moved to Canada for schooling and employment opportunities. With a degree in Applied Arts and Science (B.Sc.) specializing in advertising, marketing, communication, and public relations, including Deaf Cultural Studies, I have an interest in finding statistical information on Black Deaf Canadian Population.

Dr. Jenelle Rouse:

I am Black Deaf, Canadian-born, and raised in a hearing Caribbean, African-diaspora family. I am an experienced educator, scholar, adjunct professor, translator, consultant, presenter, and artist. In the fields of traditional and non-traditional education, I have been working with students of various grades, teacher candidates, interpreter candidates, and other professionals. As a listener and writer, I have an interest in sharing knowledge and experience with the public—academic and non-academic alike. In 2017, Danquah reached out to me during my studies, asking for my contribution to formative plans concerning

Sign Language and education. Although the timing was not a right fit in my schedule at that time, I expressed an interest in participating in turning the vision of the Black Deaf Canada into a reality after the completion of my studies. Once my studies were completed in the summer of 2020, I immediately joined Black Deaf Canada as a consultant and eventually became a co-director in 2021. Danquah teamed up with me to undertake the community-based interdisciplinary Black, Deaf-led Canadian research project, "Black Deaf History in Canada".

Amelia Palmer:

I am a history enthusiast, a community researcher, Black Deaf Canadian-born, and raised in my Caribbean family. At the time of writing, I am currently an undergraduate and paraprofessional student majoring in Deaf Studies and minoring in Linguistics. I have a keen interest in researching, observing, and documenting the linguistic perspective of Canadian Black ASL or Canadian Black Sign Language (CBSL), including Black Deaf History, with hidden lineage stories of Black Deaf Canadian individuals. While working at the university as a paraprofessional student, I noticed that the majority of Black Deaf individuals in North America are not aware of their relat(ing)[7] history during the 18th and 19th centuries. I feel the need to amplify a Black Deaf Canadian narrative as it is part of North American history.

Amy Parsons:

I am a Black deaf woman raised by two loving parents in K'jipuktuk, Turtle Island (Halifax, Nova Scotia, Canada). My roots run deep in the African Nova Scotian and Irish heritage communities. My familial roots originate from the Black communities of Lucasville and Weymouth Falls. As an activist for language, educational and economic justice, I work to dismantle hegemonies within educational systems and communities. I bring a historical perspective and scholarly analysis to the constructs of identity, disability, ableism, othering and equity in various racialized communities, particularly in Canadian contexts. Identifying as a queer woman, I continue to unpack and unlearn the effects of decades of experiencing an interpreted education through whiteness.

Simone Edwards-Forde:

I was born and raised on an island until I was three years old. Once I moved to Canada, I looked for connections with Black Deaf persons. I was also looking for information about Black Deaf history in my workplace where I am an educator. For years, I found nothing. I become an active community member of Black Deaf Canada where I learned about two main events in 2020 and 2021: panel discussions. The panel presenters were all Black and Canadian. During the second panel discussion's question and answer session, I assertively asked the research panelists if I could join their organization in order to learn more. Since January 2022, I have been an active member of the research project as a research assistant. I feel connected to this team. The atmosphere is warm, kind, respectful, and open to discussing raw feelings without a sense of dismissal, exemplifying the true meaning of teamwork.

5. Emergence of the Research Project

While the members of the research team have different upbringings, interests and motivations and live in different regions across North America, it is apparent that we came together for similar reasons. For more than a year, we met periodically via Zoom meetings and the WhatsApp platform for individual and group study sessions. At the beginning of our relationship-building period, we faced one of the key challenges: vulnerability.

Vulnerability is, as Judith Butler (2001, 2012) described, a physical and conscious act of recognizing and understanding our responsibility to identify what binds us (in terms of identity). Vulnerability also comprises interdependence, meaning we find our commonalities through specific "marks of national, cultural, religious, racial belonging" (Butler 2012, pp. 135–36). Our group is bound together by our shared characteristics, such as our nation (born and raised in or moved to Canada), culture (Sign Language, Deaf), and race (Black). However, "the bounded and living appearance of the body is the condition of being exposed to the other, exposed to solicitation, education, passion, injury, exposed in ways that sustain us but also in ways that can destroy us" (Butler 2012, p. 141). We may give our lives over, in each other's hands, and/or at each other's mercy. In a sense, vulnerability is not necessarily susceptible to violence, it is a form of relationality. It is an additional practice of developing relationships between individuals towards a sense of solidarity through, for example, actions of cultural conditioning and shaping.[8]

Once again, vulnerability, in our case, refers to our identities in terms of race, Deafness, and, for some of us, gender. We reframe vulnerability as a type of power when critically thinking about how we use specific language to portray our experience and understanding towards historical and present contexts (See Carbin 1996; for critical engagement as per collective and self-learning, see hooks 1994, 2010, 2013). While there is no adequate way of preparing to maintain control over how we share our lives with each other, our ethical relations are something we must address. In our discussions with one another, we learned that at different times we have each asked ourselves: *Do I disclose critical information or keep it to myself?* The asking of this question shows that we did not know each other well as we would have liked because we habitually practiced individualism. We opened up to one another. We developed a shared bond, respect, and understanding that led to a motivation to further each other's innate capabilities and interests (Butler 2001; Pethebridge 2016).

To support ourselves in getting to know one another and the development of our collective sense of identity in our newfound organization, we started with an "on pulse" exercise at the beginning of every online meeting, a technique inviting us to share about our lives and how we are doing. We then proceeded to discuss what we had learned from our conversations and make connections between our research interests, skills, and knowledge. Ongoing dialogue and investigation as a team influenced the process of reconstructing Black Deaf Canadian identity. Acceptance of individual vulnerability, from the moment we first had a meeting right through working together as a team, eventually allowed us to build a strong sense of collectivity. We knew that we could embrace uncertainty, because we trusted each other to be authentic and transparent.

We continued to meet and build relationships through a recruitment process that, in turn, led us to make decisions regarding our research project, "Black Deaf History in Canada". This project comes from a decision-making practice that led the team to consider the intersections in the literature between Black Deaf perspectives and vulnerability. Dr. Samantha Schalk (2014, p. 25) pushed for a better future by ensuring that all Black-related literature features, narratives, and perspectives of Black people with disabilities are acknowledged: "For marginalized people, [speculation] can mean imagining a future or alternative space where one's oppression no longer occurs or in which relations between currently empowered and disempowered groups are incredibly improved". To consciously move away from various oppressions (e.g., racism, ableism, audism), we explored different ways of presenting history and current Black Deaf narratives in a Canadian context that are iterative and attentive to our individual and collective identity. From our meetings, the following questions arose: *Where are we in history? Where are we now? Why are we not being documented?*

To address these questions, the research team voluntarily pursued a much-needed research project on a limited budget to begin and continue to amplify historical and current narratives of Black Deaf individuals. At the time of the COVID-19 lockdowns and social/physical distancing, it was difficult for the team to find specific information online that addressed both Black and Deaf/disabled experiences. It is crucial for the research team to reframe history and current narratives by getting accurate information on documented Black and Deaf/disabled Canadian individuals.

The following section presents the detailed procedures used for our data collection. Some details of our dialogue are also provided to give the reader a clear picture of the data-gathering process. The sections that follow briefly introduce our first research trip and interactions with the community, which supported us in locating Black and Deaf Canadians. Preliminary findings are highlighted, and we discuss how this scholarly experience informs a historical understanding of social identity (re)construction and provides deeper insight into how community-building practice impacts our identity development and shared history.

6. Method

Individual and collective identity development can occur when uncovering and discussing history. Although new to archival methodology, we chose to visit libraries, museums, and archives to read, reflect, discuss, and document using our exploratory approach. This exploratory method is a learning process in which we visualize, develop, and strengthen our research knowledge and skills in tracing sources. While we each have different skills and experiences, we agreed that this combined methodology of Black Deaf Gain and DisCrit is a good start for us to pinpoint significant pieces of history that allow us to redefine the meaning of Black History in Canadian contexts. Winston (2021, p. 293) suggested that we embrace "counter stories and alternate ways of knowing and performing archival work, particularly when these ways of knowing come from groups historically oppressed". This type of work requires time and effort.

Our anticipated long-term research field work was deferred to July 2022 due to the consequences of extended lockdowns and other personal/professional obligations. When we began the early stages of data collection at our own pace, multiple sources of data led us to the Atlantic provinces to visit different research sites and engage in conversations with three individual participants.

6.1. Research Sites: Libraries, Museums, and Archives

As Black Deaf Canada maintains a small collection of digital information (videos, photos), the research team gradually added to the documents we had collected prior to our research trip by choosing to visit Nova Scotia, New Brunswick, and Prince Edward Island. The team also developed clear and simple guidelines to follow when conducting conversations (see Figure 1 below).

The process of selecting participants and locations for conversations in Nova Scotia will be discussed in later sections. We started with community-building during our research trip. To practice community-building, everyone on the team was able to either take turns or work together to employ research methods and exploratory tools. We travelled together as a team to the Atlantic provinces, communicated our needs and wants to one another, found and shared information, and had in-depth conversations with participants). The different places we visited for research were as follows: (1) a self-tour of a street housing an established school for the deaf. (2) libraries. (3) archives, and (4) museums. Some of the sites were accessible to us because they provided qualified Sign Language interpreters who were supportive of our research and open to collaborations. We visited these areas to meet people, share, and learn from each other's historical and contemporary stories. Through touring and researching different areas over a three-week visit, we were able to confirm and strengthen prior knowledge gained from conversations, visits, and literature reviews.

In terms of the archival research process, we chose to use an open-ended exploratory approach. We started with libraries and then museums to see what we could learn from books, maps, and photos about where Black Deaf individuals might have been in the 19th century. We found that the sources directed us to specific archival sites for primary sources (newspaper articles, photos, and records) that may contain traces of Black Deaf local individuals of all ages, such as school records and service organizations. With the support of individuals who worked at the archival sites, we were able to compare and validate a list of hard and digital copies of history books, maps, newspaper articles, and photos before categorizing and sorting them.

Preparation Guideline

Make sure both parties (members of the research team and consented participants) are comfortable and understand that:

- Camcorders are on at all the time;
- Contribution to conversational data is voluntary and can withdraw at any time;
- New information after withdrawal will not be added unless consented

Conservation Starter(s):
1. Always make sure a consented participant signs a consent form before starting a conversation.
2. For social media purpose, ask for a verbal permission to record a separate video sharing some "sneak-peek" at, for example, artwork, social gatherings, meals, or other that may not be likely shared in print
3. At the beginning of the conversation, start with easy questions, such as their name, where and when born, names of family members
4. Allow the participant to do the talking and ask them to elaborate specific information (e.g. "Tell me more about…" "What do you remember about…")

Video-tape Setting:
- Two camcorders
  - One on participant(s)
  - Another on both conversation starters and participants (the space where they are positioned)
- Personal electronic devices (e.g., wireless phones) - Live or Story in social media

Figure 1. These Preparation Guidelines are a helpful tool for our research members to follow through prior to and during conversations with participants.

Finding specific information on Black Deaf Canadians in archival spaces using a genealogical approach is painfully challenging. Most names were not chronologically dated, nor were they distinguished as Black or non-Black in, for example, an archival handwritten census. Although we took a variety of different steps in finding information for the project, all actions required time, patience, and focus. Based on this experience, we began to develop archival methods that made sense to us. Visiting and reading history books at libraries was one of our initial steps that helped to narrow the focus. Books, such as Lawrence Hill's (2007) *The Book of Negroes* and Jim Hornby's (1991) *Black Islanders: Prince Edward Island's Historical Black Community*, offer keywords that afford parallel clues to potentially Black Deaf individuals' locations, family names, and timelines.

For example, one member of our team found maps in an atlas in the African History and Culture section at the Nova Scotia Library. The team compared the maps—one modern and another tracing back to the 19th century—and reviewed related books. This activity allowed us to identify and record the names of streets that were mentioned in the books. This information was then manually documented in our database that we refer to for review, analysis, speculation, and iterative processes about how we want to use the information In the next step, we visited museums, such as Africville Museum, New Brunswick Black History Society, and Prince Edward Island's private museum, where we were able to validate whether secondary sources were similar to what we had documented in the database. Once confirmed, we contacted archivists with a list of Black Deaf Canadians and accurate information from our research.

Developing friendly relationships and a good rapport with genealogists and experienced archivists were key to help reduce the work from months to weeks to days. The research experience is enriched by clearly explaining specific information concerning Black Deaf Canadian history to genealogists/archivists. Presenting and exchanging educational information between researchers and archivists/genealogists further inspires meaning in relationship and community-building, wherein knowledge is openly shared, developed, documented, and valued. Although this archival research is still at an early stage, our experience helped to narrow down the specific questions that we wanted to ask three community-based participants.

6.2. Participants

On the trip, the team used a snowball sampling approach to recruit Black Deaf persons with whom to talk. According to Goodman (2011), snowball sampling is an appropriate technique to use in a study such as ours, since Black Deaf Canadian individuals are foreseeably hard to reach. This snowball technique has been a consistent tool in this community-based research project, one the authors can employ to continuously deepen connections with each other and Black Canadian participants in different regions, either in-person or online. The team started with a first wave selection by asking at least two nonwhite Deaf/non-Deaf people to help us to identify Black Deaf Canadians in Nova Scotia. In total, three Black Deaf/non-Deaf people responded and contacted us.

The team engaged in individual conversations with these three Black participants—two Deaf and one hearing. At the time of writing, one participant had volunteered to help the team to recruit participants. With support from the team and participants, this study may gain a few new participants to be involved in dialogues within the next year. The more data we have, the richer the information that the team can analyze and share with the public will be.

6.3. Conversations

We sought informed consent from our participants—two local Black Deaf participants at their respective private homes and one Black hearing participant at an archival site. Three members of the team each had four semistructured questions to engage the participants in dialogue, while a fourth member recorded the conversation with one camcorder and one digital camera. The questions served as prompts for informal dialogue in the Black Deaf (and Black hearing) participants' Sign Language.

During the conversations, participants brought materials to share with the team, such as photos of classmates and extracurricular activities at the schools they had attended. One participant used their electronic device to show their history and interests (e.g., stamp collection).

6.4. Transcripts (In Process)

As seen in Figure 2, a member of the team reviewed and transcribed the recorded videos of each dialogue. That is, the member translated between a signer, ASL Gloss (verbatim), and plain English. A duplicate second transcript of plain English, as translated from Sign Language, was developed into ASL Gloss to allow for clear pictures of the members of the research team and the participants' representative cultural behavior and language use. Auto voice-to-text was used for transcription in exceptional cases when interpreting services were not available due to prohibitive costs or a limited availability of culturally appropriate interpreters (see Figure 3).

In the coming months, team members will code for recurring themes or topics as discussed from the conversations (Cohen et al. 2011). In greater detail, the practice of axial coding (open coding) with the generation of core categories (theoretical coding) may enable the team to capture, identify, and explain overall impressions and different behaviors, appearances, and Sign Languages. The collection and analysis of the data will reveal informative narratives of historical and contemporary contexts from Black Deaf individuals' perspectives and experiences.

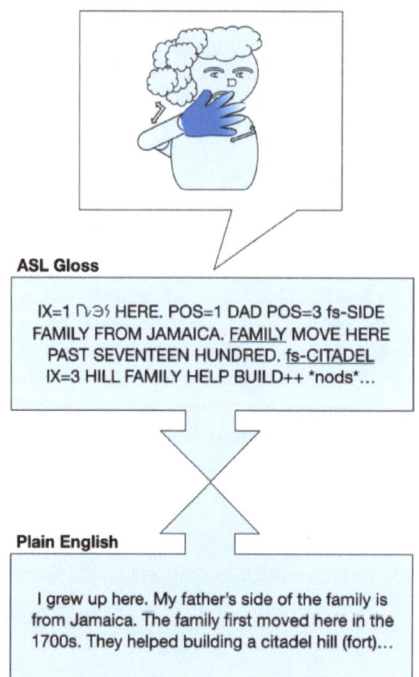

Figure 2. This is a sample of how Participant 1 was signing in a conversation, as captured from video recordings that were manually transcribed into American Sign Language (ASL) Gloss. Graphemes (i.e., symbols) are included to document any unfamiliar or unusual sign productions. For example, Participant 1 produced a word in a different palm orientation for "GROW > UP". The second box illustrates how we manually transcribed live conversations into plain English to the greatest extent possible.

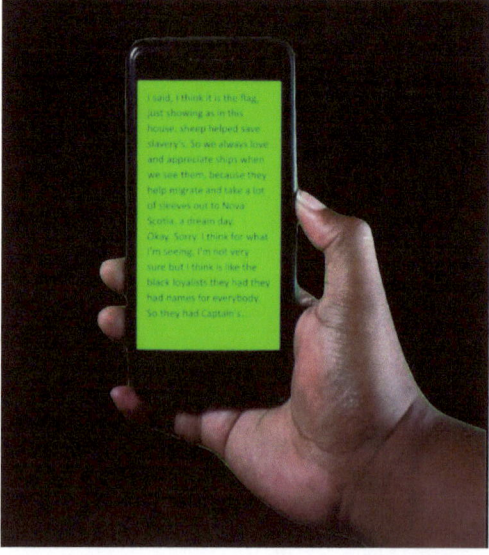

Figure 3. This is a separate sample showing spoken conversation from a tour at a museum, as transcribed by a phone's voice-to-text app. Word correction examples: sheep—ship; sleeves—slaves.

One of the many learnings from the research trip is that research requires time and patience; there is more for us to find, study, and analyze. We initially wanted to talk to at least five local Black Deaf and Black hearing participants at a social gathering (either private or public, such as a Black museum, community center, library, or park), but we ended up with only three participants. Another lesson came from the fact that during every hour-long dialogue, the battery of the camcorder ran out. This experience taught us that the research equipment needs to meet the length of our dialogues, and perhaps a professional videographer needs to be hired. A third lesson was about the relationships within the team. For some members, the research process was a new and challenging experience. The consultation with other team members throughout the process helped to deepen relationships that facilitated clearer communication. Relationship and trust building prior to the trip was helpful for inspiring that process.

7. Research Team: During the Research Trip

It is essential for the reader to know about how Canada was formed to contextualize the research trip and its findings. During the years between 1850 and 1861, Canada was not an official country as we know it today. For the decade between 1860 and 1870, Canada had two parts: West and East.

The narratives of Africville, Nova Scotia have attracted the attention of scholars and historians of all stripes. It is commonly known that, after the first Black settlement in 1794, the intergenerational community of Africville experienced racial oppression that continued for centuries. Black individuals were forced to live on uninhabitable land under difficult conditions (Clifford [1999] 2006; Nelson 2008; Rutland 2011). Despite the hardships, they managed to form a strong sense of community and thrive without governmental support (Hill 2007; Nelson 2008; Rutland 2011).

Based on the team's preliminary research findings from dialogues and archival sites in Nova Scotia, Prince Edward Island, and New Brunswick, there were several other active Black communities in East Coast cities, outside of Africville, Nova Scotia. For example, there were Black communities in Shelburne, East Preston, Annapolis Royal, Cherry Brook, Halifax, Sydney, Springhill, North Preston, and Beechville. Some Black Deaf Canadians from intergenerational Black communities within thirty kilometers of Halifax attended a school for the Deaf, which was built in 1856 on Gottigen Street (it was demolished and rebuilt in 1896 for a growing number of Deaf student enrolments from the Maritimes. The school of the Deaf in Halifax was in operation from 1896 to 1961 before it was relocated to Amherst, Nova Scotia; see (Carbin 1996)).

The terms Black Deaf, or even Deaf, rarely appeared in online archives. Instead, they are found in archival and museum sites' primary sources. The terms used by historians, surveyors, and other data collectors to identify or describe Black Deaf individuals include "Negro" and "colored". It was also a challenge to find specific and credible information on Black Deaf Canadian history, because information such as Black Deaf excellence in Canada in the distant past is ephemeral (short-lived). For example, a newspaper article in the early 20th century briefly shared a minister's recollection of a quiet Black Deaf child. The team unsuccessfully tried to find more information on the child, even with the archivists' help. A variety of documents (such as studies, reports, and censuses) typically use deficit terminology such as "deaf and dumb", "people who cannot hear", "hearing impaired", and "hearing loss". While the first term is now widely recognized to be offensive, the last three terms are still being used in audiocentric communities. The stigmatization connected to this deficit terminology further deters Black Deaf Canadians from knowing their history and from embracing their identities, languages, and other aspects of their lives.

8. Relat(ing) Identity Insights

Upon returning home from the three-week trip, we discussed and observed how we, as Black Deaf Canadians, support each other amidst community attitudes rooted in ableism. When we meticulously searched for a meaningful (re)construction of self through, for example, statistics, censuses, materials (e.g., photos), and dialogues, we uncovered unexpected information. In the past, Black Deaf Canadians experienced limited (shortened) education. They were offered prolonged and repetitive vocational training that led to the early onset of additional disabilities, underemployment, and a lack of socialization with Black hearing communities. This corresponds with the documented history of education in the United States for Black Deaf children, including a lack of access to sign language, low expectations, poorly funded resources, and prioritization of education advancement (McCaskill et al. 2011, 2022; Simms and Thumann 2007; Simms et al. 2008), and reduced livelihoods for Black Deaf adults due to the low diversity of professions, insufficient training, and medical conditions (McCaskill et al. 2011, 2022; Perrodin-Njoku et al. 2022).

Despite all of this, Black Deaf Canadians maintained optimal attitudes and strong relationships with their children. For example, a Black Deaf research participant shared that they went to a predominantly white mainstream school as a child, and their dream of becoming a judge was denied outright because they were Black Deaf. The participant was instead redirected to take vocational training when their teachers would not provide resources to ensure that their academic learning and Sign Language needs were met. The participant was whitewashed to the point where they used to believe that no Black Deaf individuals were capable of advancing their education. Not only were their future social and economic capacities suppressed by vocational education, but so were their Black Deaf identities. This participant eventually acquired Sign Language, and it is through Sign Language that they communicated their dreams to their children. Sign language is valuable for communicating dreams and, in doing so, (re)constructs history and identity. All of this participant's children are now studying human rights law, especially concerning Black Deaf lives.

9. Concluding Considerations

Black Deaf Canada and the Sign Language Deaf community are grappling with a profound lack of resources, knowledge, and opportunities. We need resources to make Black Deaf Canadian's histories visible and to foster positive cultural identities. This is especially important in the wake of the latest iteration of the Black Lives Matter movement and in the context of overt government and system-sanctioned racism.

This article shows how the authors overcame ableism and audism integrated with racism by learning, supporting, and working together. Our relationships led to the enrichment of the research project. There has been steady growth in the documentation and scholarship of Black Deaf Canadians through the application of a combined framework—Moges' (2020) Black Deaf Gain, and Annamma et al.'s (2016) DisCrit. The more people we met during our research trip, the more enlightened we became regarding Black Deaf history and identity formation. Ongoing relationship-building and decision-making helped to (re)construct Black community history and to redefine Black Deaf Canadian relatable identity/ies, changing them/us from invisible to visible. The project moved us from being buried in audism and ableism to building the community and deepening the understanding of the diversity of Black Deaf experiences in Canada. Community-building occurred among the research team, with Black Deaf Canadians, and with the museum, library, and archive personnel who we met and educated in the process of our research.

Black Deaf Canadians will benefit from gaining knowledge and community-building through our growing historical narratives. Importantly, our action research enables us to transform our identities as individual Black Deaf Canadians prior to our organization to form a collective and shared identity as we continue our research and relationship-building. Building upon the hidden history and understanding of the Black Deaf community is essential, noteworthy, and invaluable, especially when carried out with/in Black, Black Deaf, and Black disability communities.

Academic study of Deaf experiences and language has primarily focused on the white Deaf experience. Meanwhile, the academic study of Black Canadian communities has solely focused on racial experiences and not broader disabled experiences. Narratives of Black

Deaf Canadian experiences are under-documented and under-represented. Our experiences often fade into the distant past or the invisible present. Despite the omission of Black Deaf Canadians from reports, statistics, and censuses, a few mentions are documented in books, as discussed. As such, through Black Deaf Canada, we are discovering and reconstructing our history/ies.

Currently, the experience of audism is closely interwoven with ableism, racism, and other experiences of disability in Black hearing, nonsigning communities. This is a reminder of the glaring gap in the histories of Black Deaf Canadians that the research team is addressing. Our ways of tackling this gap are deeply personal, rooted in community, and challenge the status quo.

The preliminary findings from this research project provide some answers to Black Deaf Canadians of all ages. We continue to collect data, plan future research trips, and seek Black Deaf Canadians to engage in dialogue. We look forward to the analysis of the coded data from our transcripts. Despite layered oppression, narratives of Black Deaf Canadians' lived experiences, stories, and connections do live on, and—as we are discovering—are identifiable, tangible, and relatable.

While visible and/or tangible representation matters to us, identity is a vital part of the Black Deaf community because of a shared struggle to create a safe space for ourselves. Narratives of past, present, and future generations of Black Deaf Canadians are what we are fighting for: more visibility; more representation; more documentation; no more language shaming. We are centering and elevating our Black Deaf Canadian experiences in the pursuit of better education, greater access, and comprehensive resources. We broadcast with pride: We see ourselves in historical and contemporary Black Deaf Canadian narratives. Now, we know where and how to find Black Deaf Canadians in communities, in documentation, and in records. *We can finally relate.*

Author Contributions: Conceptualization, J.R.; methodology, J.R. and A.P. (Amy Parsons); validation, J.R.; writing—original draft preparation, J.R., A.P. (Amelia Palmer) and A.P. (Amy Parsons); writing—review and editing, J.R., A.P. (Amelia Palmer) and A.P. (Amy Parsons); visualization, J.R.; supervision, J.R.; project administration, J.R., A.P. (Amelia Palmer) and A.P. (Amy Parsons). All authors have read and agreed to the published version of the manuscript.

Funding: This research received no external funding.

Institutional Review Board Statement: Not applicable. The nontraditional independent research project belongs to Black Deaf Canada, as discussed in this article.

Informed Consent Statement: Informed consent was obtained from all subjects involved in the study.

Data Availability Statement: Data is not available due to privacy.

Conflicts of Interest: The authors declare no conflict of interest.

Notes

1. Considering intersectionality theory explored from two standpoints of racialized people—one hearing (Hill Collins 2000) and another deaf (Eckert and Rowley 2013), our research team has discussed and intentionally chosen to use the term, "Black Deaf", as it reflects both our individual and collective lived experiences.
2. According to McCaskill et al. (2011), racial segregation in its modern form began in the late 1800s in the United States where slavery had existed for more than two hundred years prior to the Civil War. Racial segregation resulted in public policy that banned Black people from a higher standard of education.
3. Although Black Deaf Canadian experience and narrative is omitted from the reports, statistics and censuses, it is acknowledged in a small number of documents. Examples include: McAskill et al.'s (2022) theatre arts article, "Interview with Natasha Bacchus, a.k.a. Courage", Clifton F. Carbin's (1996) years-long documented history book, *Deaf Heritage in Canada: A Distinctive Diverse and Enduring Culture*, and Evelyne Gounetenzi's (1999) hard copy report, Multiculturalism and the Deaf".
4. Eckert and Rowley (2013) further explain contextual audism in relation to discrimination of overt, covert, and aversive behaviors.
5. The remainder of responses included 17 percent reporting their experience as somewhat negative; 21 percent as somewhat positive, and 21 percent as mostly positive (Parsons 2022b).
6. This hearing activist person asked to remain anonymous.

⁷ We use the word "relat(ing)" instead of "related" to illustrate a continuous action of uncovering and relearning history that in turn evolves our identities as Black Deaf Canadians in a non-static manner—whether the history itself is distant, recent, or current.

⁸ Danielle Pethebridge (2016) discusses vulnerability in a critical framework to understand individuals' individuality-related roles in various contexts.

References

Annamma, Subini Ancy, David J. Connor, and Beth A. Ferri. 2016. Dis/Ability Critical Race Studies: Theorizing at the Intersections of Race and Dis/Ability. In *DisCrit: Disability Studies and Critical Race Theory in Education*. Edited by David J. Connor, Beth A. Ferri and Subini Ancy Annamma. New York: Teachers College Press, pp. 9–32.

Backhouse, Constance. 2017. "Bitterly Disappointed" at the Spread of "Colour-Bar Tactics": Viola Desmond's Challenge to Racial Segregation, Nova Scotia, 1946. In *The African Canadian Legal Odyssey: Historical Essays*. Edited by Barrington Walker. Toronto: University of Toronto Press, pp. 101–66. [CrossRef]

Bauman, H-Dirksen L. 2004. Audism: Exploring the Metaphysics of Oppression. *Journal of Deaf Studies and Deaf Education* 9: 239–46. [CrossRef] [PubMed]

Bauman, H-Dirksen L., and Joseph J. Murray. 2009. Reframing: From Hearing Loss to Deaf Gain. *Deaf Studies Digital Journal* 1: 1–10.

Bauman, H-Dirksen L., and Joseph J. Murray. 2014. *Deaf Gain: Raising the Stakes for Human Diversity*. Minneapolis: University of Minnesota Press.

Butler, Judith. 2001. Giving an Account of Oneself. *Diacritics* 31: 22–40. [CrossRef]

Butler, Judith. 2012. Precarious Life, Vulnerability, and the Ethics of Cohabitation. *The Journal of Speculative Philosophy* 26: 134–51. [CrossRef]

Carbin, Clifton F. 1996. *Deaf Heritage in Canada: A Distinctive, Diverse, and Enduring Culture*. Toronto: McGraw-Hill Ryerson.

Chapple, Reshawna L. 2019. Toward a Theory of Black Deaf Feminism: The Quiet Invisibility of a Population. *Affilia* 34: 186–98. [CrossRef]

Cho, Sumi, Kimberlé W. Crenshaw, and Leslie McCall. 2013. Toward a Field of Intersectionality Studies: Theory, Applications, and Praxis. *Signs: Journal of Women in Culture and Society* 38: 785–810. [CrossRef]

Clifford, Mary Louise. 2006. *From Slavery to Freetown: Black Loyalists after American Revolution*. Jefferson: McFarland and Company, Inc. First published 1999. Available online: https://archive.org/details/fromslaverytofre0000clif/page/74/mode/2up?q=hearing (accessed on 12 June 2022).

Cohen, Louis, Lawrence Manion, and Keith Morrison. 2011. *Research Methods in Education*. London: Routledge.

Eckert, Richard Clark. 2010. Toward a Theory of Deaf Ethnos: Deafnicity D/Deaf (Homaemon-Homoglosson-Homothreskon). *Journal of Deaf Studies & Deaf Education* 15: 317–33. [CrossRef]

Eckert, Richard Clark, and Amy June Rowley. 2013. Audism: A Theory and Practice of Audiocentric Privilege. *Humanity & Society* 37: 101–30. [CrossRef]

Gertz, Genie. 2008. Dysconscious Audism: A Theoretical Proposition. In *Open Your Eyes: Deaf Studies Talking*. Edited by H-Dirksen L. Bauman. Minneapolis: University of Minnesota Press, pp. 219–38.

Gillborn, David. 2015. Intersectionality, Critical Race Theory, and the Primacy of Racism: Race, Class, Gender, and Disability in Education. *Qualitative Inquiry* 21: 277–87. [CrossRef]

Goodman, Leo A. 2011. Comment: On Respondent-Driven Sampling and Snowball Sampling in Hard-to-Reach Populations and Snowball Sampling Not in Hard-to-Reach Populations. *Sociological Methodology* 41: 347–53. [CrossRef]

Gounetenzi, Evelyne. 1999. *Mullticullturalism and the Deaf*. Ottawa: Canadian Association of the Deaf.

Harder, Jenna A., Victor N. Keller, and William J. Chopik. 2019. Demographic, Experiential, and Temporal Variation in Ableism. *Journal of Social Issues* 75: 683–706. [CrossRef]

Haualand, Hilde, and Ingela Holmstrom. 2019. When Language Recognition and Language Shaming Go Hand in Hand—Sign Language Ideologies in Sweden and Norway. *Deafness & Education International* 21: 99–115. [CrossRef]

Hill Collins, Patricia. 2000. *Black Feminist Thought: Knowledge, Consciousness, and the Politics of Empowerment*. New York: Routledge. [CrossRef]

Hill, Lawrence. 2007. *The Book of Negroes*. Toronto: HarperCollins.

hooks, bell. 1994. *Teaching to Transgress: Education as the Practice of Freedom*. London: Routledge.

hooks, bell. 2010. *Teaching Critical Thinking: Practical Wisdom*. London: Routledge.

hooks, bell. 2013. *Teaching Community: A Pedagogy of Hope*. London: Routledge.

Hornby, Jim. 1991. *Black Islanders: Prince Edward Island's Historical Black Community*. Charlottetown: Institute of Island Studies.

Humphries, Tom. 1977. Communicating Across Cultures (Deaf/Hearing) and Language Learning. Ph.D. thesis, Union Graduate School, Cincinnati, OH, USA.

James, Carl, David Este, Wanda Thomas Bernard, Akua Benjamin, Bethan Lloyd, and Tana Turner. 2010. *Race and Well-Being: The Lives, Hopes and Activism of African Canadians*. Halifax: Fernwood Publishing.

Ladd, Paddy. 2003. *Understanding Deaf Culture: In Search of Deafhood*. Cleveland: Multilingual Matters.

Lane, Harlan. 1999. *Masks of Benevolence: Disabling the Deaf Community*. San Diego: Dawn Signs. First published 1992.

Leigh, Irene W., Jean F. Andrews, and Raychelle L. Harris. 2020. *Deaf Culture: Exploring Deaf Communities in the United States*. San Diego: Plural Publishing. First published 1992.

McAskill, Ash, Christopher Desloges, and Natasha Cecily Bacchus. 2022. Interview with Natasha Bacchus, a.k.a. Courage. *Canadian Theatre Review* 190: 50–52. [CrossRef]

McCaskill, Carolyn, and Joseph C. Hill. 2016. Reflections on the Black ASL Project. *Sign Language Studies* 17: 59–63. Available online: http://www.jstor.org/stable/26189128 (accessed on 2 January 2023).

McCaskill, Carolyn, Ceil Lucas, Robert Bayley, and Joseph Hill. 2011. *The Hidden Treasure of Black ASL: Its History and Structure*. Washington, DC: Gallaudet University Press.

McCaskill, Carolyn, Ceil Lucas, Robert Bayley, and Joseph Hill. 2022. Segregation and Desegregation of the Southern Schools for the Deaf: The Relationship Between Language Policy and Dialect Development. *Language* 98: 173–98. [CrossRef]

Moges, Rezenet Tsegay. 2020. From White Deaf People's Adversity to Black Deaf Gain: A Proposal for a New Lens of Black Deaf Educational History. *Journal Committed to Social Change on Race and Ethnicity* 6: 69–99. [CrossRef]

Nelson, Jennifer J. 2008. *Razing Africville: A Geography of Racism*. Toronto: University of Toronto Press.

Parsons, Amy. 2022a. (Gallaudet University, Washington, DC, USA). Personal communication.

Parsons, Amy. 2022b. Gaps in Recruiting & Retaining Black/IBPOC CDIs: Understanding and Addressing Systemic Causes. Paper presented at the Celebrating Juneteenth: The Black Deaf Experience, Washington, DC, USA, June 18.

Perrodin-Njoku, Emmanuel, Carolyn Corbett, Rezenet Moges-Riedel, Laurene Simms, and Poorna Kushalnagar. 2022. Health Disparities among Black Deaf and Hard of Hearing Americans as Compared to Black Hearing Americans: A descriptive Cross-Sectional Study. *Medicine* 101: 1–7. [CrossRef]

Pethebridge, Danielle. 2016. What's Critical about Vulnerability? Rethinking Interdependence, Recognition, and Power. *Hypatia* 31: 589–604. Available online: http://www.jstor.org/stable/44076494 (accessed on 2 November 2022). [CrossRef]

Piller, Ingrid. 2017. Explorations in Language Shaming. *Language on the Move*. Available online: https://research-management.mq.edu.au/ws/portalfiles/portal/92948453/92947702.pdf (accessed on 28 June 2022).

Renken, Maggie, Jessica Scott, Patrick Enderle, and Scott Cohen. 2021. 'It's Not a Deaf Thing, It's Not a Black Thing; It's a Deaf Black Thing': A Study of the Intersection of Adolescents' Deaf, Race, and STEM Identities. *Cultural Studies of Science Education* 16: 1105–36. [CrossRef]

Rutland, Ted. 2011. Re-Remembering Africville. *City* 15: 757–61. [CrossRef]

Schalk, Samantha Dawn. 2014. Breaking the rules: (Dis)ability in Black Women's Speculative Fiction. Ph.D. dissertation, Indiana University, Bloomington, IN, USA.

Schmitt, Shawn S. Nelson, and Irene W. Leigh. 2015. Examining a Sample of Black Deaf Individuals on the Deaf Acculturation Scale. *Journal of Deaf Studies and Deaf Education* 20: 283–95. [CrossRef] [PubMed]

Simms, Laurene, and Helen Thumann. 2007. In Search of a New Linguistically and Culturally Sensitive Paradigm in Deaf Education. *American Annals of the Deaf* 152: 302–11. [CrossRef] [PubMed]

Simms, Laurene, Melissa Rusher, Jean F. Andrews, and Judy Coryell. 2008. Apartheid in Deaf Education: Examining Workforce Diversity. *American Annals of the Deaf* 153: 384–95. [CrossRef] [PubMed]

Stapleton, Lissa. 2015. When Being Deaf Is Centered: d/Deaf Women of Color's Experiences with Racial/Ethnic and d/Deaf Identities in College. *Journal of College Student Development* 56: 570–86. [CrossRef]

Stokoe, William. 1960. *Sign Language Structure: An Outline of the Visual Communication Systems of the American Deaf*. Buffalo: Department of Anthropology and Linguistics, University of Buffalo.

Thomas, Jesse. 2021. Former Nova Scotia Orphanage for Black Children Marks 100th Anniversary—Halifax. *Global News*. Available online: https://globalnews.ca/news/7926204/nova-scotia-home-for-colored-children-anniversary (accessed on 12 June 2022).

Walker, James W. 2019. *The Black Loyalists: The Search for a Promised Land in Nova Scotia and Sierra Leone 1783–1870*. Toronto: University of Toronto Press. [CrossRef]

Winston, Rachel E. 2021. Praxis for the People: Critical Race Theory and Archival Practice. In *Knowledge Justice: Disrupting Library and Information Studies through Critical Race Theory*. Edited by Sofia Y. Leung and Jorge R. López-McKnight. Cambridge: MIT Press, pp. 283–98.

Wolsey, Ju-Lee A., Kim Misener Dunn, Scott W. Gentzke, Hannah A. Joharchi, and M. Diane Clark. 2017. Deaf/Hearing Research Partnerships. *American Annals of the Deaf* 161: 571–82. [CrossRef]

Disclaimer/Publisher's Note: The statements, opinions and data contained in all publications are solely those of the individual author(s) and contributor(s) and not of MDPI and/or the editor(s). MDPI and/or the editor(s) disclaim responsibility for any injury to people or property resulting from any ideas, methods, instructions or products referred to in the content.

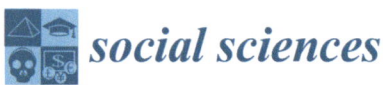# social sciences

Article

Dinner Table Experience in the Flyover Provinces: A Bricolage of Rural Deaf and Disabled Artistry in Saskatchewan

Chelsea Temple Jones [1,*], Joanne Weber [2], Abneet Atwal [1] and Helen Pridmore [3]

1. Department of Child and Youth Studies, Brock University, St. Catharines, ON L2S 3A1, Canada
2. Faculty of Education, University of Alberta, Edmonton, AB T6G 2R3, Canada
3. Independent Researcher, Saskatoon, SK S7N 0G3, Canada
* Correspondence: cjones@brocku.ca

Abstract: "Dinner table experience" describes the uniquely crip affect evoked by deaf and disabled people's childhood memories of sitting at the dinner table, witnessing conversations unfolding around them, but without them. Drawing on 11 prairie-based deaf and/or disabled artists' dinner table experiences, four researcher-artivist authors map a critical bricolage of prairie-based deaf and disabled art from the viewpoint of a metaphorical dinner table set up beneath the wide-skyed "flyover province" of Saskatchewan. Drawing on a non-linear, associative-thinking-based timespan that begins with Tracy Latimer's murder and includes a contemporary telethon, this article charts the settler colonial logics of normalcy and struggles over keeping up with urban counterparts that make prairie based deaf and disability arts unique. In upholding an affirmative, becoming-to-know prairie-based crip art and cultural ethos using place-based orientations, the authors point to the political possibilities of artmaking and (re)worlding in the space and place of the overlooked.

Keywords: disability and deaf art; dinner table experience; creative analytic practice; affirmative ethics; Canadian prairie

1. Introduction

Commonly, deaf[1] and disabled people carry childhood memories of sitting at the dinner table witnessing conversations unfolding around them but without them. The dinner table, a symbol of family experience sharing in Western hearing worlds, represents Anglo-civility, normate comportment, and the shared experience—for some, not others—of keeping up (Bahan et al. 2008). Meek (2018) describes feelings of isolation and frustration that come from being excluded from this bonding time: "The *dinner table syndrome* is a metaphor for all of the conversations that are not completely accessible when deaf people are in situations with hearing groups" (p. 2).[2] Knowing that this metaphorical experience relies on normative orientations toward the dinner table, we begin this experimental writing with one of Ahmed's (2006) opening questions in *Queer Phenomenology*: "How do we begin to know or to feel where we are, or even where we are going, by lining ourselves up with the features of the grounds we inhabit, the sky that surrounds us or the imaginary lines that cut through maps?" (p. 6).

This question is crucial to our orientations toward each other and the metaphorical dinner table because it directs our attention to what Braidotti (2018) calls the "non-negotiable politics of location" (p. 210). Taking place as both literal (where we are now) and ephemeral (the trajectories of thought we espouse), we suggest that location is a leading feature of affirmative-ethics-based process ontology and the eventual re-ordering of the world that is central to the creative and political work of deaf and disability arts. Following Chandler (2018) and this special issue's attention to (re)worlding—an affective, artful, and imaginative project guided by multiple lines of thought—we consider both the conditions of possibility for the establishment of difference in the Canadian Prairies as well as new

Citation: Jones, Chelsea Temple, Joanne Weber, Abneet Atwal, and Helen Pridmore. 2023. Dinner Table Experience in the Flyover Provinces: A Bricolage of Rural Deaf and Disabled Artistry in Saskatchewan. *Social Sciences* 12: 125. https://doi.org/10.3390/socsci12030125

Academic Editor: Nigel Parton

Received: 1 December 2022
Revised: 10 February 2023
Accepted: 14 February 2023
Published: 24 February 2023

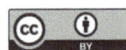

Copyright: © 2023 by the authors. Licensee MDPI, Basel, Switzerland. This article is an open access article distributed under the terms and conditions of the Creative Commons Attribution (CC BY) license (https://creativecommons.org/licenses/by/4.0/).

worldly arrangements made possible through deaf and disabled people's creative and political work. Ahmed's question points upward at "the sky that surrounds us," and is a reminder that the sky is culturally significant in Saskatchewan and for the (re)worlding that happens here. To find the "imaginary lines" that border Saskatchewan on the colonizer's map, plant your finger right in the middle of Canada. It will land on a rectangular landmass between the provinces of Alberta and Manitoba cropping a 651,000-kilometer space that engulfs six Treaty territories—Treaty 2, Treaty 4, Treaty 5, Treaty 6, Treaty 8, and Treaty 10. Much of our work takes place in Treaty 4, a negotiation between the Cree and Saulteaux in 1874 that remains important for the 11 First Nations that live in the treaty's catchment area (Stonechild n.d.). There is little to obstruct the view of the sky on this flat land, with its straight, snaking highways and Saskatchewan license plates emblazoned with the 1997 contest-winning slogan, "The land of living skies" (Romuld 2020). The livingness of the sky is sometimes characterized by bird migrations and cloudy streaks of exhaust left behind by flyover planes. Residents cheekily call Saskatchewan a "flyover province" because it is couched between urban destinations on either coast of Canada, marking an overlooked-ness that parallels the uniquely crip dinner table experience affect. Our imagined metaphorical dinner table exists beneath a wide sky on this flat, colonized land with rich but often overlooked disability art and culture.

Through this experimental writing, which draws on prairie-based deaf and disabled artists' descriptions of dinner table experience, we actively construct methods "from the tools at hand" rather than from pre-existing guidelines—an exploratory mode of scholarship Kincheloe (2005) calls bricolage (p. 324). We read bricolage as intimate scholarship because it involves process ontologies that attend to unexplored embodied knowledge through action (Strom et al. 2018), including "coming-to-know" through dialogue such as interviews, jam sessions, and creative analytic practice—methods we describe below. The process ontology represented in the writing that follows is an act of collective intimate scholarship that aims to account for the overlooked and calls for affirmative ways of becoming and (re)worlding through radical relationality amid interconnected events that shape our contexts (Braidotti 2019). Leading with location, we position ourselves as bricoleurs mapping contemporary upswells in deaf and disabled art in the northern center of Turtle Island known as the Canadian Prairies. Below, we elaborate on "coming-to-know" or, *becoming-to-know*, through a bricolage of partial, fragmented knowledges (Haraway 1988), collective memory work, and narrative—all amid settler perspectives and the intricate, un-pin-downable performative nature of rurality and voice that shapes a prairie-based crip art movement embedded in the political possibilities and (re)worlding efforts of the overlooked (Cella 2017; Hamilton et al. 2016, p. 183).

2. Positioning

Our writing collaboration includes Jones (she/her), a hearing white settler who spent much of her childhood on the Canadian Prairies growing up alongside a disabled brother; Weber (she/her), who is deaf and the artistic director of Deaf Crows Collective based in Regina, Saskatchewan; Atwal (she/her), a hearing first-generation South Asian Canadian based in the Region of Peel in Ontario; and Pridmore (she/her), a hearing first-generation British Canadian settler who is a musician based in the Prairies. We have been involved in this arts-based research collaboration since a 2019 event in Regina called "Disability Artivism in the Flyover Provinces," which began slowly mapping contemporary upswells in deaf and disabled art in Saskatchewan.

Following Braidotti (2017, 2018, 2021), who asserts that a politics of location demands accountability and new ways of thinking about processes of becoming, we situate ourselves as *becoming-to-know*. Becoming-to-know refers to practice-based processes of knowledge creation that are deeply attentive to context (Hamilton and Pinnegar 2014, 2015; Jakubik 2011) and that are "thinking alongside" rather than centering identity (Braidotti 2018, p. 210). For us, coming from fields of critical disability studies (Jones), deaf education (Weber), disabled children's childhood studies and DisCrit (Atwal), and music (Pridmore), this means tracking our transdisciplinary process ontology (Yardley 2020). To do this, we embrace non-linearity and associative thinking (what Braidotti, following Derrida, calls "zig-zag thinking" (2018, p. 210) as we ongoingly build our (inevitably partial) understanding of the disability and deaf art scene on the Canadian Prairies, beginning in Saskatchewan. Here, we meet at the intersections of disability, gender, race, place, and voice to dwell in the uniquely crip affect of not keeping up evoked by memories of being overlooked individually and culturally. Following Hardy,[3] we recast "dinner table syndrome" as "dinner table experience" (to usurp pathological connotations of "syndrome") and we bricolage three key markers of prairie-based disability culture to lend context to our research and to ground the (re)worlding work that is ongoing in this place: the 1993 killing of Tracy Latimer, the ongoing existence of a major telethon, and amidst this, the dinner table experience affect that impacts the culminating rise of deaf and disability arts and the (re)worlding work of this movement along the way.

3. Context: Research in "the Flyover" Provinces

Imagine the scene: a fowl supper, prairie gothic style. A plastic, spill-proof tablecloth covers a long fold-out table in a church basement in the town of Wilkie, Saskatchewan—a former railway station on the Canadian Pacific Railway line, today a town with a population of just over 1300 people. It is October 1993, a few days after the murder of a 12-year-old disabled girl, Tracy Latimer. Weber, a long-time resident of the community, remembers:

> It is a grey day. Farmers are continually thwarted by rain, unable to get their crops off in a timely manner. A few days ago, a farmer snapped and parked his daughter in his truck, left the ignition on in order to induce death by carbon monoxide poisoning. Despite the meager supports available to the family (who was struggling with the care for the daughter, unable to move independently, and a newborn baby), the daughter was sacrificed against the economic, social, and personal survival of the family.

Soon, this murder will make national and global headlines, escalating public debate and polarization over whose lives are worth living. In November 1994, before the case goes to court, the monthly Canadian news magazine *Maclean's* releases a full-page cover that puts readers in Robert Latimer's position by boldly asking, "what would you do?" (*Maclean's*). As the court deliberates in 1997, a *New York Times* pull quote tells readers "[a] euthanasia case becomes a cause célèbre in Canada" (DePalma 1997, p. A3). By 2009, Robert Latimer is on parole and BBC News World Service is interviewing him for a documentary broadcast that airs across the globe (*The Interview* 2009). This story will cast a long shadow on disability culture in Canada, though its rural contours will often be overlooked—flown over, in a way, as urban-based critics and scholars condemn the killing.

For now, we have gathered at this community table to reflect on, and operationalize, the setting. We wonder if "the Prairies" refers to the sky or the land or the people who live here, or to something else—perhaps a thicker, deeper affective economy rooted in a prairie aesthetic. Marler (2011) describes "the Prairies" as "a landscape perceived, paradoxically, as both edenic and utopic as well as dystopic—foreign, empty, abject" (p. 9). Or, put another way, "the Prairies" operate in a culture of crisis despite its vividly romantic and picturesque living skies (Kaye 2005). Aware that power and place are coproduced (Tuck and McKenzie 2015), we know that the temporal and spatial dimensions of this work leave their mark on our bodies, and it is our bodies that move us through our *becoming-to-know* methodology and methods.

In our findings below, we situate our research processes in a Western, prairie-entangled cultural logic whose dominant narratives of deafness and disability result in a gendered, ableist, audiocentric, and rural cultural mix. Despite the perception that "nothing happens" while we occupy this space and place, what emerges as grievable is determined as that which is "culturally living" in the minds, memory, and events perceived by others (Massey 2005; Pullman and Nichols 2015, p. 29). Yet, given that non-normative lives have been recognized as lives to be grieved, disability and deaf cultural production is always bound up in the complex politics of grief—grief is a line etched into the dinner table (Ahmed 2015; Piepzna-Samarasinha 2022). In building a bricolage deaf and disability artistry on the Prairies, the lingering grief around Tracy Latimer's murder serves as a useful foundation. This event flags a particular apprehension of space and time that frames our research: what sets Latimer's murder apart from other disability rights propellors in Canada is the gendered nature of this violence and its subsequent excusability based on white settler logics willing to overlook the killing of a disabled girl.

3.1. "A Perfectly Nice Guy": Convergences of Race, Gender, and Disability

To understand the conditions of possibility for Tracy Latimer's murder, we consider the construction of prairie-based white femininity in the late nineteenth century that helped sustain concepts of racial and cultural difference by establishing the vulnerable white woman and girl. Euro-American settlement began on the prairies over a century earlier through farming, which was—and remains—a patriarchal activity (Bye 2005; Corman and Kubik 2016). However, women have long been "deeply intertwined" with farming communities writ large, even across racial divides (Fletcher 2016, p. 261). During early settler contact, Indigenous women assisted newcomers with their knowledge of medicine, thereby strengthening community bonds between themselves and white women (Carter 1997). Yet, this history tends to be overshadowed by gendered colonial stories (Faye 2006). As Carter (1997) chronicles in *Capturing Women: The Manipulation of Cultural Imagery in Canada's Prairie West*, dominant tropes of white prairie women as frail and delicate contributed to settlement and civility work; the pure, pious woman's free labor was useful in "[emphasizing] the frailty and delicacy of the white woman, as well as her dependence on males" (p. 8). To compound matters, white women's perceived frailty paired well with an imagined threat of Indigenous people, alienating Indigenous and white women from one another (Carter 1997, p. 6). This resounding imaginary of the fragile, white prairie woman contributes to Saskatchewan's "unique mythology" of settler aesthetic that both influences subjectivity production and supports Canadian nation building (Marler 2011, p. 1).

Tracy was not exempt from this settler aesthetic. A farmer's daughter, she was also bound up in patriarchal myths that bind male farmers to the land—part of the great "Canadian outdoors" (Laurendeau et al. 2021)—and an inherently colonial impulse to tame it. In a chapter called "The Tantalizing Possibility of Living on the Plains," Kaye (2005) describes the prairie farmer when he is positioned as neighbor:

> It would be easy to play our neighbour as the heavy—the big John Deere tractor loafing diesel fumes as he goes home for lunch, passing a petition the first year we were here to close down the village school because the cost of accommodating a child who used a wheelchair might raise taxes too high. A big landowner, a successful farmer, bent on passing to his children a farm homesteaded by ancestors a century ago ... It would be easy to say that the greed ... that would refuse ramps to a child in a wheelchair (that would suggest, in fact, that the child should have his legs amputated so he could be fitted with prosthesis and taught to climb stairs) is monstrous greed ... but such a metaphoric reading is itself cramped and cruel, no better than scapegoating. My neighbour is a perfectly nice guy. (p. 30)

Kaye's (2005) description of this neighbour-farmer demonstrates how ableism layers into the highly gendered and colonial characteristics of this man, whose violent thoughts and actions are excused on the basis that he is a "perfectly nice guy" (p. 30). By Kaye's account, the "perfectly nice guy" is a character who embodies a cultural ethos where white male dominance settles both lands and disputes over personhood. To observe how this ethos translates into reality, we recall that in 2018 white male farmer Gerald Stanley was found not guilty of second-degree murder by a jury in Battleford, Saskatchewan after shooting Indigenous man Colten Boushie as he sat in the back of a parked vehicle. In a *New York Times* op-ed, Saskatchewan-born Indigenous writer Scrimshaw called out "the century-long history of systemic racism that led to Colten Boushie's killing" (Scrimshaw 2018).

If conditions of possibility for Boushie's recent murder and the decided innocence of his killer have roots in over a hundred years of racism, then it is possible that the conditions of possibility for Tracy Latimer's killing also lay in the historic legacy of the "perfectly nice guy" insofar as this imagined subject is contingent on the intersection of disability, gender, race, and place. After all, Janz (2009) argues that early-aughts media coverage of Tracy's killing overemphasized unwarranted descriptions of pain conflated with cerebral palsy so thoroughly that Tracy's personhood was subsumed by ableist presumptions of suffering (p. 46).[4] Today, Robert Latimer's ambition of having his earlier conviction for second-degree murder overturned is supported by a public that describes him as a "simple" man up against "irrational" critics (Issa 2019; Janz 2018; Bauslaugh 2010). By contrast, Tracy was on a trajectory toward becoming a disabled white woman in a Western context, where gender and coloniality are significant forms of cultural capital (Thobani 2018; Fletcher et al. 2020) and where the work of social reproduction may be inaccessible for some disabled women. The risks of not contributing to capitalist production are high for disabled folks (Goodley et al. 2014). And, in Canada, a country that actively relies on the reproduction of inspirational disability tropes to uphold settler dominance (Peers 2015), Tracy's white, rural femininity/fragility also overlapped with tropes of innocence already etched into childhood (Dyer 2019). This case lays bare the collision of well-entrenched prairie tropes at the intersection of disability, gender, race, and place: the absence of Tracy's personhood combined with the apparent criminal immunity afforded to some white prairie men positions Robert Latimer as a "perfectly nice guy" intervening in the life, and ultimately the death, of a frail prairie girl.

However, prairie-based disabled artists have narrativized Tracy's case differently Following deaf and disability arts traditions of offering multiple representations of existent events, Enns's (1999) writing draws on excerpts from a communication book written about Tracy by her mother. Even earlier, Alberta-based playwright Heidi Janz wrote a performance called *Return to Sender* with a similar storyline. In a 1997 media interview, Janz explained that the purpose of this play was to "counteract the general mindset of focusing on the disability rather than on the person" (D. Johnston 1997, n.p.). These arts-based (re)worldings of Tracy Latimer's personhood as a lived human experience rather than a prairie-based trope complexify the conditions of possibility for our work in a posthumanist context wherein the politics of location are foundational (Braidotti 2018; Kincheloe 2001); it is possible to think of place as not only where we are, but as an intergenerational network we carry in our bodies through ongoing processes of becoming, which can include enacting different worlds (Simpson 2017). As Lee reminds us (McGregor 2020), art created by and for disabled folks punctures normative ideas of how disability is lived including, in this case, the enactment of mainstream ableism that asserts disability should not be *lived* and ongoingly condones the killing of a rural, disabled girl. Both Enns' and Janz's art insist on reimagining this event in ways that challenge the culturally contingent ableism; their work is a grievous reminder that where "inclusion into the world as it is currently arranged is not possible" for many, including those who have been killed, disability and deaf art delivers new worldly arrangements amid this grief (Chandler 2018, p. 462).

If we are to follow Tuck and McKenzie's (2015) directive to work toward decolonizing research by moving beyond place as a neutral backdrop to our inquiry (p. 18), we must attend to the backdrop of this case; to consider the place of Tracy's murder to be of little or no consequence requires an "erasure of the body" that assumes the body can move, and can *become*, in just any space or place (Cella 2017, p. 285). This assumption is alive today, including through audiocentric assumptions of place neutrality for deaf people To date, the provincial government has released one set of recommendations concerning deaf education—a 1990 report that asserts that the even distribution of programs and services throughout Saskatchewan is possible (*Preliminary Report on Deaf Education* 1990) Yet, deaf cultural histories in the province tell a different story. These histories include the 1991 closure of the R. J. D. Williams School for the Deaf which led to an "exodus" of signing deaf leaders, teachers, and professionals from the province (Weber 2021; Weber and Snoddon 2020, p. 602). As a result, the current primary approach to teaching deaf children today is to include them in mainstream systems such as schools, where parents and advocates report being discouraged against using ASL (Saskatchewan Human Rights Commission 2016, pp. 5–7). In reports published in 2016 and 2021, respectively, the Saskatchewan Human Rights Commission acknowledged the isolation of deaf students amid an uneven patchwork of programs for deaf people fueled by conflicting ideologies about the acquisition of speech and language.[5] Concurrently, in recent years, the province's capital city, Regina, has received an inflow of deaf newcomer youth who represent a "fragile beginning of a new generation of deaf community members" (Weber and Snoddon 2020, p. 615). This unique combination of people has been described as a deaf diaspora (p. 615). Some of the folks who make up this diaspora are involved in Weber's Deaf Crows Collective, including through the Collective's flagship performance, *Apple Time*. Described as a "bridge to all realms," *Apple Time* is a production that blends traditional deaf storytelling, puppetry, props, costumes, clowning, and ASL poetry "to create entire new worlds" using no spoken English (Artesian 2018). Such liminal (re)worlding reimagines and reorders the traditional prairie-scape into an evolving setting that includes knowledge and aesthetics from other countries, hybrid translanguaging, and the new, emergent affect and aesthetic that is the result of cultural fractures combined with diasporic assemblage. The works of Enns, Janz, and Deaf Crows Collective remind us that deaf and disabled artists' becomings persistently resist ableist and audiocentric erasures of difference specific to this place in ways that are anything but neutral.

3.2. "Ring Those Phones!": Rurality, Charity, and Sanism

The identarian category of "rural" is elusive. Broadly, rurality takes on vastly different shapes and descriptions worldwide, and the contemporary rural–urban dichotomy is contentious (Dymitrow and Brauer 2017, p. 29). To label someone as "rural"—as we do in our labelling of Tracy Latimer as a rural, disabled girl and in our conception of research participants (below) as rural artists—risks imposing a performative identity on someone without their consent (Edensor 2006; Dymitrow and Brauer 2017). Yet, embodiment plays a role in our interaction with space (Cella 2017), and place has a significant impact on our sense of identity (Massey 2005; Stehlik 2017). What is more, disability is constructed differently in different places and spaces (Short et al. 2018). In Saskatchewan, rural disability is constructed through charity.

Since 1976, the Kinsmen Foundation has been hosting a telethon in Saskatchewan called TeleMiracle. As a teenager in the early 2000s, Jones attended a TeleMiracle telethon taping in Regina. On stage was a line-up of volunteers, ready to answer landline telephones. Between performances by (mainly) Canadian talent, hosts would chant "Ring those phones! Ring those phones!"—a jingle familiar to many Saskatchewanians—to urge the live and at-home television audience to call in and donate.[6] Today, the 20-h event continues to follow charity traditions of launching widespread advertising campaigns featuring objectifying images of disabled people. The prominence of whiteness and childhood in these promotional campaigns is a reminder of how infantilization and "inspiration porn" (Young 2014) collude to reassert white dominance, repeating a pattern earlier noted in Tracy Latimer's killing (Peers 2015). Decidedly unpolitical, Tracy's legacy as a person whose access to medical treatment was cut off in childhood through her father's decision to end her life is not acknowledged by TeleMiracle, even though it is plausible that Tracy would have qualified for this charity's funding had she lived. TeleMiracle raises millions of dollars to fund medical treatment and mobility/communication equipment for qualifying Saskatchewanians (TeleMiracle 2022). The telethon's profits fill a glaring social service gaps and represent a necessary route to accessing medical care for disabled adults with few other supports in the province (Loeppky 2022).

The necessity of the telethon for disabled people's survival in the province is also a testament to the dominance of charity tropes in Saskatchewan's cultural milieu. Being charitable is, for many, a necessary condition toward sustaining a rural life (Gibson and Barrett 2018). In their study of small rural missionary hospitals in Canada during the early twentieth century, Vandenberg and Gallagher-Cohoon (2021) report on the legacy of medical missionary work as social welfare in the Canadian Prairies that was foundational to colonial nationhood expansion. The link between medical and social care rooted former premier Tommy Douglas's 1961 introduction of universal health care legislation.[7] Mythology around this achievement is laced with sanism. In a biography of Douglas, writer Margoshes (1999) begins a chapter called "The Battle Over Medicare" with some local folklore:

> ... [Douglas] pays a visit to the mental hospital at Weyburn, where he meets a patient walking along on the grounds.
>
> 'How are you sir, and what is your name?'
>
> 'Oh fine,' the patient said. 'My name is Bob. Who are you?'
>
> 'Oh I'm Tommy Douglas. You know, the premier of Saskatchewan.'
>
> The patient gives him a suspicious glance, then replies: 'That's all right, you'll get over it. I thought I was Napoleon when I came here.' (p. 129)

Douglas reportedly did visit the Souris Valley Extended Care Centre in Weyburn, Saskatchewan (Davies 2019). Prior to its demolition in 2009, the center was one of the largest institutions in Canada (Leung n.d.). Known for its "psychedelic" legacy of experimental research including LSD treatments (Dyck 2010; Marcotte 2015), the center is a rich starting point for prairie-based mad people's history (Davies 2019; Dyck and Deighton 2017; Leung n.d.; Melville Whyte 2012). In 2002, community members and artists "took over one wing of the derelict [institution]" to stage (The Weyburn Project n.d.), a six-week performance that cast a reflexive view on the hospital as a less-than-charitable institution (Irwin 2019, p. 134). The Knowhere Productions performance began with artists and community members "camping" in one of the site's buildings and rummaging through archival material (abandoned patient records and medical devices) as they contrived a performance in the abandoned building:

> During the two-hour-long performance ... audiences of 25 individuals walked through the once-locked wards, corridors, electric shock treatment rooms, and holding cells. ... Escorted by former psychiatric nurses, they were taken on a journey through 100 years of mental treatment in Saskatchewan. The materiality of the experience (the smells, sounds, textures and light) ... underscored the ... horrible details of medical successes and failed experiments. (Irwin 2019, p. 135)

Such arts-based interventions add context to our bricolage of prairie-based *becomings* and suggest that disability arts movements have a legacy of disrupting and (re)worlding prairie-based colonial ethos, such as that which links charity to care in rural contexts. By offering a new interpretation of prairie-based institutionalization to audiences, the performance centered local experience of difference in an imaginative, affect-evoking way designed to turn our attention toward regional mad histories.

More recently, artists have begun speaking out against the charitable connotations of their lives: Loeppky (2021), a disabled artist-activist, describes today's rendition of this phenomenon as a "crip tax"—extra costs imposed upon disabled Saskatchewanians, who must pay out-of-pocket for much care unless charity projects like TeleMiracle supplement these costs. In contrast to pervasive charitable rhetoric that is so taxing for disabled people, Saskatchewan's first and only disability-led disability arts organization, Listen to Dis (LTD) Community Arts Organization, hosts online cultural events geared toward disabled people's political right to exist and gather. In a 2021 online "Pajama Party Politics" event, LTD members launched a "crip declaration." This ongoing declaration responds to and reimagines disabled Saskatchewanian's place-based experiences. These experiences are described in the organization's annual report as those which position disabled artists as "crashing headlong into barriers that some claim we've moved past," including but not limited to longstanding charitable tropes and the pervasive crip tax (Listen to Dis 2022, p. 5). The continued legacy of disability arts and culture amid a resoundingly charity-driven ableism demonstrates another mode of (re)worlding well underway on the Canadian Prairies.

4. Methodology

Our interdisciplinary artivist research bricolage engages outward-facing intimate scholarship that lends itself to the numerous contexts in which we operate—real, imagined, or otherwise. Our respective disciplines intersect at the nexus of art and activism, offering what Leduc (2016) describes as an "artivist" perspective: a research-laden collision of art, activism, and community as a possible positionality. Specifically, all the research is deeply connected to the prairie-based performers in both the Deaf Crows Collective and Listen to Listen to Dis (2021), the only deaf- and disability-led arts organizations in Saskatchewan. Perhaps it is the action implication of "artivist" that compels us to build something via the process of *becoming-to-know*, which brings us to the multi-method move of bricolage (Kincheloe 2001). Explaining his support for thorough research that spans beyond the limitations of any singular discipline or method, Kincheloe (2001) describes the process ontology (ruptures and insights) one must embrace during the longevity of scholarly work wherein "[w]e occupy a scholarly world with faded disciplinary boundary lines" (p. 683). Rather than bending to methodologies established by a colonial, ableist academe, bricolage responds to interdisciplinary shifts in knowledge production, validation, and rigor. Kincheloe (2001) compares traditional, discipline-bound praxis to worship at a temple: "My argument . . . is that we must operate in the ruins of the temple, in a postapocalyptic social, cultural, psychological, and educational science where certainty and stability have long departed for parts unknown" (p. 681).

We replace Kincheloe's (2001) temple with our own imagined dinner table. Here, too, we might be amid the ruins. Who ever said the table was functional, intact, and inclusive? We can imagine the table as untidy, wobbly, and even overturned; we can allow the table to impress upon us the sinister baggage of "the Prairies" by being a gathering place where there are pieces to pick up, absences to notice, and (re)worlding to observe. We bring our identities, carved as they are in space and time. We layer into these questions about "what we are capable of becoming" amid the impression of "the Prairies" we have gathered thus far (Braidotti 2018, p. 207).

4.1. Methods

4.1.1. Interviews

Our research team conducted interviews with 11 rural-identified deaf and/or disabled artists using Zoom and Google Hangouts. Interviewees were recruited in 2021 through the distribution of an email invitation to participate. The invitation included a link to an American Sign Language (ASL) vlog and an English, text-based translation of the invitation. The email was sent by the lead author to 24 deaf- and disability-related organizations across all the provinces and territories. A Qualtrics-based, digital consent form was available to all invitation recipients. The form consisted of ASL vlog sections that were translated into English text to make the consent form accessible in both languages. Through the form participants were given the option to use their real names or pseudonyms. The participants interviewed for this article indicated a preference to use their real first names, and decisions about naming were also confirmed during the interviews. The researchers conducted one-on-one interviews in ASL or English, using a semi-structured interview method. Following Brinkmann (2022), semi-structured interviews are part of a continuum of interview method that fluctuates between structured (with some questions thought through in advance, a designated start and end time, and a decided focus on the participant's story), flexibility (with the researchers' willingness to change course, respond, and be in-relation with participants as the story unfolds), and improvisation (which, Price (2012) argues, is an essential ingredient to disability-related research that must always be concerned with access). Interviews typically lasted 45 min to one hour. Following the interviews, the research team developed a coding book to conduct a thematic analysis using NVivo. Codes included childhood experiences, community, conceptions of voice, COVID-19, experiences with jam sessions, identity descriptions, rural experiences or experiences of place, and dinner table experiences.

4.1.2. Jam Sessions

Sonic improvisation is emerging as a social and artistic practice that resists the "rarefied and exclusive world" (Morris 2022, para. 5) of traditional music composition (Born 2017; Bobier and Ignagni 2021; Lewis 2008; Warren-Crow 2018). The possibilities for interaction, collaboration, and expression in improvisation focus on "not knowing what you will find on the way" (Mattin 2017). A method of sound- and movement-based improvisation that embraces "harsh noise-based research" (Warren and Hopkins 2021) and notes the ableist assumptions around contemporary music composition (Carlson 2016), jam sessions were developed by Pridmore in 2018 for expressing "voice" in different ways. The purpose of jam sessions has evolved in recent years, in tune with emergent incorporations of multisensory experiences in sound-based performances (Morris 2022). Drawing on Alper (2017) and Jones et al.'s (2022) critiques of "giving voice" as well as crip linguistics and disabled languaging (Henner and Robinson 2021), we suggest that jam sessions have drifted away from a concentration on vocality to refer, simply and separately, to expression. Even so, for deaf groups in particular, the conflation of vocality with expression is problematic: in audiocentric cultures, "voice" is a weighty form of cultural capital and a tool used in ongoing attempts to assimilate deaf people into the speaking world, interfering with their vibrant carnivalesque cultural production that does not center on vocal expression (Peters 2009; Weber and Snoddon 2020). For deaf folks, "voice" takes on different meaning than that found in hearing worlds. "Our hands are our voices", Weber (2022) once explained ahead of a jam session. Jam sessions, then, are the act of getting together either online or in person for improvisational expression in a group setting where harmonic, melodic, and rhythmic elements merge to create a whole (Sawyer 2007, p. 2). We create our own unique compositions in many ways, including through embodied actions (e.g., gurgling, clapping, vocal sounds, signing words) and by using technology (e.g., sound-producing software on iPads, mobile phone ringtones, the clanging together of pots and pans). Pridmore (2022) refers to this as "jamming." Between July 2021 and August 2021, Pridmore led four one-hour jam sessions via Zoom with up to 10 participants in each session. Participants in these jam sessions also completed informed consent forms. Jam session participants chose to identify themselves in many ways including by their real first names, by pseudonyms, and by no name (in which case they are known simply as "Participant").

4.2. Creative Analytic Practice (CAP)

Creative Analytic Practice (CAP) is a method of knowing via writing in ways that are both creative and analytical and describes our method of experimental writing thus far (Richardson 2000). From the perspectives of four people taking in one another from different sides of the table, from different perspectives, we gather the pieces of our collective knowledge and develop our bricolage through CAP. Foregrounded by feminist poststructuralism's and postmodernism's challenge to rationalism, CAP offers new narratives about the contexts in which writing is produced—from family ties to social movements to disciplinary constraints—that emphasize the critical reflexivity, grounding, and danger of such narratives as "they nest [our] projects ethically" (Richardson 1999, p. 665). Following CAP's imaginative edge, which embraces all forms, including metaphor, we offer both the dinner table and the bricolage as metaphors that uphold this transversal of thought and meet the limits between "what we do" (Greene 2011, p. 3) and the affirmative ethics of "opening outward to the world" (Braidotti 2018, p. 210). CAP invests in multiple, intertextual methods of inquiry and their theoretical underpinnings. Concerned with the connections between textual data—including textual creation and interpretation of research accounts—bricoleurs become "methodological negotiators" who must step back from traditional ways of knowing and instead make space for the fragmented, layered, and multiple textual representations of something else (Kincheloe 2005, p. 325; Markham 2005). Our "something else" is a constellation of methods, represented through the intimate artivist research we bring to the CAP-anchored imagined dinner table.

5. Findings

5.1. Jam Sessions as Dinner Table "Flourishing"

During one jam session, participants were invited to imagine a dinner table. The game expanded when they were asked to imagine a potluck to which they brought a dish. A moment later our imagined feast was abundant with layers of sound: popping popcorn, hissing fizzy water, and the slurping licks of eating ice cream. Participants also shared their dinner table experiences. They reported "not being able to keep up with multiple conversations" and experiencing sensory overload. When invited to express these feelings, one participant rocked back and forth, another began hitting their head, and groans filled the air:

> **Participant 1:** [releases a throaty groan]
>
> **Maria:** [speaking] "I'm just frustrated right now"
>
> **Participant 2:** [speaking] "uuuhhhh . . . ." [begins groaning]
>
> **Lee Hope:** [speaking] "inhale, exhale to try and calm down"

In this jam session moment, improvisation was paramount to telling the sound-based story of the dinner table. Each person offered something intimate to the scene, whether through embodied noises or through spoken words. The result is a chorus of agony—a moment of guttural, groaned frustration mixed in with a delicious potluck spread, which lets us in on the mixed feelings some folks carry to the dinner table.

We discovered that it is possible to gain insight into dinner table experience through sound-based improvisation. Despite its absence in high art traditions (Sawyer 2007; Varvarigou 2017), music improvisation is an important method for engaging in collaboration, interdependence, and "flourishing" that involves experimental sound, movements, and meanings (Kuppers 2019, p. 138). We emphasize "flourishing" following Carlson's (2016) connections between musical experience and intellectually disabled people's human flourishing. By this, Carlson refers not to therapeutic musical interventions, but to the ethical significance of letting go of attempts to explain and analyze music and disability in the interest of new modes of solidarity that come with the embodied experience of music making—or, more simply, making sound for the sake of making sound. If part of the problem with mainstream arts is that it emerges from an unspoken agreement between audiences and creators that the output be in some way understandable (Kuppers 2019), we follow in crip arts traditions of usurping understandability in our jam session rendition of dinner table experience. By choosing cacophony over composition, possibilities for new understandings emerge, highlighting the experiences of those who would be excluded from the dinner table.

5.2. Dinner Table Experience as Being Overlooked

In research moments where we engaged in word-based inquiry, such as through ASL or English interviews, we were met with narrative dinner table experiences that fluctuate between the metaphoric and the literal. One hearing interviewee, Victor, recalled their experience growing up in the Prairie Provinces in the late 1950s, witnessing a gendered division between those who occupied the metaphorical dinner table in their household:

> The table is an important metaphor in my life . . . for [my mother], the dinner table was always a challenge and very seldom a pleasure, because of course she was expected to do it all and though my dad was helpful, usually at that time we

still had, you know, we had three acres outside of town and my dad had chores. My dad took care of the outside. There is another traditional literary metaphor that goes back to the last century about house and horse, the female perspective is supposedly and this argument uh, embodies by what's inside the house like a dinner table, where a man is outside in the garden, say, or in the barn, or riding a horse or riding to the damsel's rescue or whatever.

Multiple applications of the dinner table as a metaphor allowed for a varied, rich explication of the experiences of deaf and disabled members. By contrast, Mustafa, a deaf participant, explained that many deaf people refer to the literal deferral by loving, hearing members of their families who promise future explanations of family dynamics and tensions, relay of jokes, and explication of arguments, mostly encapsulated in the phrase, "I will tell you later." Only, later never comes as the conversation shifts, its threads forgotten in the effort to keep up. Mustafa elaborates:

> I love my family but its so frustrating . . . so many times I have asked my family member what they are talking about at the table . . . and often they will say 'hold on' and make me wait and wait. . . . But that's what my family does . . . they will not accept the fact that I cannot hear them at all. I have been Deaf since birth . . . my family has asked that I get the cochlear implant and I told them that I can't, I am much too old and it would not work for me.

For Mustafa, the crip affect of missing out is punitive, compounded by familial expectations or normativity that he somehow strive to hear (perhaps through cochlear implants). This example reminds us that dinner table experience is not only the affect of not fitting in because, in part, some bodies do not fit the shape of the imagined dinner table exchange. The impact is the cutting off of deaf family members' access to incidental learning, such as overlapping conversations. This example also reflects research elsewhere that suggests dinner table experience is most prevalent among those from hearing families whose first language is not a signed language (Listman and Kurz 2020).

A hearing interviewee, Kelsey, opened up about the dinner table experience by first describing a meal with other arts-engaged peers who tried to support her eating, but did not think to bring a knife to cut an apple into bite-sized portions that would make the meal more accessible. Later, she expanded on the affect of missed accessibility gestures:

> And also on the other side of things it's like people might, people might be cracking a joke and I might not get it right away because of cognitive processing. So it might take me three days later I'll get that joke but in the moment it's like Oh, I don't know. I don't know what they've said . . . or what it was, right? So that's kind of weird in a sense because you don't know if they are making jokes about you or the people around you.

If mealtime should be an opportunity to both eat and participate in larger group conversations (Meek 2020), the above example illustrates that divisions of labor and expectations of normate comportment related to Western eating rituals pose barriers to equitable participation, even in contexts that mean to be supportive of disability and deaf art. Indeed, disabled and deaf people often "violate" the rules of normate and hearing etiquette (Meek 2020, p. 1690), and our participants' experiences reveal that mealtimes tend to mark a moment where their previously desired, arts-based "disruptions" come to halt, when possible (re)worlding is abruptly grounded by an existent worldly ritual rife with barriers.

More ephemerally, Kelsey expressed concern about not understanding the rhetoric circulating at mealtime until a few days later—a common retrospective element of dinner table experience that comes with the realization of having missed out on conversations. This timelapse reminds us that dinner table experience is a uniquely crip temporal affect of overlooked-ness that lingers after mealtime is over (Meek 2020, p. 1688). As a reviewer of this article pointed out, the grip that dinner table encounters have on experiences may stay with us throughout our lives. This staying power is productive for re-imagining our sense of understandings of events and everyday moments that shape our subjectivities.

Further, the sticky temporal facets of the dinner table experience—its emergence both in-the-moment and as potentially long-held memory—offer new connections to the rubric of crip time.[8] Along with being a "wry reference to the disability-related events that always seem to start late", crip time as affective temporality points to the challenges of normative, linear pacing when we are faced with a combination of ableist barriers and slowness that characterizes the non-normative engagement with an ableist world (Kafer 2013, p. 26). Kafer (2021) suggests we think less about what crip time is and more about what it does (p. 421). To this end: crip time does the work of making space for grief, including grief over lost experiences (Samuels 2017); crip time also encompasses waiting—in Kelsey's case, waiting for meaning to emerge; crip time encompasses the affective, temporal flux of dinner table experience and reminds us that this experience does not end when the table is cleared and the guests depart. We know about the intersections of crip time and dinner table experience because the affective remnants of this phenomenon stretch into other facets of our work, including jam sessions (above) filled with the noises of groans and reminders to breathe.

This cultural disavowal of difference at the dinner table extends to larger arts movements: as LTD artistic director Traci Foster recently pointed out in a public conversation about cripping art and access in Saskatchewan as compared to its urban Canadian counterparts, "We are currently incapable of keeping up, and therefore, of course, we can't catch up" (Listen to Dis 2022). This incapability seems predicated on the major milestones that bring us to the present, including Tracy Latimer's killing and an ongoing telethon that sustains harmful charitable tropes. These important events are exclusive to Saskatchewan and are imprinted on the lives of all prairie people and the backdrop to the collective work disability and deaf artists must do to establish and sustain their presence in this place.[9] Foster's words, then, succinctly characterize the distinctly crip affect of "not keeping up" as something more politically willful than simply being left behind. Disabled and deaf artistry in an overlooked context refuses to operate in parallel to its more highly resourced urban counterparts because it cannot. Instead, prairie-based deaf and disability arts' propulsion happens amidst a uniquely paced, place-contingent resistance and (re)worlding laced with a crip failure (Mitchell et al. 2014) toward "keeping up" or "catching up", and through a deeply experienced enactment of this crip affect, the rural, prairie movement offers something that urban centers cannot.

6. Reflection

The findings above offer a glimpse into prairie-based artists' dinner table experience. We note that apart from the golden sheaves and canned harvest vegetables and fruits that made their way to our metaphorical dinner table on some research occasions, the prairie aesthetic is fraught with grave discourses of overlooked-ness that pop up in imagined dinner table settings: a prairie brand of ableism, sexism, racism, and audism that is exacerbated by charity tropes and leaves artists feeling set apart from deaf and disability movements in other places. Through this bricolage of dinner table experience, we reflect on what we and others (deaf and disabled artists) are *becoming* beneath the open prairie sky and amid the highly gendered expectations of rural labor and the charity-riddled community ethos that routinely overlooks their work and results in a sense of being unable to keep up (Braidotti 2018). Places and our orientation to deaf and disabled persons are informed by context; our attempt to understand both disability and deafness as complex processes of becoming is difficult even as the deaf and disability arts sector experiences growth in Saskatchewan (Weber 2013; Weber and Snoddon 2020; Canada Council for the Arts 2021).

Beginning with Tracy Latimer's murder, we map how the world is arranged for deaf and disabled artists in this place, and we assert that the context of artists' work is embedded in challenges about whose life is valuable and therefore grievable (Pullman and Nichols 2015). In other words, the dinner table experience is a useful metaphor in pointing us toward the worthiness emanating from the task of embracing difficulties, collaborating, and recognizing subjectivity as a collective assemblage. The dinner table can also stand as a representative of the jam session, in that each guest brings an individual "voice" to the jam session's "table", adding to and collaborating with the cacophony in a unique experience of sound making amid crip time, one that is broader than the prescribed limitations of composed music and that allows for communication above organization. From the vantage points of people who have pulled up a metaphorical seat with us and reflected on their lived dinner table experiences, perhaps with the televised cheers and music of TeleMiracle filling the background with noise, we assert that prairie-based deaf and disability art is on a long-time trajectory of becoming that which is rooted in a politics of the overlooked—an affective "flyover" positioning that remains written on the bones of those of us who engage with it, even in varying degrees, and whose history is recalled by the living and memorialized by the dead.

In the spirit of affirmative ethics, overlookedness need not be an affect of mourning or melancholy (Braidotti 2017). For instance, our emphasis on Tracy Latimer through storied fragments is an attempt to nurture an intergenerational connection symbolized by the imagined dinner table as a gathering place that clocks both presence and absence (Braidotti 2018). In part, Braidotti (2017) describes affirmative ethics as a way of being worthy of what happens to us. As bricoleurs we lean into non-linearity and associative thinking and leave our construction of prairie-based deaf and disabled arts decidedly incomplete; we do not consider our partial knowledge to be a blockage (Guyotte and Flint 2021; Thrift 2008). The purpose of experimental bricolage writing, a form of CAP, is to better understand our positioning as people involved—each to different degrees—around the prairie dinner table. This means understanding multiple perspectives as "humble artisan[s]" not as "master thinker[s]" who are part of the dinner event, to borrow Braidotti's (2021) phrase (p. 531). As such, the question of what we want to become is one that spans far beyond our writing—fittingly, given the context of a land whose horizon point can be too far away to spot with human vision. Here, we acknowledge the work of disabled and deaf artists, including Listen To Dis, Deaf Crows Collective, and several disabled artists who remain committed to the political and artistic work of challenging an oppressive prairie ethos and (re)worlding through their uniquely generative positioning as overlooked.

7. Conclusions

To close, we return to Ahmed's (2006) question that directs us to the sky and asks "[h]ow we begin to know or feel where we are" (p. 6). We approached this question in a *becoming-to-know* position à la Braidotti (2018) that critically notes the Canadian Prairies' reputation as a pastoral, apolitical backdrop as an ableist, colonial construction. Massie (2010) reminds us of how picturesque biomes on yearly calendars—"an astonishing sunset or skyline framing a golden field of wheat" (p. 172)—offer an "epistemic wallpaper" difficult to peel away from foundational Western imaginaries (Massie 2010; Thrift 2004, p. 585). This is where the significant (re)worlding of deaf and disabled artists takes place. Writing as a bricolage from this place is an experiment in *becoming-to-know* deaf and disability art in the "flyover provinces" over time, through disciplinary combinations (Kincheloe 2005; Yardley 2020). The intimacy of this scholarship is tied up in process ontologies which take place—in this case, beneath the living prairie sky in a place called Saskatchewan—as a starting point for a cumulative bricolage of arts-based knowledge pulled both from our own and others' experiences as we know these so far. We acknowledge that there are several artists and cultural producers doing significant work in prairie-based disability, deaf, and mad arts beyond the scope of this writing. Our bricolage refuses picturesque reductionism, asserting "the frontiers of knowledge work rest in the liminal zones where disciplines collide" and expand complexly, in multiple ways that might transcend disciplinary borders (Kincheloe 2005, p. 689; Thrift 2008). Here, we have offered the metaphor of the dinner table and the memories and temporalities it evokes as representations of that liminal zone to which Kincheloe (2005) refers, where the overlookedness of this place's disability and deaf art ensues an emergent and unique (re)worlding. Though we know that disabled, deaf, and mad people have always made art, we acknowledge that their contemporary (re)worlding in prairie contexts remains place-based and liminal—often overlooked in, or on the periphery of, the wider world of urban crip artmaking which has gained much attention in Canada in the last decade (Chandler 2019; Chandler et al. 2021; K. Johnston 2012; Orsini and Kelly 2016; Watkin 2022). Ultimately, this nonlinear collection of findings around deaf and disabled art on the Canadian Prairies represents a blend of memory, testimony, and forecasting around the understated political force of deaf and disability arts in an overlooked "flyover" zone.

Author Contributions: Conceptualization, C.T.J.; data collection, C.T.J., J.W., A.A. and H.P.; methodology, H.P.; writing—original draft preparation, C.T.J.; writing—review and editing, A.A., J.W. and H.P. Funding acquisition, C.T.J. and H.P. All authors have read and agreed to the published version of the manuscript.

Funding: This research was funded through The Social Sciences and Humanities Research Council (SSHRC) Insight Development Grant titled, "Troubling Vocalities: Disability and Deaf Art on the Canadian Prairies" (430-2020-00189). Funding was also provided by The Council for Research in the Social Sciences (CRISS) of the Faculty of Social Sciences at Brock University (October 2020) and by the Social Justice Research Institute (SJRI) through an SJRI Community Engagement Grant (Beyond Niagara) at Brock University (336-242-071).

Institutional Review Board Statement: The study was conducted in accordance with the Declaration of Helsinki, and approved by the Institutional Review Board (or Ethics Committee) of Brock University (protocol code 20-261-JONES), approved 21 March 2021.

Informed Consent Statement: Informed consent was obtained from all subjects involved in the study.

Data Availability Statement: Not applicable.

Conflicts of Interest: The authors declare no conflict of interest.

Notes

[1] Commonly lowercase "deaf" is used to refer to audiological impairment while uppercase "Deaf" refers to a cultural group who share beliefs, practices, and a language (American Sign Language). Here, however, we lean into lowercase "deaf" to reflect the recommendation by Friedner and Kusters (2015) to eschew binarization between groups of deaf people and to reflect the notion of deafhood (Ladd 2003) as a state of becoming in which traits belonging to both realities noted by the use of "d" and "D" are often used according to shifting circumstances.

[2] The dinner table phenomenon is metaphorical because it represents not only something that happens at dinner time but also the experience of missing out on overlapping conversation that can happen, for example, while a radio is playing during a car ride, children are playing on the playground, and people are gathering during holiday gatherings. Meek (2020) is clear that dinner table experience happens in most any "other instances where a deaf individual interacts with a group of people" (p. 1676), and this experience is especially prominent in the lives of deaf people with hearing families (Listman and Kurz 2020).

[3] We acknowledge the work of Monte Hardy for bringing the idea of "dinner table experience" to this project in early 2020 during his work as a research assistant for the The Social Sciences and Humanities Research Council (SSHRC) Insight Development Grant titled, "Troubling Vocalities: Disability and Deaf Art on the Canadian Prairies." At Hardy's suggestion, we orchestrated an ASL-first methodology that was later translated into English.

[4] The cultural erasure of Tracy's personhood is also well documented elsewhere (Heavin 2001; Sobsey n.d.). Notably, in a 2003 book chapter describing national reaction to the Latimer case as that which aligns with representational patterns of disability in Canadian literature, Truchan-Tataryn (2003) points to an episode of the Canadian Broadcasting Corporation radio show *Ideas* wherein Hingsburger described a drama class improvisational activity centered on the scene of Tracy's death. The actors initially portrayed Robert Latimer "as a loving father" in a scene about parenthood. When asked to portray Tracy, the actors struggled. "What would she think?" Hingsuberg asked one actor. "Tracy was retarded", the actor replied, "Do they think?" (p. 11).

[5] The Saskatchewan Human Rights Commission (2016) report, called *Access and Equality for Deaf, deaf, and Hard of Hearing People: A Report to Stakeholders*, noted that preschool opportunities for deaf children are rare, and services for deaf children entering elementary school are problematic (p. 8). In Saskatchewan Human Rights Commission (2021), an update to the report was published. The update, *Access and Equality for Deaf, deaf, and Hard of Hearing People: Update to Stakeholders 2021*, names actions undertaken to address disparities in programs and services for deaf persons: universal newborn hearing screening (p. 22), implementation of visual bus announcements on City of Saskatoon Transit Service (p. 22), and new provisions around university-

6   based notetaking support (p. 25) among others. That these actions are brand new offer a glimpse into the audiocentric world deaf folks are navigating in the province.

6   Years later, while teaching an introductory course in critical disability studies, Jones's students were surprised to learn that telethons still existed. United States-based writing on telethons often describes them as events of the past that spectacularized charity-based tropes (Haller 2010) and offered a "'new' freak show" (Smit 2003, p. 689) and left and imprint on our cultural understandings of disability in ways that tend to be oblivious to artistic and cultural movements crafted by disabled folks (Shapiro 1994).

7   Tommy Douglas is widely credited as being the "father of Canada's health-care system" and in 2004 was awarded the honour of "greatest Canadian" by the Canadian Broadcasting Corporation (2004).

8   We wish to thank the editors of this special issue for pointing out that the temporal aspects of the dinner table experience are alive in Kelsey's account. The editors thoughtfully suggested that Kelsey's experience points to new facets of crip time "entangled with audiocentric experiences".

9   In a follow-up email conversation with Foster about this quotation, she explained: "We individually and collectively understand that without the collective presence, our presence is weakened and the fights that we have fought and have made some tiny wins within, will be once again be lost to the community. That is to say, without the onerous work of 'keeping up' with what the funders and other organizations are doing, the shifts we have instigated and insisted on being sustainable will drift back into the ethos of the living skies" (Foster, personal communication, 2 February 2023).

References

Ahmed, Sara. 2006. *Queer Phenomenology: Orientations, Objects, Others*. Durham: Duke University Press.
Ahmed, Sara. 2015. Queer Feelings. In *The Cultural Politics of Emotion*. New York and London: Routledge, pp. 144–67.
Alper, Mary. 2017. *Giving Voice: Mobile Communication, Disability, and Inequality*. Cambridge: MIT Press. [CrossRef]
Artesian. 2018. Deaf Crows Collective: Apple Time. Available online: https://artesianon13th.ca/event-calendar/post/deaf-crows-collective-apple-time (accessed on 30 November 2022).
Bahan, Ben, H-Dirkson Bauman, and Facundo Montenegro. 2008. *Audism Unveiled*. San Diego: DawnSign Press.
Bauslaugh, Gary. 2010. *Robert Latimer: A Story of Justice and Mercy*. Toronto: James Lorimer & Co.
Bobier, David, and Esther Ignagni. 2021. Interview with David Bobier (Dispatch). *Studies in Social Justice* 15: 282–87. [CrossRef]
Born, Georgina. 2017. After Relational Aesthetics: Improvised Music, the Social, and (Re)Theorizing the Aesthetic. In *Improvisation and Social Aesthetics*. Edited by Georgina Born, Eric Lewis and Will Straw. Durham: Duke University Press, pp. 33–58.
Braidotti, Rosi. 2017. Posthuman critical theory. *Journal of Posthuman Studies* 1: 9–25. [CrossRef]
Braidotti, Rosi. 2018. Affirmative Ethics, Posthuman Subjectivity, and Intimate Scholarship: A Conversation with Rosi Braidotti. In *Decentering the Researcher in Intimate Scholarship*. Edited by Kathryn Strom, Tammy Mills and Alan Ovens. Bradford: Emerald Publishing Limited, vol. 31, pp. 179–88.
Braidotti, Rosi. 2019. A Theoretical Framework for the Critical Posthumanities. *Theory, Culture & Society* 36: 31–61. [CrossRef]
Braidotti, Rosi. 2021. Postface. *Postcolonial Studies* 24: 528–33. [CrossRef]
Brinkmann, Svend. 2022. *Qualitative Interviewing: Conversational Knowledge through Research Interviews*. Oxford: Oxford University Press.
Bye, Cristine Georgina. 2005. "I Like to Hoe My Own Row": A Saskatchewan Farm Woman's Notions about Work and Womanhood during the Great Depression. *Frontiers: A Journal of Women Studies* 26: 135–67. Available online: http://www.jstor.org/stable/4137376 (accessed on 30 November 2022).
Canada Council for the Arts. 2021. *Deaf and Disability Arts Practices in Canada*. Research Report. Montreal: Canada Council for the Arts.
Canadian Broadcasting Corporation. 2004. Tommy Douglas Crowned 'Greatest Canadian'. Available online: https://www.cbc.ca/news/entertainment/tommy-douglas-crowned-greatest-canadian-1.510403 (accessed on 30 November 2022).
Carlson, Licia. 2016. Music, Intellectual Disability, and Human Flourishing. In *The Oxford Handbook of Music and Disability Studies*. Edited by Blake Howe, Stephanie Jensen-Moulton, Neil William Lerner and Joseph Nathan Straus. New York: Oxford University Press, pp. 37–53.
Carter, Sarah. 1997. *Capturing Women: The Manipulation of Cultural Imagery in Canada's Prairie West*. Montreal: McGill-Queen's University Press.
Cella, Matthew J. C. 2017. Retrofitting Rurality: Embodiment and Emplacement in Disability Narratives. *Journal of Rural Studies* 51: 284–94. [CrossRef]
Chandler, Eliza. 2018. Disability Art and Re-Worlding Possibilities. *Auto/Biography Studies* 22: 458–63. [CrossRef]
Chandler, Eliza, ed. 2019. Cripping the Arts in Canada Special issue. *Canadian Journal of Disability Studies* 8: 1–14. [CrossRef]
Chandler, Eliza, Katie Aubrecht, Esther Ignagni, and Carla Rice, eds. 2021. Cripistemologies of Disability Arts and Culture: Reflections on the Cripping the Arts Symposium Special issue. *Studies in Social Justice* 15: 170–79. [CrossRef]
Corman, Amber J., and Wendee Kubik. 2016. Who's Counting . . . on the Farm? In *Women in Agriculture Worldwide: Key Issues and Practical Approaches*, 1st ed. Edited by Amber Fletcher and Wendee Kubik. New York: Routledge, pp. 23–38. [CrossRef]
Davies, Megan J. 2019. Managing Madness Review of *Weyburn Mental Hospital and the Transformation of Psychiatric Care in Canada* by Erika Dyck and Alex Deighton. *Canadian Bulletin of Medical History* 36: 203–5. [CrossRef]

DePalma, Anthony. 1997. Fathers Killing of Canadian Girl: Mercy or Murder? *The New York Times*. p. A3. Available online: https://www.nytimes.com/1997/12/01/world/father-s-killing-of-canadian-girl-mercy-or-murder.html#:~:text=Robert%20Latimer%20admits%20that%20he,farmer%20of%20second%2Ddegree%20murder (accessed on 30 November 2022).

Dyck, Erika. 2010. Spaced-Out in Saskatchewan: Modernism, Anti-Psychiatry, and Deinstitutionalization, 1950–1968. *Bulletin of the History of Medicine* 84: 640–66.

Dyck, Erika, and Alex Deighton. 2017. *Managing Madness: Weyburn Mental Hospital and the Transformation of Psychiatric Care in Canada*. Winnipeg: University of Manitoba Press.

Dyer, Hannah. 2019. *The Queer Aesthetics of Childhood: Asymmetries of Innocence and the Cultural Politics of Child Development*. New Brunswick: Rutgers University Press.

Dymitrow, Mirek, and René Brauer. 2017. Performing Rurality. But Who? *Bulletin of Geography* 38: 27–45. [CrossRef]

Edensor, Tim. 2006. National Temporalities: Institutional Times, Everyday Routines, Serial Spaces and Synchronicities. *European Journal of Social Theory* 9: 525–45. [CrossRef]

Enns, Ruth. 1999. *A Voice Unheard: The Latimer Case and People with Disabilities*. Halifax: Fernwood Publishing.

Faye, Lisa M. 2006. *Redefining 'Farmer': Agrarian Feminist Theory and the Work of Saskatchewan Farm Women*. Ann Arbor: ProQuest Dissertations Publishing. Available online: https://research.library.mun.ca/10478/ (accessed on 30 November 2022).

Fletcher, Amber J. 2016. Conclusion: What Works for Women in Agriculture? In *Women in Agriculture Worldwide: Key Issues and Practical Approaches*, 1st ed. Edited by Amber Fletcher and Wendee Kubik. New York: Routledge, pp. 257–68.

Fletcher, Amber J., Nancy Sah Akwen, Margot Hurlbert, and Harry Diaz. 2020. "You Relied on God and Your Neighbour to Get through It": Social Capital and Climate Change Adaptation in the Rural Canadian Prairies. *Regional Environmental Change* 20: 61. [CrossRef]

Friedner, Michele, and Annelies Kusters. 2015. *It's a Small World: International Deaf Spaces and Encounters*. Washington, DC: Gallaudet University Press.

Gibson, Ryan, and Joshua Barrett. 2018. Philanthropic Organizations to the Rescue? Alternative Funding Solutions for Rural Sustainability. In *Service Provision and Rural Sustainability: Infrastructure and Innovation*. Edited by Greg Halseth, Sean Markey and Laura Ryser. New York: Routledge, pp. 109–22.

Goodley, Dan, Rebecca Lawthom, and Katherine Runswick-Cole. 2014. Dis/ability and Austerity: Beyond Work and Slow Death. *Disability & Society* 29: 980–84.

Greene, Maxine. 2011. Releasing the Imagination. *NJ: Drama Australia Journal* 34: 61–70. [CrossRef]

Guyotte, Kelly W., and Maureen A. Flint. 2021. Pedagogical Impasses: Posthuman Inquiry in Exhaustive Times. *Qualitative Inquiry* 27: 639–49. [CrossRef]

Haller, Beth A. 2010. *Representing Disability in an Ableist World: Essays on Mass Media*. Louisville: The Advocado Press.

Hamilton, Mary Lynn, and Steffinee Pinnegar. 2014. Intimate Scholarship in Research: An Example From Self-Study of Teaching and Teacher Education Practices Methodology. *Learning Landscapes* 8: 153–71. [CrossRef]

Hamilton, Mary Lynn, and Steffinee Pinnegar. 2015. *Knowing, Becoming, Doing as Teacher Educators: Identity, Intimate Scholarship, Inquiry*. Bingley: Emerald Publishing, vol. 26.

Hamilton, Mary Lynn, Steffinee Pinnegar, and Ronnie Davey. 2016. Intimate Scholarship: An Examination of Identity and Inquiry in the Work of Teacher Educators. In *International Handbook of Teacher Education*. Edited by John Loughran and Mary Lynn Hamilton. Singapore: Springer, pp. 181–237.

Haraway, Donna. 1988. Situated Knowledges: The Science Question in Feminism and the Privilege of Partial Perspective. *Feminist Studies* 14: 575–99. [CrossRef]

Heavin, Heather. 2001. Perspectives on the Latimer Trial: Human Rights Issues in R. v. Latimer and Their Significance for Disabled Canadians. *Saskatchewan Law Review* 64: 613. Available online: https://www.facebook.com/notes/1125902324536168/ (accessed on 15 November 2022).

Henner, Jon, and Octavian Robinson. 2021. *Linguistic Discrimination in U.S. Higher Education: Power, Prejudice, Impacts, and Remedies*, 1st ed. Edited by Gaillynn Clements and Marnie Jo Petray. New York: Routledge, pp. 92–109.

Irwin, Kathleen. 2019. Performative Mapping. In *Artistic Approaches to Cultural Mapping: Activating Imaginaries and Means of Knowing*, 1st ed. Edited by Nancy Duxbury, W. F. Garrett-Petts and Alys Longley. New York: Routledge, pp. 127–42.

Issa, Omayra. 2019. 25 Years after Conviction, Robert Latimer Still Believes He Was Right to Kill His Daughter. *CBC News*. November 17. Available online: https://www.cbc.ca/news/canada/saskatoon/robert-latimer-25-years-later-1.5360711 (accessed on 30 November 2022).

Jakubik, Maria. 2011. Becoming to Know: Shifting the Knowledge Creation Paradigm. *Journal of Knowledge Management* 15: 374–402. [CrossRef]

Janz, Heidi. 2009. The Unkindest Cut of All: Portrayals of Pain and Surgery in the Tracy Latimer Case. *Developmental Disabilities Bulletin* 37: 45–62.

Janz, Heidi. 2018. Opinion: Latimer Pardon Request Stirs Up Nightmare for Disabled. *Edmonton Journal*. July 20. Available online: https://edmontonjournal.com/opinion/columnists/opinion-latimer-pardon-request-stirs-up-nightmare-for-disabled (accessed on 30 November 2022).

Johnston, Deborah. 1997. Latimer Case Inspires Student to Write "Return to Sender". *Folio*. May 30. Available online: https://sites.ualberta.ca/~publicas/folio/34/19/09.html (accessed on 30 November 2022).

Johnston, Kirsty. 2012. *Stage Turns: Canadian Disability Theatre*. Montreal: McGill-Queen's University Press.
Jones, Chelsea Temple, Randy Johner, Anna Lozhkina, and Rachel Walliser. 2022. Voice, Communication Technology, Disability, and Art: An Interdisciplinary Scoping Review and Reflection. *Disability & Society*, 1–20. [CrossRef]
Kafer, Alison. 2013. Time for Disability Studies and a Future for Crips. In *Feminist, Queer, Crip*. Bloomington and Indianapolis: Indiana University Press, pp. 25–46.
Kafer, Alison. 2021. After Crip, Crip Afters. *The South Atlantic Quarterly* 120: 415–34. [CrossRef]
Kaye, Frances W. 2005. The Tantalizing Possibility of Living on the Plains. In *History, Literature and the Writing of the Canadian Prairies*. Edited by Alison C. Calder and Robert Alexander Wardhaugh. Winnipeg: University of Manitoba Press, pp. 25–42.
Kincheloe, Joe L. 2001. Describing the Bricolage: Conceptualizing a New Rigor in Qualitative Research. *Qualitative Inquiry* 7: 679–92 [CrossRef]
Kincheloe, Joe L. 2005. On to the Next Level: Continuing the Conceptualization of the Bricolage. *Qualitative Inquiry* 11: 323–50. [CrossRef]
Kuppers, Petra. 2019. *Community Performance: An Introduction*, 2nd ed. Abingdon: Routledge.
Ladd, Paddy. 2003. *Understanding Deaf Culture: In Search of Deafhood*. Clevedon: Multilingual Matters.
Laurendeau, Jason, Tiffany Higham, and Danielle Peers. 2021. Mountain Equipment Co-Op, "Diversity Work", and the "Inclusive" Politics of Erasure. *Sociology of Sport Journal* 38: 120–30. [CrossRef]
Leduc, Vero. 2016. "It Fell on Deaf Ears": Deafhood through the Graphic Signed Novel as a Form of Artivism. In *Mobilizing Metaphor: Art, Culture, and Disability Activism in Canada*. Edited by Michael Orsini and Christine Kelly. Vancouver: UBC Press, pp. 118–37.
Leung, Colette. n.d. Weyburn Mental Hospital. Available online: https://eugenicsarchive.ca/discover/institutions/map/519b32ec4d7d6e000000000b (accessed on 30 November 2022).
Lewis, George E. 2008. Improvisation and Pedagogy: Background and Focus of Inquiry. *Critical Studies in Improvisation*. 3. Available online: https://www.criticalimprov.com/index.php/csieci/article/view/412/658 (accessed on 30 November 2022).
Listen to Dis. 2021. *Pajama Party Politics: There is No Justice without Access*. Online Event. Regina: Saskatchewan Arts Alliance, May 31
Listen to Dis. 2022. *Annual Report*. Regina: Listen to Dis.
Listman, Jason D., and Kim B. Kurz. 2020. Lived Experience: Deaf Professionals' Stories of Resilience and Risks. *The Journal of Deaf Studies and Deaf Education* 25: 239–49. [CrossRef]
Loeppky, John. 2021. The "Crip Tax": Everything Has a Cost, But for People with Disabilities That's Quite Literally the Case. *CBC*. April 15. Available online: https://www.cbc.ca/news/canada/saskatchewan/crip-tax-opinion-1.5856848 (accessed on 30 November 2022).
Loeppky, John. 2022. We Need to Design, Fund Our Social Systems around the Idea That Disabled Children Turn into Disabled Adults *CBC*. May 31. Available online: https://www.cbc.ca/news/canada/saskatchewan/taking-a-sitting-stand-cradle-to-grave-1.6465975?fbclid=IwAR09yWIXRwTMS1qmtTrkuYeTscU8C4Xs6MxSXLPj3xhh6-AixxcDQHdXd1U (accessed on 30 November 2022).
Marcotte, Amanda. 2015. Did You Know Saskatchewan Is "Psychadelic"? *CBC News*. June 19. Available online: https://www.cbc.ca/news/canada/saskatchewan/did-you-know-saskatchewan-is-psychedelic-1.3120921 (accessed on 30 November 2022).
Margoshes, Dave. 1999. *Tommy Douglas: Building the New Society*. Toronto: Dundurn.
Markham, Annette. 2005. "Go Ugly Early": Fragmented Narrative and Bricolage as Interpretive Method. *Qualitative Inquiry* 11: 813–39 [CrossRef]
Marler, Regena Lynn. 2011. *(Un) Wanted Foreign Bodies: The Colonization of Psychic Space in Saskatchewan as Place*. (Order No MR79885). ProQuest Dissertations & Theses Global. Available online: https://ourspace.uregina.ca/handle/10294/13805?show=full (accessed on 30 November 2022).
Massey, Doreen. 2005. *For Space*. London: Sage.
Massie, Merle. 2010. When You're Not from the Prairie: Place History in the Forest Fringe of Saskatchewan. *Journal of Canadian Studies* 44: 171–92. [CrossRef]
Mattin. 2017. Going Fragile. In *Audio Culture: Readings in Modern Music*, rev. ed. Edited by Christoph Cox and Daniel Warner. New York: Bloomsbury Academic, pp. 403–6.
McGregor, Hannah. 2020. Disability Art Is the Last Avant-Garde with Sean Lee. *Secret Feminist Agenda*. episode 4. June 12 Available online: https://secretfeministagenda.com/2020/06/12/episode-4-22-disability-art-is-the-last-avant-garde-with-sean-lee/ (accessed on 30 November 2022).
Meek, David R. 2018. Experiences of Family Dinner Conversations in the Lives of Deaf Adults. Ph.D. dissertation, Lamar University, Beaumont, TX, USA.
Meek, David R. 2020. Dinner Table Syndrome: A Phenomenological Study of Deaf Individuals' Experiences with Inaccessible Communication. *The Qualitative Report* 25: 1676–94. [CrossRef]
Melville Whyte, Jayne. 2012. *Pivot Points: A Fragmented History of Mental Health in Saskatchewan*. Regina: Canadian Mental Health Association (Saskatchewan Division), Inc.
Mitchell, David, Sharon L. Snyder, and Linda Ware. 2014. "[Every] Child Left Behind": Curricular Cripistemologies and the Crip/Queer Art of Failure. *Journal of Literary and Cultural Disability Studies* 8: 295–313. [CrossRef]
Morris, Hugh. 2022. When Technology Makes Music More Accessible. *New York Times*. Available online: https://www.nytimes.com/2022/11/03/arts/music/technology-disability-music.html (accessed on 30 November 2022).

Orsini, Michael, and Christine Kelly. 2016. *Mobilizing Metaphor: Art, Culture, and Disability Activism in Canada*. Edited by Michael Orsini and Christine Kelly. Vancouver: UBC Press.

Peers, Danielle L. 2015. From Eugenics to Paralympics: Inspirational Disability, Physical Fitness, and the White Canadian Nation. Ph.D. dissertation, The University of Alberta, Edmonton, AB, Canada.

Peters, Cynthia. 2009. *Deaf American Literature: From Carnival to the Canon*. Washington, DC: Gallaudet University Press.

Piepzna-Samarasinha, Leah Lakshmi. 2022. Introduction: Writing a Disabled Future, in Progress. In *The Future Is Disabled: Prophecies, Love Notes and Mourning Songs*. Vancouver: Arsenal Pulp Press, pp. 17–50.

Preliminary Report on Deaf Education. 1990. *Preliminary Report on Deaf Education to the Honourable Ray Meiklejohn Minister of Education, Government of Saskatchewan*. Regina: Saskatchewan Ministry of Education and Minister's Advisory Committee on Deaf Education.

Price, Margaret. 2012. Disability Studies Methodology: Explaining Ourselves to Ourselves. In *Practicing Research in Writing Studies*. New York: Hampton Press, pp. 159–86.

Pullman, Ashley, and Chris Nichols. 2015. "Framing Peace by Piece": How to Teach Peace to a Subject that is Continually in Crisis. In *Framing Peace: Thinking about and Enacting Curriculum as "Radical Hope"*. Edited by Hans Smits and Rachel Naqvi. New York: Peter Lang, pp. 29–41.

Richardson, Laurel. 1999. Feathers in our Cap. *Journal of Contemporary Ethnography* 28: 660–68. [CrossRef]

Richardson, Laurel. 2000. Writing: A Method of Inquiry. In *The Handbook of Qualitative Research*, 2nd ed. Edited by Norman K. Denzin and Yvonna S. Lincoln. Thousand Oaks: Sage, pp. 923–48.

Romuld, Darrell. 2020. #JustCurious How Did Sask. Get the Slogan "Land of the Living Skies". *CTV News Regina*. June 23. Available online: https://regina.ctvnews.ca/just-curious/justcurious-how-did-sask-get-the-slogan-land-of-the-living-skies-1.4996888 (accessed on 30 November 2022).

Samuels, Ellen. 2017. Six Ways of Looking at Crip Time. *Disability Studies Quarterly* 3: 37. Available online: https://dsq-sds.org/article/view/5824/4684 (accessed on 30 November 2022).

Saskatchewan Human Rights Commission. 2016. *Access and Equality for Deaf, Deaf, and Hard of Hearing People: A Report to Stakeholders*. Saskatoon: Saskatchewan Human Rights Commission. Available online: https://saskatchewanhumanrights.ca/wp-content/uploads/2020/03/20160512_SHRC_DdHoH_Report.pdf (accessed on 30 November 2022).

Saskatchewan Human Rights Commission. 2021. *Access and Equality for Deaf, Deaf, and Hard of Hearing People: Update to Stakeholders 2021*. Saskatoon: Saskatchewan Human Rights Commission. Available online: https://saskatchewanhumanrights.ca/wp-content/uploads/2021/10/SHRC_DdHoH_Website.pdf (accessed on 30 November 2022).

Sawyer, Keith. 2007. Improvisation and Teaching. *Critical Studies in Improvisation* 3. [CrossRef]

Scrimshaw, Gabrielle. 2018. A Killing in Saskatchewan. *New York Times*. February 15. Available online: https://www.nytimes.com/2018/02/15/opinion/colten-boushie-killing-saskatchewan.html (accessed on 30 November 2022).

Shapiro, Joseph P. 1994. *No Pity: People with Disabilities Forging a New Civil Rights Movement*. New York: Times Books.

Short, Monica, Murray Seiffert, Rob Haynes, and Leanna Haynes. 2018. Church, Disability, and Rurality: The Lived Experience. *Journal of Disability & Religion* 22: 63–88. [CrossRef]

Simpson, Leanne Betasamosake. 2017. *As We Have Always Done: Indigenous Freedom through Radical Resistance*. Minneapolis: University of Minnesota Press.

Smit, Christopher R. 2003. "Please Call Now, Before It's Too Late": Spectacle Discourse in the Jerry Lewis Muscular Dystrophy Telethon. *Journal of Popular Culture* 36: 687–703. [CrossRef]

Sobsey, Dick. n.d. The Latimer Case: The Reflections of People with Disabilities—Media. Council of Canadians with Disabilities. Available online: http://www.ccdonline.ca/en/humanrights/endoflife/latimer/reflections/media (accessed on 15 November 2022).

Stehlik, Daniela. 2017. Rurality, Disability and Place Identity. In *Disability and Rurality: Identity, Gender and Belonging*. Edited by Karen Soldatic and Kelly Johnston. New York: Routledge, pp. 69–80.

Stonechild, Blair. n.d. Treaty 4. Indigenous Saskatchewan Encyclopedia. Available online: https://teaching.usask.ca/indigenoussk/import/treaty_4.php (accessed on 30 November 2022).

Strom, Kathryn, Tammy Mills, and Alan Ovens. 2018. Introduction: Decentering the Researcher in Intimate Scholarship. In *Decentering the Researcher in Intimate Scholarship*. Edited by Kathryn Strom, Tammy Mills and Alan Ovens. Bradford: Emerald Publishing Limited, vol. 31, pp. 15–24.

TeleMiracle. 2022. TeleMiracle Kinsmen Foundation. Available online: https://telemiracle.com/ (accessed on 30 November 2022).

The Interview. 2009. Robert Latimer. *BBC News World Service [The Interview Archive]*. February 20. Available online: https://www.bbc.co.uk/programmes/p03qtqst (accessed on 30 November 2022).

The Weyburn Project. n.d. Mental Hospital at Weyburn: An Archaeolgoy of Madness. YouTube Video. 32:10. Available online: https://www.youtube.com/watch?v=FxSqaqO_Cv0 (accessed on 30 November 2022).

Thobani, Sunera. 2018. Neoliberal Multiculturalism and Western Exceptionalism: The Cultural Politics of the West. *Fudan Journal of the Humanities and Social Sciences* 11: 161–74. [CrossRef]

Thrift, Nigel. 2004. Movement-Space: The Changing Domain of Thinking Resulting from the Development of New Kinds of Spatial Awareness. *Economy and Society* 33: 582–604. [CrossRef]

Thrift, Nigel. 2008. *Non-Representational Theory: Space, Politics, Affect*. New York: Routledge.

Truchan-Tataryn, Maria. 2003. Life sentences of death? Disability in Canadian literature. In *Culture and the State: Disability Studies and Indigenous Studies*. Edited by James Gifford and G. Zezulko-Maillouz. Saskatoon: University of Saskatchewan, pp. 207–18.

Tuck, Eve, and Marcia McKenzie. 2015. *Place in Research: Theory, Methodology, and Methods*. New York: Routledge.

Vandenberg, Helen, and Erin Gallagher-Cohoon. 2021. Health, Charity, and Citizenship: Protestant Hospitals in Rural Saskatchewan, Canada 1906–1942. *European Review of History (Revue Européene D'histoire)* 28: 718–39. [CrossRef]

Varvarigou, Maria. 2017. Group Playing by Ear in Higher Education: The Processes that Support Imitation, Invention and Group Improvisation. *British Journal of Music Education* 34: 291–304. [CrossRef]

Warren, S., and Sami Hopkins. 2021. Harsh Noise-Based Research. Paper presented at 2021 SDS@OSU Multiple Perspectives on Access, Inclusion, and Disability, Virtual Conference, April 17.

Warren-Crow, Heather. 2018. '[I]t Seizes [sic] To Be Heard': Sound Art, Music, and Disability Aesthetics. *Parse Journal, Exclusion* 8. Available online: https://parsejournal.com/article/it-seizes-sic-to-be-heard-sound-art-music-and-disability-aesthetics/ (accessed on 30 November 2022).

Watkin, Jessica. 2022. *Interdependent Magic: Disability Performance in Canada*. Edited by Jessica Watkin. Toronto: Playwrights Canada Press.

Weber, Joanne. 2013. *The Deaf House*. Saskatoon: Thistledown Press.

Weber, Joanne. 2021. Plurilingualism and Policy in Deaf Education. In *Critical Perspectives on Plurilingualism in Deaf Education*. Edited by Kristin Snoddon and Joanne Weber. Bristol: Multilingual Matters.

Weber, Joanne, and Kristin Snoddon. 2020. Intelligibility as a Methodological Problem in the Rehearsal Spaces of Apple Time, a Signed Play. *Sign Language Studies* 20: 595–618. [CrossRef]

Yardley, Ainslie. 2020. *Bricolage as Method*. Edited by Paul Atkinson, Sara Delamont, Alexander Cernat, Joseph W. Sakshaug and Richard A. Williams. New York: SAGE Publications Ltd.

Young, Stella. 2014. I'm Not Your Inspiration, Thank You Very Much. TedxSydney Video. 9:03. Available online: https://www.ted.com/talks/stella_young_i_m_not_your_inspiration_thank_you_very_much?language=en (accessed on 30 November 2022).

Disclaimer/Publisher's Note: The statements, opinions and data contained in all publications are solely those of the individual author(s) and contributor(s) and not of MDPI and/or the editor(s). MDPI and/or the editor(s) disclaim responsibility for any injury to people or property resulting from any ideas, methods, instructions or products referred to in the content.

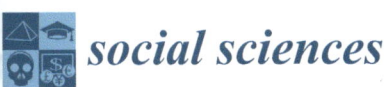

Article

Crip Time and Radical Care in/as Artful Politics

May Chazan

Department of Gender & Social Justice, Trent University, 1600 West Bank Drive, Peterborough, ON K9L 0G2, Canada; maychazan@trentu.ca

Abstract: This article brings together critical disability scholarship and personal narrative, sharing the author's pandemic story of disruption, caregiving, grief, burnout, cancer, and post-operative fatigue. It offers critical reflection on the limits of the neoliberal academy and possibilities for practicing liberatory politics within it, posing two central questions: What does it mean to crip time and centre care as an arts-based researcher? What might a commitment to honouring crip time based on radical care do for the author and their scholarship, and for others aspiring to conduct reworlding research? This analysis suggests that while committing to "slow scholarship" is a form of resistance to ableist capitalist and colonial pressures within the academy, slowness alone does not sufficiently crip research processes. Crip time, by contrast, involves multiply enfolded temporalities imposed upon (and reclaimed by) many researchers, particularly those living with disabilities and/or chronic illness. The article concludes that researchers can commit to recognizing crip time, valuing it, and caring for those living through it, including themselves, not only/necessarily by slowing down. Indeed, they can also carry out this work by actively imagining the crip futures they are striving to make along any/all trajectories and temporalities. This means simultaneously transforming academic institutions, refusing internalized pressures, reclaiming interdependence, and valuing all care work in whatever time it takes.

Keywords: crip time; radical care; slow scholarship; reworlding; crip futures; ableism

Citation: Chazan, May. 2023. Crip Time and Radical Care in/as Artful Politics. *Social Sciences* 12: 99. https://doi.org/10.3390/socsci12020099

Academic Editors: Nadine Changfoot, Eliza Chandler, Carla Rice and Barbara Fawcett

Received: 12 December 2022
Revised: 2 February 2023
Accepted: 6 February 2023
Published: 13 February 2023

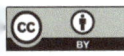

Copyright: © 2023 by the author. Licensee MDPI, Basel, Switzerland. This article is an open access article distributed under the terms and conditions of the Creative Commons Attribution (CC BY) license (https://creativecommons.org/licenses/by/4.0/).

1. Introduction

This article is full of disclosures, all of them vulnerable. As María Elena Cepeda suggests, being a tenured academic comes with a responsibility, "a moral obligation," to disclose the ways in which, as disabled academics, we experience academic institutions as further disabling (Cepeda 2021, p. 312). She advocates for us to disclose "because [we] hold the potential to propel us past the current framework of invisible disability . . . as individual aberration and 'problem' to a more collective approach" (Cepeda 2021, p. 316). I hope my own disclosures might help, somehow, in ditching damaging frameworks and working toward collectivity and compassion.

I share my own pandemic story of disruption, caregiving, grief, burnout, cancer, and post-operative fatigue, as a kind of artful praxis—wherein critical disability theory meets personal narrative—with the hope of thinking through both the limits of the neoliberal academy and some possibilities for holding onto the liberatory politics within it. In reflecting on my own changing bodymind[1] and, by extension, my changing understanding of crip time and radical care, I draw together my lived experience with brilliant scholarship (e.g., Kafer 2021; Meyerhoff and Noterman 2019) to offer insights for navigating community-based, arts-based, and/or storytelling research in these complicated times.

By crip time, I mean the non-linear, unpredictable, ever-changing, or multiply enfolded temporalities of being disabled (Kafer 2021). I understand these shifts in tempo as necessary in order to survive, resist, and transform abled modes (Samuels 2017; Krebs 2022). By radical care, I mean the practice of taking care of ourselves as interwoven with taking care of each other (Piepzna-Samarasinha 2018a); this valuing of interdependence confronts the individualism at the core of capitalism and its self-care industry.[2] Crip time and radical care are co-creations of crip existence, necessary for both survival and transformative reworlding toward just, livable, crip, decolonial, anti-capitalist futures (Hobart and Kneese 2020; Piepzna-Samarasinha 2022). I understand reworlding as generating alternative ways of being, knowing, and relating, outside of existing colonial structures, and making future worlds in the present moment through the ways we relate, imagine, and act (Carter et al. 2018). Reworlding research reaches toward making the next world through practices of sharing stories, listening, and visiting, in old and new ways.

A queer settler of Jewish ancestry in my late 40s, I have been a Canada Research Chair (CRC) in gender studies at Trent University, located in Michi Saagig Anishinaabe territory (currently known as Peterborough, Canada), for almost a decade.[3] The focus of my CRC is leading Aging Activisms, an intergenerational activist research collective seeking to challenge capitalist, colonial, ableist understandings of aging, futures, and social change (Chazan 2020; www.agingactivisms.org, accessed on 12 December 2022). With a team of dedicated academics, students, and community researchers, we facilitate arts-based and storytelling workshops, centring the experiences of local changemakers who are most often omitted from academic study due to being racialized, Indigenous, gender-diverse, LGBTQ2IA+, and/or disabled.

As a methodological inquiry, Aging Activisms strives to resist extractive practices, cultivate care, and circulate critical counter-normative stories. It is built on "slow scholarship"—a revolutionary tempo change that encourages building relationships of care against neoliberal academic currents and capitalist, colonial, ableist temporalities of productivity (Meyerhoff and Noterman 2019; see also Cole 2019)—as well as on notions of crip time, valuing multiple temporalities as resistance to ableist norms (Kafer 2021). In building Aging Activisms as a (then/temporarily) able-bodied person, I often equated slow scholarship with crip time, understanding both as necessary ethical–political commitments in anti-oppressive research. While these concepts have been part of my work since long before COVID-19, my understanding and practice of them have changed.

Specifically, I circle two scholarly questions in this article. First: what does it mean to meaningfully crip time and centre care as an arts-based researcher in uncertain and tumultuous times? In the past, we slowed the pace of Aging Activisms to care for participants, but not necessarily in ways that allowed us to care for ourselves (i.e., myself or my research team); there are indeed institutional barriers to practicing such radical care. Through isolation and illness, I have come to believe that while slowness is necessary, it alone cannot sufficiently crip our processes. Like Alison Kafer, I am learning "how easily crip time has been reduced to, narrowed to, more time—more time as a way of mobilizing disabled people into productivity rather than transforming systems" (Kafer 2021, p. 419). Kafer challenges us to examine the insufficiencies and complexities of slowing down, the possibilities for harm and exploitation, and the question of "what crip time does."

Kafer's reflection frames my second question: What might a commitment to honouring crip time based on radical care do for me, for Aging Activisms, and for others aspiring to reworlding research? In telling my story, I explore what I have been learning: that crip time is not something we commit to; it is something imposed upon (and perhaps reclaimed by) us. However, we can commit to recognizing it, valuing it, and caring for those living through it, including ourselves. In doing so, I believe we are called on not only/necessarily to slow down, but, collectively, to actively imagine the crip futures we are striving to make along any/all trajectories and temporalities available to us. We are challenged to simultaneously transform academic institutions, refuse our own internalized capitalist–ableist pressures, reclaim interdependence, and value all care work in whatever time it takes (Cepeda 2021; Medak-Saltzman et al. 2022; Krebs 2022).

I am a changed person from the one who embarked on an academic career a decade ago, and even from the one who proposed to be part of this Special Issue last year. So many of us are struggling from the fallout of this mass-disabling and alienating pandemic (Barbarin 2021). I find myself unable to "return to normal" following clinical burnout, breast cancer, and multiple pandemic upheavals (Krebs 2022). I struggled to even write this article as I am often horizontal or experiencing brain fog. Writing this was only possible with the support and care of my long-time research assistants (RAs), Melissa Baldwin and Ziysah von Bieberstein, who offered discussions, literature review, editing, and transcription of my voice memos. Like others, I am re-committing to crip, queer, decolonize, and unsettle my own research practices, creative pursuits, and artful politics (Changfoot et al. 2022; FitzGibbon 2021). I am doing my best to refuse the capitalist aspiration of "return", often "breaking time" by collapsing into a nap, allowing my students to rest, leaning on trusted relationships, keeping my mask on in public, or avoiding large events (Cepeda 2021). I commit and refuse in these ways because "I want freedom and survival for all of us" (Cepeda 2021, p. 307).

2. Aging Activisms in the Before-Times

By just visiting—mawadisidiwag // they visit each other—we are already doing and making in important ways.

(Miner 2019, p. 133)

In the years leading up to the pandemic, I was learning about the complexities of slowing down, about crip time and radical care. Between 2015 and 2019, my research team led seven research arts-based and storytelling gatherings, bringing together multi-age groups of artists and activists to share, listen, eat, and create together. We facilitated embodied theatre workshops, music-making, poetry-writing, zine-making, collage, and art installation co-creation. This led to hundreds of creative pieces and dozens of "media capsules," short videos that captured intimate group storytelling processes, collectively offering an oral history of social change in our community.[4]

These events focused on relationship-building that reverberated into the world in many generative ways (Chazan 2020). We spent time caring for participants before, during, and after each workshop with a ratio of one facilitator to every two or three participants. In addition to carrying the heart-work of the project, research tasks included facilitating, documenting, making tea, listening attentively, ensuring access to food, supporting accessibility needs, arranging participants' transport, strengthening relationships with and among participants, and attending to complex group dynamics, emotions, and energies. We also collaborated on participants' endeavours in the broader community, including symposia, seminars, rallies, teach-ins, film screenings, and poetry readings.

Slowing down to centre community care was meaningful, rewarding, even transformative. Participants reported a sense of connection and validation. Many contrasted the care and slow listening in our project with the extractive, contractual, and/or time-pressured encounters they experience in other community spaces (such as meetings, events, workshops, etc.). Participants' reflections suggested that this slowing-together became a collective practice of sowing-together, making livable futures in real time at the micro-scale of our gatherings (Carter et al. 2018; Miner 2019).

The project had challenges, of course; most significantly, its uneasy fit within an academic institution. I preface this critique by crediting the CRC position at Trent University. When I began in this role, I was parenting a still-nursing one-year-old and an autistic five-year-old. By funding my research and research time (affording me a reduced teaching load) for ten years, the CRC allowed me to undertake slow, care-centred research and to simultaneously prioritize care in my family/community, even if neither were always easy to justify. Still, working and parenting together is a more-than-full-time job. And, working explicitly in feminist scholarship, it was never lost on me that I was managing the ever-expanding, often-gendered, dual-load of caretaking both within academia and working-motherhood (Medak-Saltzman et al. 2022; Mitchell-Eaton 2020).

There were institutional challenges that I faced even before COVID-19. In short, academic structures and funding policies are not designed to support care-centred scholarship; choosing this path comes with costs—mostly for me, but also for my research team (FitzGibbon 2021). For example, as part of an activist research practice, I directed much of my research funding to the community via honoraria, food, paid positions, gifts from local vendors, sponsorships, etc. This meant justifying "non-traditional" research expenses that were not listed on institutional forms. Submitting and defending expense claims added significantly to the already time-intensive work; I regularly gave up on accessing research funds for even basic expenses, instead paying out of pocket. This felt worthwhile and fair in the context of income disparity between me and many participants, even as it illustrated the extent to which academic funding structures are not designed for community research.

Then, there was the ongoing pressure to enumerate outputs through annual reports, tenure portfolios, etc., which prioritized particular products (publications and conferences), and did not offer space to describe or value care-centred research processes. There were less overt costs, too. For instance, focusing on accessible video creation instead of peer-reviewed publication could decrease my chances of being promoted or receiving future research grants. And, in a small department in a small Canadian university, I was navigating the bureaucratic dimensions of my research with no administrative support. In my research log in 2019, I wrote: "working against the grain, even when it is so care-filled, is exhausting." I was sick with my fourth round of strep throat that year.

What I am describing is a paradox. In the university environment, caring so intensively for others was at odds with caring for myself, largely because the care that is central to my research was deemed an add-on to my job expectations (Bailey 2021). When I shared this reflection with my team, I realized they faced a similar paradox, too; RAs were intensively caretaking for participants while unable to properly care for themselves during or after workshops due to lack of adequate support, compensation, and job security. My team included many diverse bodyminds—introverted, neurodivergent, and chronically ill. Recovery time required after an intensive workshop was elusive and unpaid. Without structural change, my efforts to increase hours and pay rates were never adequate; to academic funding bodies, RA rest and recovery time is not a justifiable expense.

Before COVID-19, I often felt filled up—in a good way—by the reciprocal care of Aging Activisms, and my RAs echoed these sentiments. But the bureaucratic pieces were depleting, as was the assumption that community care and relationship-building are extraneous to metrics of productivity. These complexities and tensions exploded for me, as they did for many others, in COVID-19's first wave.

3. Forced Stop

> What are the temporalities that unfold beyond, away from, askance of productivity, capacity, self-sufficiency, independence, achievement?
>
> (Kafer 2021, p. 420)

This story is about being propelled to crip time, accept loss, and care radically in a society desperate to maintain the capitalist status quo. While my experiences of the past few years have been exceptional in the context of my own life, I was certainly not the only one to suffer. Most were propelled to crip time with far less structural privilege and support; where I have had ongoing job, housing, and food security and a supportive partner and family, many lost access to their livelihoods, struggled for basic needs, and were far more isolated. Those already disabled faced ever-narrowing chances of survival (Barbarin 2021; Medak-Saltzman et al. 2022). In my case, experiences of trauma, illness, and disability burst the bubble of many comforts in my life, revealing the fragility and facade of institutional support; I was exposed to harsher tempos of loss, grief, and disability already commonplace to many; I experienced the disposability of care. My story is about these converging crises and what they revealed, from the context of my significant financial and societal privilege as a tenured academic. I will highlight both the crises and the privilege, illustrating the urgency to attend to the story's unexceptionality, particularly for those of us aspiring toward reworlding from academic positions.

When COVID-19 hit our community in March 2020, I promptly cancelled all Aging Activisms events without knowing if/how Trent and the CRC would accommodate. In a global emergency, my primary concern was to protect the most vulnerable, many of whom were central to our research. The first wave and lockdown came very abruptly. By public health orders, universities were to stop all in-person teaching and research; students were asked to vacate residences; we scrambled to move our teaching online. Mostly, I stopped teaching and just met virtually with students, who were scared and isolated, exempting them from their final assignments. I also delivered food packages to ill students.

Working in this period was extremely disorienting. The forced research hiatus was not accompanied by any communication from the CRC, nor with any immediate reassurance from Trent that the academic clock would be paused. I was grateful for my secure income and my ability to stay home. Still, the necessity to stop, the uncertainty around institutional accommodation, the fear of contagion, and the inaccessibility of so many spaces were destabilizing experiences. This type of disorientation has long been part of regular life for many in the crip community. It resonated when Emily Krebs, like others, explained that COVID-19 was imposing aspects of crip time onto non-disabled bodyminds: "What many non-disabled people experienced as a 'collective disorientation' was, in many ways, a reorientation toward crip/sick ways of life" (Krebs 2022, p. 19). The immediate shift in tempo alongside the stark inequities of the pandemic threw into sharp relief the tensions between slow care and urgent liberation (Kim and Schalk 2021; Piepzna-Samarasinha 2018b).

Initially, I sought to keep as many of my RAs employed as possible and to offer support and care to the Aging Activisms community. In April and May, I had my team phone, email, and drop off essentials to the most vulnerable in our networks, justifying this pandemic care as research—that is, maintaining relationships we would come back to. My team created a virtual Aging Activisms space for sharing creative pursuits and student work while in isolation.[5]

As public health measures were extended, I further cancelled two immersive workshops for the late summer and fall. We explored, briefly, moving to a virtual format, but participants were focused on their basic physical and emotional needs and did not have the capacity for virtual gatherings or creative endeavours. At this point, most SSHRC grants were automatically extended, but my research office at Trent informed me that the CRC did not intend to extend or pause my grant in any way (I assumed this to be the case for all CRC grants). In this moment, I recognized how little some academic structures would accommodate the collective crip experience (Krebs 2022). It was unsafe, even illegal, for me to continue the research that I was funded to conduct, but my funder would not accommodate a pause in the work. This was a clear example of institutional inflexibility reinforcing productivist/abled temporalities.

Through that first pandemic spring, I leaned into radical slowness in a different part of my life—parenting—learning lessons about care and crip time that I would only come to recognize later. The abrupt cancellation of school, supports, and therapies, alongside expectations to pivot to online learning, was challenging for my children, who have learning, sensory-processing, and communication disabilities. I took on the role of teacher, counsellor, speech therapist, recreational coordinator, tech support, and parent. Even with the privilege of a partner to lean on, we could not keep up with all the responsibilities.

In mid-April, we decided to scale back—not just a slowdown, but a shift in expectations. We made schoolwork optional, offering instead rest time, creative projects, gardening, and being on the land. Although de-schooling required justification to the school and alternative activities, it significantly cut back the teacher and tech support roles. The turn toward meaningful care was healing for all of us. I was present, rested, and attentive, in ways I could not be while also working outside of the home. For my children, it was an unprecedented break from capitalist/ableist pressures to keep up and perform. Anxiety decreased, sleep improved; they were content and calm despite the global upheaval.

What I was learning in my previous research was reinforced at home. I understood anew how capitalist pressures are disabling; in letting go of those pressures, we no longer needed most of the therapies and supports we previously relied on. This shift depended on dedicated caregiver time, energy, and presence, none of which are typically valued or compensated in our society.

4. Care Time

> We reassemble ourselves through the ordinary, everyday, and often painstaking work of looking after ourselves, looking after each other.
>
> (Ahmed 2017, p. 240)

Radical care and uneven economies of care are not new to me, but during the pandemic, I lived them ever more acutely. In July 2020, both my parents experienced acute medical crises, the details of which are beyond the scope of this article. In one particularly traumatic instance, I received a call in the middle of the night that my mother had been rushed to hospital with heart failure and it was uncertain whether she would survive. COVID-19 protocols and best practices had prevented us from visiting her for months, and now we were not permitted at her bedside. It was a terrible moment of panic, grief, and helplessness. Miraculously, she pulled through, but she could no longer climb the stairs in her house, and there were several further 9-1-1 calls due to congestive heart failure.

We were experiencing the pandemic reality of crip time for elders with underlying conditions; precarious and vulnerable, their required care remained critically unsupported and inflexible (Tsai 2022). The lockdowns exacerbated ongoing challenges of care availability, access, and safety. Driving to Toronto to care for my parents multiple times per week (a minimum 3-hour return trip) jostled me abruptly out of my quiet child-filled routines. And I worried that my in-person care might put my parents at risk of COVID-19.

My parents and I decided to sell their house and find them an accessible, single-level residence close to us. The asset of a long-ago purchased house in an urban centre was another tremendous privilege that allowed my parents to relocate. The move was a mammoth undertaking amidst repeated hospitalizations. Formal supports were scarce; we organized close friends and family to provide access to medical care, house cleaning, and grocery delivery.

Danika Medak-Saltzman et al. (2022, p. 9) describe the compounding, though unexceptional, pressures of caregiving during the pandemic, and the ways in which academic institutions failed to adapt:

> Colleges and universities [did not] adapt to the tremendous increase in labor for workers with caregiving responsibilities, who suddenly faced homeschooling and childcare, elder care or care for the disabled when their carefully crafted care networks broke apart as schools closed, living facilities for the elderly became particularly dangerous, and poorly paid in-home care workers now suddenly were both particularly vulnerable to infection and seen as a potential source of transmission.

I expected that my parents would gradually need more intensive, perhaps palliative, care. Being their primary caregiver would be challenging, but I believed it was the best option for their dignity and survival.

Though physical schools re-opened in September, we decided to homeschool in order to (more) safely "bubble" with my parents. This was not a decision made lightly; we knew there were social, emotional, academic, and therapeutic experiences we could not provide nor access from home. We hired some part-time childcare and tutoring support for my children to allow me to continue working without overburdening my partner. The media was reporting on the pandemic toll of caregiving, especially on working mothers. Medak-Saltzman et al. noted how academics acting as caregivers through this time risked impacting their capacities to keep up with the academic clock of tenure and promotion (Medak-Saltzman et al. 2022, p. 3).

My own fall teaching term was taught entirely online. Trent faculty were now expected to also find ways to continue research amidst public health restrictions. Colleagues were turning to writing and virtual presentations. I felt these productivity pressures. However, it did not make sense to start writing or presenting about the community-intensive research I was still so much in the middle of. Plus, I was exhausted.

Then, my mother fell in the night and broke her hip. For two months, in addition to teaching, supporting students, and homeschooling, I spent a minimum of eight hours per day physically caring for her as she convalesced at home. I learned a lot about crip time at my mother's bedside. While days were repetitive and one blurred into the next, I was keenly aware of her care and survival as a tremendous collective effort. Life went something like this: I spent early mornings with my children, leaving them with a basic plan for their day. My partner did most of the daily household care: childcare, shopping, cooking, and laundry. Meanwhile, I tended to my mother's basic needs: I helped with dressing, bathing, and moving; I made food, managed medical appointments, and assisted with physiotherapy. I taught my courses and attended departmental meetings from my parents' home, sometimes from their bedside. In the evenings, my brother attended to my mother while I caught up on work emails, read books with my children, and made sure to get to bed early.

We lived in this care-time rhythm for six weeks without one single day off. I was deeply ensconced in what Sarah E. Stevens calls "care time" or the "liminal space between crip time and abled time" (Stevens 2018). It would have been impossible for me to run workshops in that time, even if we were not restricted by the pandemic. My paid work was pared down to absolute essentials. As Mei-Yu Tsai describes, "care work is slow work, and care time requires slow and consistent effort to resist ableist emphases on independence, productivity, efficiency, and speed" (2022 p. 12). I tried to accept my crip temporalities, but the institutional pressures weighed on me. I once again explored the possibility of a pause on my research funding, but the CRC was unreachable, and Trent's research office was very sympathetic to my situation but had no way to assist. The irony of not being able to adapt the very position that awarded my care-centred, slow scholarship was ever-present:

5. Grief Time

To whose normal are we returning? Who is going back? And who will be left behind?

(Krebs 2022, p. 121)

The academic funding institution would not bend; there would be no accommodation for the crip time imposed on me and my research. I felt demoralized and depleted by what this would cost in terms of Aging Activisms; I was quite devastated at the continued devaluation of care.

On the advice of a dear friend, I sought counselling. Maybe I could figure out how to cope better, how to manage my time, how to fold myself back into productivity while caring full-time. But my counsellor said there was simply no magic way through the unmovable stresses I faced. Since abandoning my children or my parents at the height of a pandemic was not an option, I would have to take something else—i.e., work—off my plate to make space for caring for myself. "If you want everyone to survive this," she said, "you have to put your own oxygen mask on first."

I had trouble accepting this. I may have fully embraced the sentiment, but I did not believe I could add additional tasks of self-care to my already-packed days. Tasks such as exercise and rest would take time; they seemed impossible and tiring. In retrospect, I could have turned to more radical notions of interdependence and community care rather than turning the burden of self-care back on myself. But self-care did not (yet) feel necessary to my survival; I was coping. I was too tired to imagine how to take a break, so I just continued along.

Then, almost overnight, my mother started to walk again. Her pain subsided as her body healed. She still needed me, but not nearly as consistently or urgently. Suddenly, I felt I had copious amounts of time, which is interesting given that I was still teaching and homeschooling. I was coming to understand that crip temporalities operate in unpredictable ways. I did not collapse into a heap and rest, although I probably should have. Rather, a week opened for me in which I could think; I accelerated into a burst of worktime.

I quickly reached out to my former team, relieved and even excited to be in this rapid thinking/planning space. I have since come to understand this kind of energetic burst as another dimension of crip time, an unexpected acceleration (Kafer 2021). I felt excited to devise a new, community-informed plan for the final years of Aging Activisms. This was partly underpinned by those tentacles of productivity; I thought if I worked quickly enough, I could have a plan in place by March to align with my annual reporting requirements and funding cycles.

I spoke to my counsellor again, excited to tell her about the shift. Thoughtfully, she asked whether I might turn my momentary energy toward my own care, given my state and all who were depending on me. She also encouraged me to allow myself some space in the planning to grieve; to begin letting go of Aging Activisms as it was in the before-times. While I did not yet understand the scope of what she was suggesting, I did take her advice to shelve the planning temporarily and take a two-week winter break "off" to rest and reconnect with my partner and children. In retrospect, I have come to understand that both the burst to accelerated time and the deliberate pacing (with a self-imposed break) were elements of crip time, both complicated. Neither was imposed on me to the extent that the previous "care time" had been; yet both were, in part, responses to feeling pressure to produce amid ongoing constraints (resulting from pandemic-related restrictions and caregiving). The acceleration was driven by my genuine desire and excitement to imagine my research into a future on the one hand, and, on the other, by a looming pressure to comply with institutional reporting requirements. The decision to pause—to "rest" (or at least turn to more focused care for my children while navigating our first pandemic holiday season)—was similarly conflicted. This was, in part, me reclaiming crip time, resisting productivist work pressures, and recognizing my own and my family's needs; it was also me pacing myself, knowing that I would need to come back from this "break" with even more energy and readiness to reinvent my research.

What happened next, however, was not rest or recovery. On the night of 25 December, the strictest lockdown thus far in Ontario was announced. That same night, my family faced another middle-of-the-night crisis: my partner's father fell backward down the stairs, leading to a coma and, two weeks later, death. This would have been devastating in any context; during COVID-19, the tragedy was deepened by not being able to say goodbye or gather with family.

In our home, time swelled and stilled. Ellen Samuels' statement, "crip time is grief time" resonates. Like for Samuels, time stopped; we were unprepared for "the way the days slowed and swelled unbearably" around death (Samuels 2017). My partner was spiralling through shock, anger, pain, and loss, all while tending to logistics. My care for him felt inadequate, so I focused on the children and cooking. We were all in a fog of shock and sadness.

Heading into the new year, we remained in an intensified lockdown. My partner would be away intermittently for months, closing his father's apartment. The cumulative strains were now causing me insomnia, body aches, and anxiety. Reaching out again for some relief from my work responsibilities, my Department Chair generously went to the Dean on my behalf. It is worth noting the additional privilege I had here; my Chair and the Dean were both extremely supportive of me throughout this time. However, my Chair was told there was "no precedent" for paid caregiving support or to postpone my teaching to the spring term. With sympathy, my Dean offered two options: to apply for a reduction to part-time or to take full unpaid leave. As my family's primary income-earner, neither seemed viable. I would push through.

I had just moved foggily into the winter teaching term when we were faced with yet another family medical emergency: my sister was admitted to hospital in Chicago. Like my mother, her congenital heart condition had intensified; she needed a heart transplant. I knew that few in this condition survive beyond months. I wanted desperately to visit her, but travel was not possible. As she worked through trauma, I spent many late nights supporting her remotely. Then, in February, by which time I understood she likely had only days to live, she received the transplant. In the lead up to the operation, I was fully on "grief time"; the days and nights went on forever and without break.

The time spent caring for my mother with her broken hip was repetitive but passed quickly. Now, I was mired in emotional paralysis. The compounding grief and anxiety at a time of so much isolation became debilitating and disabling. I was cycling through so many crip temporalities, all without the supports I needed to care for myself.

6. Broken Time

Caring for myself is not self-indulgence, it is self-preservation, and that is an act of political warfare.

(Lorde [1988] 2017, p. 130)

The breakdown in my own mental and physical health was a rupture of sorts. My counsellor called it "clinical burnout brought on by compounding, exceptional stresses, resulting in cognitive impairment, insomnia, fatigue, emotional numbing, and body pain." In practical terms, I could not focus on anything; I felt as if I was watching someone else through a movie camera. I was unable to keep track of my own schedule and regularly missed meetings. I could not make sense of my own teaching notes nor make it through the readings I had assigned my students. I was still feeling tension regarding Aging Activisms—I had no creative plan to offer on my annual report—but I stopped caring. I did not have the focus for any form of self-care; even trying to drink water felt like a challenge. By early March, I reached out to my doctor in desperation; I asked her to prescribe sleeping pills, which turned out to be of little use. My counsellor urged me to apply for medical leave.

My counsellor and department Chair graciously took me through the initial application process for the maximum of 6 months paid sick/stress leave provided for in my collective agreement. My Dean fully supported this and offered additional accommodations (support with marking) to help tide me over until the leave would begin. With this, the CRC was required to pause my grant for six months. However, my research was already one year behind; even with support from my research office (and the advocacy of the VP of Research at my university), the CRC refused any further extension. Meanwhile, the internalized pressures of productivity and student care continued. How could I hand over a course I barely had a grip on? What about my students set to defend dissertations? My research team? As Samuels explains, neoliberalism demands we navigate inaccessible bureaucratic steps before we might be afforded time for recovery; I would have to "work hard to earn the time to be sick" (Samuels 2017). This was "broken time." While I had collapsed, I still had to rally any remaining productivity to achieve medical leave.

I moved toward further crip temporalities and self-care. I needed to do less and be responsible for less. The ableist assumption embedded in my leave was that "reduced capacities are one-time temporary conditions" (Medak-Saltzman et al. 2022, p. 6), and that I would return "back to normal." While six months is more paid leave than most are entitled to, it is nonetheless a rigid deadline for recovery; it did not hold enough space for the brokenness I was experiencing, the compounding illness I was about to experience, or the ongoing pandemic disruptions. As Samuels writes:

> [Crip time] requires us to break in our bodies and minds to new rhythms, new patterns of thinking and feeling and moving through the world. It forces us to take breaks, even when we don't want to, even when we want to keep going, to move ahead. It insists that we listen to our bodyminds so closely, so attentively, in a culture that tells us to divide the two and push the body away from us while also pushing it beyond its limits. Crip time means listening to the broken languages of our bodies, translating them, honoring their words. (Samuels 2017)

I was about to learn this even more deeply.

7. Cancer Time

Survival can thus be what we do for others, with others. We need each other to survive; we need to be a part of each other's survival.

(Ahmed 2017, p. 235)

In March 2021, a mammogram as part of a high-risk screening revealed a small abnormality—in the month that followed, I learned I had breast cancer. Many have written powerfully about their journeys with breast cancer (Lorde 1980; Lin 2016). While I will not go into depth here, I do want to highlight how the stress of the cancer diagnosis, compounded by the pandemic, exacerbated my burnout. The cancer added significantly to my recovery time, but it also went essentially unnoticed by the institutions at play in my work life. In other words, the arbitrary six months allotted for my full and complete recovery from my existing clinical burnout remained static. This offered another clear insight into structural inflexibility and the need for systemic transformation. I also started to understand in a more embodied way that crip time entails multiple, unpredictable temporalities, and that surviving these temporalities within capitalist systems depends on care as a reciprocal practice.

The experience of cancer is not only physical; it is also the worry, fear, and worst-case-scenarios, and the work of protecting those around you (i.e., my children). The cancer jogged me out of my numbness; I cried a lot at night when everyone else was sleeping. The most stressful part was the waiting. Time suddenly went very slowly again. It was nine very long weeks from my first abnormal mammogram to the pathology report; thankfully, the cancer was caught early and had not spread. These two months were spent anxiously as I scheduled, re-scheduled, modified, and attended various procedures, tests, surgeries, pandemic-related delays, and consultations. In the limited options of pandemic healthcare, I underwent an outpatient double mastectomy with sparse aftercare, and waited three more weeks for a pathology report.

As Kafer (2021) writes, the slowness and endless waiting of crip time can be punishing, unrelenting. In the isolation of a third wave of lockdowns, a few close friends held me virtually through the waiting, reminding me that I needed community. In the week or so before surgery, I gathered the courage to send a group email to select friends and colleagues. It felt odd to reach out with this narrative of personal trauma, but I was immediately showered with gifts of community care. The afternoon before my surgery, three friends showed up on my street, despite the stay-at-home orders. They brought drums, a hand-made basket full of medicines from the land, and their children. They drummed and sang songs of strength as I sat on my front step crying. My children held me, and then ran around with the other children, a rare opportunity in lockdown. I felt vulnerable yet also strengthened enough to reach out even more. One friend, Ziysah in fact, told me that my reaching out provided them with the opportunity to care; it was reciprocal. This realization of our interdependence was another turning point for me.

The physical toll of the cancer was significant. The weeks following my surgery were painful and incapacitating as I had tubes draining from my chest. It took months of hard work to (mostly) regain the strength and mobility of my upper body. I was told I made an excellent recovery, though I continue to have a limited range of motion and pain in one shoulder. During my initial recovery, my family and community showered me with every kind of care. And—uncharacteristically—I accepted it. Porch visits, home-made meals, chocolate, books, and gifts for the children. My partner's mother and Melissa provided childcare while I rested in a way that I had not previously nor have since. It took this extreme scenario for me to finally prioritize self-care. I was able to do so because of the care from our community and the institutional support of paid leave.

Healing, like crip time, is never linear. As I came out of recovery that summer with four months left of leave, my body was still straining and my mind remained foggy. Wearily, I continued the work of self and family care, while many community supports faded.

I contacted my family doctor mid-summer. When was I going to feel better? She noticed then that, in the COVID-19 chaos, I never had routine pre-surgical bloodwork to check for underlying conditions; I also had not had post-operative care, nor been informed that there was significant blood loss in my surgery, making me prone to anemia. Bloodwork revealed very low iron levels and I was prescribed iron supplements. But the fatigue continued. Was it lingering burnout, iron deficiency, or something else?

The next medical surprise was another cancer scare as an "irregular mass" was found in a pelvic scan. With six weeks left of paid leave, I was thrown deeper into that elongated experience of cancer time. There was more waiting and out-of-town testing. Fortunately, the mass was benign, but other, non-life-threatening issues were detected that were likely compounding my fatigue. Suffice it to say, these last months of my leave were not restful.

I turned to the possibility of long-term disability via my health benefits. There were many barriers: the system was based on the idea of a worsening condition, but I had a new condition; it required a medical professional to have approved my first leave, and my counsellor did not qualify; the six-month maximum applied regardless of any new condition. My colleagues advised that I would likely be declined; one called it "denial by design." Apparently, it was just bad luck that the cancer did not wait 18 months to appear, when I would have been afforded more time for recovery.

In these moments, I experienced the drag of crip time. Like Samuels:

> I moved backward instead of forward; not into a state of health, but further into the world of disability, a world I was increasingly coming to understand as my own. I moved from being someone who kept getting sick to someone who was sick all the time, whose inner clock was attuned to my own physical state rather than the external routines of a society ordered around bodies that were not like mine (Samuels 2017).

Mired in fatigue, I did not have the emotional wherewithal for bureaucracy. It felt easier to return to work than to wade through institutional barriers.

8. Gentle Methodologies

The times are urgent, so let us slow down.

(Akomolafe 2020, p. 49)

Despite everything, I felt a bit hopeful about returning to work in fall of 2021, at least pandemic-wise. Vaccine uptake was high in my community, and they were about to begin rolling out vaccines for children. It was still "Delta times." There was hope that vaccines would curb transmission; mask mandates and limitations on indoor gatherings remained. Our children went back to school after being home for a year and a half. As a family with vulnerable members, we were especially cautious, even as we welcomed the opportunity to be somewhat less isolated.

As I returned to work in November, my primary task was to get Aging Activisms running again. I knew I was not well enough to start organizing workshops and caring for others, nor was it safe or legal to gather in the ways we had been used to. The wisdom I gained over the previous year led me to look more seriously at the internalized pressures of academia/capitalism. What might crip time mean for me now and what might it do for my return, my research? I knew the underpinning capitalist ableism I was up against (Krebs 2022). But what to do? Leaning into my privilege as a tenured professor, I knew I did not need to be productive by someone else's definition or metric, or at least that the stakes were not dire. But, in the productivity-obsessed culture of academia, I also felt lost and anxious.

A feminist academic writing coach with a deep understanding of academic structures and remarkable criticality in her approach to work asked me: "What is the worst that could happen if you do nothing more with the CRC grant, but let it run out with the research not completed?" I considered this carefully. I did not like the idea, on principle. But the only tangible repercussions I could identify were financial: impacts on my future promotion to full professor and a decreased likelihood of success in future funding competitions. Although these scenarios were significant losses, they gave me huge assurance. I did not need a promotion, raise, or more research funding. What I needed was continued healing. I wanted to be able to complete the work I had proposed years ago, but the proposal had come from a different time and a different bodymind. I had to release the shame of letting this research go in order to ensure the wellbeing (and maybe survival) of myself, my family, and my team.

It was a reckoning to realize that Aging Activisms' commitment to radical care rather than community care would have to start with honouring my own crip temporalities and disabled bodymind. I needed to approach the question of 'what next?' with genuine curiosity, not panic or pressure to produce a new plan. What could we do, gently, with the remaining time and funding left on my grant, in the pandemic context? There would be losses, but maybe also unexpected possibilities.

In my first term back at work, my departmental colleagues asked almost no service of me, and my Chair (with the support of my Dean) managed to shield me from teaching for that full academic year, on the basis that I needed to get Aging Activisms re-started. They were caring for me so I could care for myself.

I stepped slowly back into the work. I hosted a campfire on campus, inviting former research team members to visit and re-connect. I walked with grad students, exchanging ideas. From my bed, I watched some of our earlier media capsules, and called some participants to ask how they were doing. I started an email conversation with my research team—Ziysah, Melissa, and dear friend and colleague Jenn Cole—about "gentle methodologies." We came up with ideas such as river walks and campfire conversations as research methods. We discussed what we obtain—what care is turned back onto us as researchers—in our research relationships, and how we might further honour this interdependence and reciprocity in/as intrinsic to our collective reworlding practices. Ziysah raised the joy they derived from visiting with a participant at her home, a remarkable woman of then 99 years old, to allow her to accessibly sign a consent form. On this visit, they took the time to fix a vacuum and have tea—such activities were not unusual in our research encounters. They reflected that, even if they had not billed out these hours (which they did, upon our mutual agreement), this visit would have been deeply nurturing and worthwhile for them both. How often do we have opportunities to visit with likeminded folks six decades older/younger than ourselves? This was such an important reminder; clearly, I could not have expressed this within institutional reporting requirements or on a CV, but the mismatch between these structures and the essence of the work did not diminish such moments of mutual care.

I leaned on the team to help me think through the question I was pondering: what do radical care and crip time mean for Aging Activisms? I was reminded that Aging Activisms had long been grappling with these very questions. RAs asked how we might, even amidst institutionalized capitalism, practice decolonial, crip, caring futures in real time, in practical, grounded ways; make the lines of care and sharing within the work more reciprocal in all directions; and maybe even push the university to count things such as healing, sharing, recovering, growing, and grieving in their metrics of productivity. Their questions helped seed this article.

We began to plan in a non-labour-intensive way, with minimal energy required from me, and the bulk of the organizing taken on by my RAs. We planned a series of "miniworkshops" for early winter: campfire conversations and virtual "crafternoons." In these "easeful" gatherings, as Ziysah called them, we would revisit our questions from our final workshop in 2019: How do we imagine livable/just futures in this community? We would also ask if and how thinking about futures had changed over the pandemic, and consider what, in COVID-times, gentle, care-oriented research might involve. I felt lifted to be returning to this work in a more relaxed way.

9. Creative Time

Radical care can present an otherwise.

(Hobart and Kneese 2020, p. 13)

Omicron arrived just over a month after my return to work, evading vaccines and shattering hopes. By mid-December, we were heading into renewed lockdowns. Another holiday season in isolation. The one-year anniversary of my father-in-law's tragic death. I was not the only one struggling; the anti-lockdown occupations that followed in Canada (and elsewhere) were evidence of widespread unhinging. While I appreciated that public health leaders and politicians were continuing to take measures to protect the most vulnerable, looping back into imposed hiatus just as I was finding my way to a gentle return came as a blow. I crashed: intensified fatigue, insomnia, body pain. It reminded me again that crip time—whether a result of bodily healing or collective disorientation—is never linear or predictable (Kafer 2021).

Schools did not re-open for several weeks after winter break. We were privileged to be able to keep our children home until we could all be fully vaccinated and boosted, and we were acutely aware that other families did not have such options. As the spring approached, I felt helpless that provincial policies were set to abandon the most vulnerable. This round of homeschooling was also exponentially more difficult. Where the first stint at home was a much-needed break for my children, this time, it was a palpable loss of community. We leaned on friends who had made the same choice.

At work, our plans for fireside workshops were shelved. We paused and entered another cycle of slow, grief-filled time, yearning for connection but afraid to gather. I was not well enough to dig into scholarly activities such as reading or writing at that point, but something low-pressure and creative might help me stay connected. On a whim, I registered for an eight-week online digital storytelling course to learn a technique and methodology that had long intrigued me.[6] Making space for my own creative practice was an unexpected bit of self-care, and I recognized the privilege of having a family and job that supported this practice.

Each student was required to make a film. I decided to turn the question of how we imagine futures in these times back on myself, as a kind of reflexive practice. In one rapid burst of energy, I answered my research question in the form of a letter to my younger child about her climate grief. Less explicitly, I was also writing a letter to Aging Activisms and to Michi Saagiig land and territory, sharing what I was learning in our work together. With the help of photos stored on my phone, this letter became a 5-minute digital story, called *Dream Beautiful Futures*.[7] The story moves from the helplessness of the apocalypse toward the possibility of alternative world-making through daily acts of connecting, caring, and creating. The piece felt vulnerable; I started by sharing it with a few people close to me, who received it with love. Jenn even said she received it as "heart-medicine." In the writing exercises and creation process involved in that course, I realized anew that the work of making liveable futures is deeply connected to the work of caregiving and intergenerational continuance. All the caring for myself and my loved ones was radical reworlding (Hobart and Kneese 2020; Tsai 2022).

In the spirit of the unpredictability and never-finishing nature of crip time, I will end the story here, with the completion of the only thing I have "produced" in this pandemic (other than this article!). This creative practice pulled me back to the broader project of Aging Activisms: to actively imagine crip, decolonial, just, liveable futures; to enact collective survival; and to make these futures in the present through creative, care-filled, loving practices.

If I had more space (both within the word limits of this publication and within my own capacity), I would continue the story with how I bumbled along through the term; eventually held two virtual gatherings with Aging Activisms participants, which included screening my digital story; and continued to creatively, if not unproblematically, navigate care, chronic symptoms, and work expectations. I would write, too, about the ironies of trying to write this article along the multiple temporalities of crip time. I would send a shout-out to the editors of this Special Issue for their flexibility, enabling my process in the time it took, and caring for me along the way. I would tell you that I am at a critical juncture: with no more leave available to me and one year of CRC funding left, I have yet to substantively resume my research. I miss Aging Activisms, my community, and the creative intellectual work, but my bodymind continues to struggle. I want to resume research in even more caring ways. I want to de-program from the looming sense of "time running out." I know that neither the world nor my work nor my bodymind can go back.

I am working to accept and imagine otherwise. As I write this article, I am coming to understand a radically different world.

10. Crip Time, Radical Care, and Beautiful Futures: Conclusions

We will leave no one behind as we roll, limp, stim, sign and create the decolonial living future. [...] I am dreaming like my life depends on it. Because it does. And so does yours.

(Piepzna-Samarasinha 2018b)

To conclude, I return to the questions I set out in the introduction and suggest what my narrative might contribute to ongoing scholarship. What does it mean to meaningfully crip time and centre care in artful research in these tumultuous times? What might a commitment to crip time based on radical care do for me, for Aging Activisms, and for others aspiring to reworlding research?

Like Kafer (2021), I have learned that slowing down is, at times, necessary, revolutionary, ethical, and care-filled. But I have also learned that a political and ethical commitment to slow scholarship does not always or necessarily equate with crip time. I learned this the hard way, through my own changing bodymind in a rapidly shifting global emergency. The slow scholarship at the core of Aging Activisms originally allowed my research team to care for community members. Incredible activists, artists, and organizers, many of whom are marginalized within society, felt validated and held in ways they rarely experienced within the academy; researchers, too, were nurtured by the care shown to them by participants. The relationships that formed still reverberate in beautiful ways through the community and the reciprocity of care in this research holds intrinsic value. Still, there were significant institutional hurdles involved; slowing down to centre community care often meant more work and less care for me and my team. A commitment to crip research, to resisting timelines based on pressures for productivity and efficiency, requires more than community care; if structural issues remain intact, it can only mean greater strain on researchers (Bailey 2021).

The pandemic experience, for me and many others, was deeply disorienting, out of our control, and exposing of capitalist–colonial fissures everywhere in society, including in academia (Krebs 2022). Crip time is not the same as political–ethical imperatives to slow down, care, and resist ableism, though these are important anti-oppressive commitments. I came to this revelation not by choice, but by having crip time imposed on me. The hiatus in my work, which began in the first wave of the pandemic and, in many ways, continues, was imposed, much as changes in temporality and possibility were experienced widely, and wildly unevenly, around the world (Barbarin 2021).

I have come to appreciate in new and ever-evolving ways how crip time always entails multiple temporalities and trajectories, always imposed (and sometimes reclaimed) differently upon (or by) different people. The story I tell is full of shifting tempos, from the slow, elongated temporalities of cancer time to the drawn-out, swollen periods of grief. They include the moments of full hiatus when it was safer not to gather and when my bodymind felt too broken to push through (Samuels 2017). Sometimes, this was care time, all-encompassing and repetitive (Tsai 2022); sometimes, it was accelerated bursts of energy and work time (Kafer 2021). Our ethical–political commitment must be to resist ableism by honouring and valuing all versions of crip time, by supporting our own and others' multiple and ever-changing circumstances, bodyminds, and care needs.

My story illustrates the ways institutions, including academic institutions, are inflexible and pose barriers to care-centred practices. Even when the individuals involved are generous and supportive, the setup of the institution denies the possibility of care in structural ways. From the "denial by design" of medical leave that could not be extended even for a breast cancer diagnosis, to the research grant that cannot be paused, even when the proposed work becomes unsafe and illegal, there is a disjuncture between crip realities and institutional pressures for "productivity at all costs" (Cepeda 2021).

My immediate family survived against this cracked backdrop, through continuous, interconnected, active care, and thanks to immense systemic privilege.[8] Upon reflection, this radical care that sustained me and my family may also be the stuff of reworlding. Cripping time in a capitalist–colonial world means understanding, reclaiming, and practicing radical care as part of our work of always actively imagining and making the futures we are striving for. Many, such as Leah Lakshmi Piepzna-Samarasinha (Piepzna-Samarasinha 2022) and Hi'ilei Julia Kawehipuaakahaopulani Hobart and Tamara Kneese (Hobart and Kneese 2020), have offered brilliant visions around care and survival, and even around the liberatory potential of radical care. But what I had not connected before my pandemic experience, or at least not in an embodied way, was how radical care is both necessary to survival *and* the key to how we might make the next world, the one I want to be part of.

I am learning (like Kim and Schalk 2021; Piepzna-Samarasinha 2018a) to lean into interdependence, to value the work of caregiving in the time it takes, and (like Cepeda (2021) and Krebs (2022)) that part of my own self-care is refusing the internalized pressures of capitalism and the tentacles of the "return to." This refusal is not without costs and it is not about my own individual resilience; refusal, and even loss, can be generative too, opening new possibilities, new collective possibilities outside of ongoing oppressions. Grieving the loss of what Aging Activisms once was opened a space for me to turn inward in creative practice. This emergent, unplanned detour led to a small offering of heart-medicine and future-making for my family, my research community, and myself.

In my experience of the pandemic, crip time imposed different temporalities, realities, and trajectories, even while strengthening colonial, capitalist, ableist systems. But crip time also pushes us to reclaim radical care. This hard work is imbued with the generativity of our refusals, our grief, our creativity, our imaginations, and the wisdom we are gaining. This radical care is a reworlding practice; it orients us to the future, propelling us to imagine and make beautiful worlds.

In closing, a final thought about the beauty and urgency of slowness. My commitment to slower ways never came from thinking that the work I do is leisurely or untimely. My work is about intergenerational continuance at a time of growing inequalities, violence, and ecological collapse; it is anything but leisurely or low-priority. There is a "complexity of claiming time for ourselves to slow down, to take care, while also understanding the real urgency of our contemporary moment" (Kim and Schalk 2021, p. 327). In times of desperation and doom, Aging Activisms has been dreaming otherworlds and shifting cultural imaginaries (Chazan and Whetung 2022). Research for the next world must find other ways beyond fast-paced, high-production extraction. As Bayo Akomolafe offers, "times are urgent, so let us slow down" (Akomolafe 2020, p. 49). But I understand now that slowing down, on its own, is not enough; we must also shift to radical self- and community care. In our care-filled, artful practices, we slowly make our next world.

Funding: I gratefully acknowledge funding provided by the Canada Research Chairs program, through the Social Sciences and Humanities Research Council of Canada, grant number CRC231791.

Institutional Review Board Statement: The author's research program, Aging Activisms, has undergone institutional review by Trent University's Research Ethics Board annually from 2013 to 2023, in accordance with Canada's Tri-Council Policy for Research on Human Subjects. This article offers primarily the author's personal narrative and experience and thus falls largely outside the purview of this ethical review. The institutional review is nevertheless relevant because the article states some participants' reflections on their experiences of the research, as share during research workshops.

Informed Consent Statement: Informed consent was obtained from all participants in this study.

Data Availability Statement: Not applicable.

Acknowledgments: First and foremost, Ben, Cam and Alex Hodson have been caring for, inspiring, and sustaining me through all the moments; I would not be here without you. I would also like to express my deep thanks and gratitude to so many other family members, friends, colleagues, and to my health team. I cannot name you all, but in many different ways you (my community) are teaching me about radical care within and outside of academia: Melissa Baldwin, Ziysah von Bieberstein, Jessi Dobyns, Karine Rogers, Jenn Cole, Ashley Street, Gabrielle Chackal, Emily Root, Natalie Whiting, Urpi Pine, Kerry Bebee, Heidi Burns, Richard Brooks, Shane Patey, Tasha Lackman, Kelly McGuire, Karleen Pendleton-Jimenez, Sally Chivers, Madeline Whetung, Lisa Boucher, Dana Capell, Nael Bhanji, Nadine Changfoot, Elizabeth Russel, Janet Miron, Jean Koning, Lisa Clarke, Cheri Patrick, Dreda Blow, Velvet Lacasse, Shan Culkeen, Alison Thomas, and Kim Curtin. I am truly grateful for the unconditional love of my family; thank you for being so much part of this story: Beverly Kraft, Eric Kokish, Gayle Trupish, Elyse and Lori Chazan, Marion Little, Ted Hodson, and Luna. There are so many others who are quietly present in this article—omissions here are purely my own brain fog! Thank you to everyone who has been part of Aging Activisms from 2013 to 2023 (too many incredible people to name), and to Michi Saagiig land and territory—for all the care and teachings. I acknowledge the support of Trent University, its administration, and the CRC. I leaned heavily on Melissa and Ziysah in writing this—thank you! Any oversights in my retelling of this story are purely my own memory errors and I take full responsibility.

Conflicts of Interest: The author declares no conflict of interest.

Notes

[1] The term bodymind "emphasize[s] that although 'body' and 'mind' usually occupy separate conceptual and linguistic territories, they are deeply intertwined" (Price 2011, p. 240, in Krebs 2022). Like Cepeda (2021), I understand this as resistance to the ableism of neoliberal university demands for a productive mind detached from bodily needs.

[2] Many disability scholars describe crip time as nonlinear slowing down of abled modes or shifting of the tempo of engagement to centre "rest, care, and honouring our bodyminds' needs" (Krebs 2022, p. 122; Changfoot et al. 2018). It is a way of being that "embraces the anti-normative chronotropic rhythms of disabled bodyminds" while resisting "capitalist rhythms that debilitate people through the demands of productivity" (Krebs 2022, p. 120). In its multiple, messy, broken, and wayward paces, crip time both encompasses transgressive, resistant, and liberatory possibilities, and manifests an urgent and worldmaking tempo of survival (Kafer 2021; Samuels 2017). Crip time and radical care are interconnected. Many scholars articulate radical politics of caring—self-care, care for each other, and care for the collective—rewriting care out of capitalist dismissal, exploitation, and co-optation, and into an otherwise (Hobart and Kneese 2020; Kim and Schalk 2021). Relational, interdependent care is what we owe to each other and ourselves, and it unsettles ableist individualism (Piepzna-Samarasinha 2022). As both a critical survival strategy and collective making, radical care can remake worlds beyond the strictures of this one.

[3] A CRC is a research-intensive professor position funded by the Canadian government (mine through the Social Sciences and Humanities Research Council of Canada, SSHRC). I have been funded for 10 years as an emerging scholar (2013–2023); I started as Assistant Professor in 2013 and was promoted to Associate and awarded tenure in mid-2018, 1.5 years before the pandemic was declared.

[4] See: www.agingactivisms.org and https://digitalcollections.trentu.ca/collections/stories-resistance-resurgence-and-resilience-nogojiwanong-peterborough (Accessed on: 12 December 2022).

[5] See: www.agingactivisms.org/creativity-connection-covid (Accessed on: 12 December 2022).

[6] Offered through StoryCenter in Berkley, USA; see: https://www.storycenter.org/ (Accessed on: 12 December 2022).

[7] See: www.agingactivisms.org/dream-beautiful-futures/ (Accessed on: 12 December 2022).

[8] Many others did not survive. Governmental disregard for the immunocompromised and for the safety of precariously employed essential workers in Ontario led to escalating rates of death and severe illness, which are highest among already-disabled people. This has included influential disabled thinkers who have been a part of shaping the crip wisdom I am learning from, such as Stacey Park Milbern, who passed in the early months of the pandemic.

References

Ahmed, Sara. 2017. *Living a Feminist Life*. Durham: Duke University Press.

Akomolafe, Bayo. 2020. I, Coronavirus. Mother, Monster, Activist. Self-Published. Available online: www.scribd.com/document/466902311/I-Coronavirus-Mother-Monster-Activist-by-Bayo-Akomolafe (accessed on 12 August 2022).

Bailey, Moya. 2021. The ethics of pace. *The South Atlantic Quarterly* 120: 285–99. [CrossRef]

Barbarin, Imani. 2021. Death by a Thousand Words: COVID-19 and the Pandemic of Ableist Media. Refinery29. Available online: www.refinery29.com/en-us/2021/08/10645352/covid-19-and-the-pandemic-of-ableist-media (accessed on 5 September 2022).

Carter, Jill, Karyn Recollet, and Dylan Robinson. 2018. Interventions into the maw of old world hunger: Frog monsters, kinstellatory maps, and radical relationalities in a project of reworlding. In *Canadian Performance Histories and Historiographies*. Edited by Heather David-Fisch. Toronto: Playwrights Canada Press, pp. 205–31.

Cepeda, María Elena. 2021. Thrice unseen, forever on borrowed time: Latia feminist reflections on mental disability and the neoliberal academy. *The South Atlantic Quarterly* 120: 301–20. [CrossRef]

Changfoot, Nadine, Carla Rice, Sally Chivers, Alice Olsen WIlliams, Angela Connors, Awnna Barrett, Mary Gordon, and Gisele Lalonde. 2022. Revisioning aging: Indigenous, crip and queer renderings. *Journal of Aging Studies* 63: 100930. [CrossRef] [PubMed]

Changfoot, Nadine, Mary Anne Ansley, and Andrea Dodsworth. 2018. Strengthening our activisms by creating intersectional spaces for the personal, the professional, disability, and aging. In *Unsettling Activisms: Critical Interventions on Aging, Gender, and Social Change*. Edited by May Chazan, Melissa Baldwin and Patricia Evans. Toronto: Canadian Scholars' Press.

Chazan, May. 2020. Ode to Odenabe: Intergenerational storytelling and the art of making. *Anthropology & Aging* 41: 95–106.

Chazan, May, and Madeline Whetung. 2022. 'Carving a future out of the past and the present': Rethinking aging futures. *Journal of Aging Studies* 63: 100937. [CrossRef] [PubMed]

Cole, Jenn. 2019. Relinquishing expertise: Notes on feminist Indigenous performance methodology. *Canadian Theatre Review* 178: 68–71. [CrossRef]

FitzGibbon, Ali. 2021. Just because you can doesn't mean you should. In *Qualitative and Digital Research in Times of Crisis: Methods, Reflexivity, and Ethics*. Edited by Helen Kara and Su-Ming Khoo. Bristol: Policy Press.

Hobart, Hi'ilei Julia Kawehipuaakahaopulani, and Tamara Kneese. 2020. Radical care: Survival strategies for uncertain times. *Social Text* 38: 1–16. [CrossRef]

Kafer, Alison. 2021. After crip, crip afters. *The South Atlantic Quarterly* 120: 415–34. [CrossRef]

Kim, Jina B., and Sami Schalk. 2021. Reclaiming the radical politics of self-care: A crip-of-colour critique. *The South Atlantic Quarterly* 120: 325–42. [CrossRef]

Krebs, Emily. 2022. A sour taste of sick chronicity: Pandemic time and the violence of 'returning to normal'. *Communication and Critical/Cultural Studies* 19: 119–26. [CrossRef]

Lin, Lana. 2016. The queer art of survival. *WSQ* 44: 341–46. [CrossRef]

Lorde, Audre. 1980. *The Cancer Journals*. San Francisco: Spinsters | Aunt Lute.

Lorde, Audre. 2017. *A Burst of Light: And Other Essays*. Mineola: Ixia Press. First published 1988.

Medak-Saltzman, Danika, Deepti Misri, and Beverly Weber. 2022. Decolonizing time, knowledge, and disability on the tenure clock. *Feminist Formations* 34: 1–24. [CrossRef]

Meyerhoff, Eli, and Elsa Noterman. 2019. Revolutionary scholarship by any speed necessary: Slow or fast but for the end of this world. *ACME* 18: 217–45.

Miner, Dylan A. T. 2019. Mawadisidiwag miinawaa wiidanokiindiwag // They visit and work together. In *Makers, Crafters, Educators: Working for Cultural Change*. Edited by Elizabeth Garber, Lisa Hochtritt and Manisha Sharma. New York: Routledge.

Mitchell-Eaton, Emily. 2020. Postpartum geographies: Intersections of academic labor and care work. *Environment and Planning* 39: 1755–72. [CrossRef]

Piepzna-Samarasinha, Leah Lakshmi. 2018a. *Care Work: Dreaming Disability Justice*. Vancouver: Arsenal Pulp Press.

Piepzna-Samarasinha, Leah Lakshmi. 2018b. To Survive the Trumpocalypse, We Need Wild Disability Justice Dreams. *Truthout*. Available online: https://truthout.org/articles/to-survive-the-trumpocalypse-we-need-wild-disability-justice-dreams/ (accessed on 6 May 2022).

Piepzna-Samarasinha, Leah Lakshmi. 2022. *The Future Is Disabled: Prophecies, Love Notes and Mourning Songs*. Vancouver: Arsenal Pulp Press.

Price, Margaret. 2011. *Mad at School: Rhetorics of Mental Disability and Academic Life*. Ann Arbor: University of Michigan Press.

Samuels, Ellen. 2017. Six ways of looking at crip time. *Disability Studies Quarterly* 37. [CrossRef]

Stevens, Sarah E. 2018. Care time. *Disability Studies Quarterly* 38. [CrossRef]

Tsai, Mei-Yu. 2022. Aging, crip time, and dependency care in Joyce Farmer's Special Exits. *Graphic Medicine Review* 2: 1–14.

Disclaimer/Publisher's Note: The statements, opinions and data contained in all publications are solely those of the individual author(s) and contributor(s) and not of MDPI and/or the editor(s). MDPI and/or the editor(s) disclaim responsibility for any injury to people or property resulting from any ideas, methods, instructions or products referred to in the content.

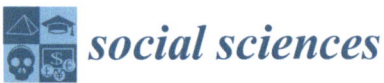

Article

Epistemological Weaving: Writing and Sense Making in Qualitative Research with Gloria Anzaldúa

Luis R. Alvarez-Hernandez [1,*] and Maureen Flint [2]

1. Department of Clinical Practice, School of Social Work, Boston University, Boston, MA 02215, USA
2. Department of Lifelong Education, Administration, and Policy, Mary Frances Early College of Education, University of Georgia, Athens, GA 30602, USA
* Correspondence: lrah@bu.edu

Abstract: How is writing a part of creatively understanding ourselves, research questions, data, and theory? Writing is a critical form of connecting concepts, exploring data, and weaving knowledge in qualitative research. In other words, writing is integral to theorizing. However, writing is not an individualistic process. Writing is a relational and creative epistemological weaving of thoughts and embodiments constructed by researchers and their interactions with mentors and instructors, participants, and theoretical proponents. In this paper we discuss this creative process by paying attention to each co-constructor of knowledge and the ways in which the weaving of knowledge was constructed through our shared and different journeys as doctoral student and instructor. Grounded in Gloria Anzaldúa's borderland and *nepantla* work, we will present our positionalities, interactions, and suggestions for fellow qualitative writers struggling to make sense of their writing and theorizing. Our hope is that doctoral students and veteran academics alike can benefit from this exploration.

Keywords: epistemology; theory; Chicana feminism; critical feminism; Latinas; pedagogy; teaching qualitative methods; creative writing

---

Citation: Alvarez-Hernandez, Luis R., and Maureen Flint. 2023. Epistemological Weaving: Writing and Sense Making in Qualitative Research with Gloria Anzaldúa. *Social Sciences* 12: 408. https://doi.org/10.3390/socsci12070408

Academic Editors: Nadine Changfoot, Eliza Chandler and Carla Rice

Received: 13 December 2022
Revised: 7 July 2023
Accepted: 13 July 2023
Published: 16 July 2023

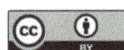

Copyright: © 2023 by the authors. Licensee MDPI, Basel, Switzerland. This article is an open access article distributed under the terms and conditions of the Creative Commons Attribution (CC BY) license (https:// creativecommons.org/licenses/by/ 4.0/).

1. Introduction

Writing is like pulling miles of entrails through your mouth. Why the resistance? Because you're scared that you won't do it justice. Because it'll take time, and there's no guarantee that you'll be able to pull it off. Because it is stressful and exhausting. [...] Writing also involves envisioning and conceptualizing the work and dreaming the story into a virtual reality. The different stages in embodying the story are not clearly demarcated, sequential, or linear; they overlap, shift back and forth, take place simultaneously. (Anzaldúa 2015, p. 102)

Writing is an often-overlooked aspect of the doctoral journey, an act that does not often cross the mind of students as they apply for and enter doctoral programs. Writing is understood and turned to as just the output, the necessary vehicle for communicating the interesting, provocative, and world-changing research that is the 'actual point' of doctoral work. This is reinforced by the fact that often what we see in terms of finished writing products is only a small part of the larger writing process (Cannon and Cross 2020). Yet, many doctoral students and their mentors focus only on the outcome. This is the case even as writing is a critical part of the doctoral journey. Throughout that journey, as part of the constant cycle of thinking and scholarly work, doctoral students receive feedback, advice, and notes on their writing. Some of this feedback is explicit: notes in the margins and comments via tracked changes, suggestions from peers, faculty, or advisors. Other writing feedback is more subtle: reading a scholarly work that plays with form or says something in a poetic way and realizing, "oh, I can do that." Reading a theorist and being inspired by an idea; taking a prompt from an assignment and following it down a rabbit hole; creating a completely unexpected and yet beautiful piece of writing and thinking—these are all additional ways a writer works with feedback. Through writing, researchers become engaged with discussions, debates, and scholarly circles in their discipline. Writing—far from a peripheral task—is an integral part of being and becoming an academic (Sword 2017). Writing is a critical form of connecting concepts, understanding data, and weaving knowledge (Richardson and St. Pierre 2005). Writing is a part of the creative process of inquiry, how we come to know ourselves in the world (Colyar 2009). This process is cyclical, iterative, and far from linear. The output does not reflect the many steps and materials used. We see a beautiful tapestry, but we do not see the selection of the thread, the hands of the weaver, the redrafting of patterns, the conversations had over the weaving process, let alone the grass grazed on by the sheep that grew the wool that was sheared, then carded and spun for yarn. Writing, like a tapestry, is a multilayered and creative process that brings together diverse inspirations, sources, and influences.

Others in qualitative inquiry have explored the possibilities of writing and inquiry. Richardson and St. Pierre's (2005) writing as inquiry has been echoed by Colyar (2009). Others have explored the creative potential of writing (Helin 2019; Ulmer 2018; Ulmer et al. 2017) and writing nonlinearly with theoretical concepts (Bright 2017; Hein 2019; St. Pierre 1997; Zapata et al. 2018), along with those who have written on writing as an embodied practice (Evans-Winters 2019; Foster 2010; The Latina Feminist Group 2001). There is a significant stream of research on collaborative writing practices (Alexander and Wyatt 2018; Gale and Jonathan 2017; Mazzei and Jackson 2013; McKnight et al. 2017). Still others have explored writing and the doctoral journey from the experiences of doctoral students (Cisneros 2018; Moore 2017) and from the collaborative perspective of advisor and student navigating the doctoral journey (Mazzei and Smithers 2020; Tierney and Hallett 2010). This scholarship on writing in the field of qualitative inquiry emphasizes the creative and generative potential of writing for thinking theoretically and conceptually.

Writing and theorization often happen collectively. We, the authors, co-construct knowledge in this manuscript similar to how many Latina and Chicana feminists have written papers and books. The Latina Feminist Group (2001), for example, theorized and made meaning of their lives, struggles, and joys by meeting regularly and sharing their "*papelitos guardados*" (writings tucked away) with their thoughts. These notes and conversations led them to feel seen and empowered by the other women in the group—their book *Telling to Live: Latina Feminist Testimonios* is an outcome of these co-constructions. Anzaldúa also wrote in community, co-constructing knowledge with other Chicana feminists like Moraga (Moraga and Anzaldúa 2021). Even after Anzaldúa's death, Keating (Anzaldúa 2015) and Cantú and Hurtado (Anzaldúa 2012) continued to highlight and build on Anzaldúa's books; in each new edition of her texts, they offer new readings, new thinkings with one another and with Anzaldúa. This practice of thinking and writing collectively, co-constructing knowledge, is one that is oriented toward relationality, a shift from the individual to the collective, disrupting traditional conceptions of knowledge production (Alvarez-Hernandez and Bermudez forthcoming).

Building from this scholarship on writing practices, this paper follows the writings of a doctoral student (Luis) as he navigates a series of courses in qualitative inquiry facilitated by an instructor (Maureen). Our epistemological weaving began when Luis, as a doctoral student, was in the process of writing an assignment for a qualitative course taught by Maureen. Luis began to think about the process of creating/finding/producing/co-constructing knowledge. Over the course of several semesters, he began to experiment and play with his style of writing through different assignments, continuing to reconceptualize the relationship(s) between writing, theory, and research. Through these processes, Luis realized that his writing and theorizing were not *only his*. Writing had become an epistemological weaving of thoughts and embodiments constructed by himself, his qualitative instructor Maureen, his participants, and his theoretical proponent Gloria Anzaldúa.

In this manuscript, we discuss this weaving process between learning qualitative inquiry and creative writing through paying attention to each co-constructor of knowledge and the ways in which the weaving of knowledge was constructed. We zigzag between

Luis's reflections and excerpts from assignments, Maureen's feedback and notes on those assignments, our (shared and individual) narratives of the courses, and assignment provocations. As we weave together our reflections and thoughts, we also note that we do not make causal claims—that something Maureen did produced something Luis thought, or something Luis asked produced something Maureen taught. Instead, we offer our entwined writing around doing~teaching~thinking~becoming to explore the creative process of learning and thinking qualitatively and methodologically. As Luis noted in a writing meeting composing this paper, this is a paper he would have liked to have read on his own doctoral journey—a paper that peels back the layers of learning qualitative inquiry to show the reader what the process might look like. Throughout, we center the process and act of writing as one essential to learning and teaching qualitatively, and one that is inherently creative. We explore how writing, and writing feedback, is entangled with the process of grappling with questions of ethics and responsibility in qualitative research. We present a brief introduction to Anzaldúa's work, and our positionalities, interactions, and suggestions for fellow qualitative writers struggling to make sense of their writing. As we present these sections, we weave in some of Anzaldúa's quotes where she ponders on the process of writing as storytelling and embodiment, and as a form of transforming and creating our realities. We add these quotes as a way to frame our epistemological processes. We invite the readers to also ponder on the meaning these quotes may have for their own theorizing and writing processes. Our hope is that doctoral students and veteran academics alike can benefit from this exploration.

2. Gloria Anzaldúa's Theorizations

Anzaldúa, a Chicana–lesbian–feminist–writer–theorist–philosopher, discussed the experiences with positionality and identity of Chicanas through her development of *frontera* or borderlands theory and, later, through the concept of *nepantla*. For Anzaldúa (2012), being and becoming was a matter of physical and spiritual embodiment. According to Keating (2015), "[...] for Anzaldúa, epistemology and ontology (knowing and being) are intimately interrelated—two halves of one complex, multidimensional process employed in the service of progressive social change" (p. xxx). Therefore, Anzaldúa saw knowing and being as a process in which the writer feels the tensions between the colonial ways of knowledge development while weaving their multiple identities and experiences into this ever-changing knowledge.

After borderlands theory, Anzaldúa engaged in exploring her identities and experiences from a spiritual standpoint. In this theorization, Anzaldúa (2015) speaks about her body as a source of data and epistemology. She wrote, "My feminism is grounded not on incorporeal abstraction but on corporal realities. The material body is center, and central. The body is the ground of thought. The body is a text" (Anzaldúa 2015, p. 5). For Anzaldúa, the body and the spirit are interconnected.

The spiritual Aztec terms *Coyolxauhqui*, *nepantla*, and *nepantleras* are introduced in Anzaldúa's writing. Through *Coyolxauhqui*, we construct and deconstruct knowledge and experiences (Anzaldúa 2015). In *nepantla*, we inhabit in-between spaces (Anzaldúa 2015). The *nepantleras* are the women who choose to inhabit *nepantla* (Anzaldúa 2015). According to Anzaldúa (2015), the *nepantleras* are "threshold people, those who move within and among multiple worlds and use their movement in the service of transformation" (p. xxxv). It is in these liminal spaces that change and action occur.

3. Our Positionalities

We begin by introducing ourselves and our positionalities in the qualitative classroom, an academic world of thinking and doing. Then, we weave through assignments and reflections. These conversations are constructed as three epistemological assignments and are woven with the feedback from the qualitative instructor for each exercise. For the purposes of this paper, we amalgamate provocations from different assignments facilitated by Maureen in her classes and writing by Luis in response to these assignments. We created these amalgamations to tell the story of our becomings together as student and instructor, rather than offer a linear narrative of participation in a class. We are guided by a narrative ethic, which "is governed by the intentions I have towards my audience and towards those whose lives are entangled in the story" (Yardley 2008, p. 23). In the writing of this paper, as we engaged with past assignments, writing, and memories from our shared time in the classroom, we particularly paid attention to moments of co-construction between student–instructor–research–Anzaldúa. Specifically, we were interested in the relationships, questions, and connections between us as "we imagine the space in-between as a relational space where stories to live by are composed. The 'in-between' spaces, [are] spaces where we ask[ed] one another 'who' and not 'what' we are" (Caine and Steeves 2009, p. 8). Lingering in these in-between spaces, we conclude by providing suggestions that emerged from our work together, provocations for doctoral students and instructors thinking, writing, and researching qualitatively that could be applicable to a variety of educators and researchers.

3.1. The Doctoral Student

An image is a bridge between evoked emotion and conscious knowledge; words are the cables that hold up the bridge. Images are more direct, more immediate than words, and closer to the unconscious. Picture language precedes thinking in words; the metaphorical mind precedes analytical consciousness. (Anzaldúa 2012, p. 91)

I walk into the classroom—a Brown–Queer–doctoral student ready to learn. I bring in with me a multiplicity of experiences as a Spanish-speaker, a clinical social worker, an eager learner, an advocate for recognizing the importance of identity and resistance, and the first person in my family to become a doctoral student. I walk into the classroom ready to put into practice what I know, what I think I know. We are learning how to design qualitative research in this course. I am asked to explain the connection between theory and my interview data. I had interviewed Latina community health workers, *promotoras de salud*, who were part of a community-based participatory project (CBPR). I was curious to know what meanings these Latina immigrants made about their leadership roles in their communities in the southeastern U.S. See (Orpinas et al. 2020, 2021) for more about the work of these *promotoras de salud* and their project.

3.2. The Qualitative Instructor

The ability of story (prose and poetry) to transform the storyteller and the listener into something or someone is shamanistic. The writer, as shape-changer, is a *nahual*, a shaman. (Anzaldúa 2012, p. 88, *emphasis in original*)

I walk into the classroom. A white cisgender woman. I am nervous with this new group of students, hoping that together we can do justice to their projects and the questions they want to ask, the answers they seek. As we move through discussing the readings for the semester, the syllabus during that first class, I am aware of my whiteness and my gender. How my identities mirror the history of qualitative research, one that as Denzin (2017) noted, has a "complicity with colonialism and the global politics of White, patriarchal capitalism" (p. 9). I want to teach research and research design in a way that pushes back against the "small set of beliefs" of objectivism, neutrality, extraction, and proceduralism that mark the history and present of qualitative inquiry (Denzin 2017, p. 9; see also Bhattacharya 2021; Kuntz 2015). As an instructor of qualitative inquiry, my role is to facilitate students' individual development of their study, while also challenging and complicating simplistic ideas of what constitutes research. As they each plan out a ministudy, a series of encounters with places and people and topics, we think together about questions of ethics and power and knowledge and agency and representation. Teaching, like writing, is about dreaming potential into reality. Like writing, teaching often begins with an idea, a spark, and then leads you somewhere unexpected. Sometimes you do not know where teaching will take you. I take a deep breath and introduce the first assignment for the course.

4. Assignment #1: Emerging Research Interests and Subjectivities Statement

At the beginning of the semester, Maureen encouraged students to conceptualize their research proposal by writing a statement of the problem, purpose of the study, theoretical underpinnings, and subjectivities . Luis's study sought to gain insight into the leadership experiences of the Mexican women he worked with in the CBPR project who were *promotoras de salud*. More specifically, Luis's study sought to describe the process that *promotoras* experienced developing their roles as leaders, list examples of their leadership, and understand the meaning that they make of their leadership roles and experiences. The research questions that guided Luis's work were:

1. What are *promotoras'* perceptions of their role as leaders?
    a. What meanings do *promotoras* attribute to their roles as leaders?
2. How do the *promotoras* of a CBPR project enact their leadership?
    a. How do *promotoras* develop their role as leaders?

4.1. The Doctoral Student: Reflections on First Assignment

As I concluded my first exercise, I was struck that after reviewing the leadership literature among Latinas, most of it was based on the experiences of executives and academics, not on community health workers or Latinas engaged in other community-based roles. I found myself in need of theories that went beyond a production-based understanding of leadership. As Latinas leading their communities and navigating their multiple identities, I thought of understanding their experiences through the theoretical lenses of Gloria Anzaldúa. Anzaldúa's work seemed to be able to describe the experiences of the *promotoras* from the standpoint of their identities, the context of their experiences, and their process of *becoming* leaders as Latinas.

4.2. The Qualitative Instructor: Feedback on First Assignment

Nice job on this emerging research statement, Luis. Some things to think about as you go forward: First, Chicana feminism is more than just explaining dynamics of oppression—what does this mean for the way that you understand power, agency, representation, voice, etc., in your work? I also wonder what member checking might look like following your epistemological framework, why does this matter? Does your bias matter in the context of the theories you are bringing to the table (or might these relationships strengthen your research?) Keep thinking about how you might communicate what you describe as the "badassness" of the *promotoras* (and your tension with insider/outsiderness) in your writing/representation.

Finally, I would love to see you draw more lines between your identities and the identities of the *promotoras*. What do the similarities and differences do to the research process? What tensions do you notice?

4.3. The Doctoral Student: Weaving Theory and Writing

> "We're going to have to do something about your tongue," I hear the anger rising in his voice. My tongue keeps pushing out the wads of cotton, pushing back the drills, the long thin needles. "I've never seen anything as strong or as stubborn," he says. And I think, how do we tame a wild tongue, train it to be quiet, how do you bridle and saddle it? How do you make it lie down? (Anzaldúa 2012, p. 75)

What does Chicana feminism mean for the way I understand power, agency, representation, and voice in my work? How can I weave myself, the theory, the data, and my participants? I learned about Anzaldúa during my doctoral studies. I was fascinated by the fact that I had learned about theory by White European men before I was given the opportunity to meet Anzaldúa.

Scholars of color are not always included in research communities, including qualitative research spaces (Evans-Winters and Esposito 2018). Like other Latinx doctoral students (Sánchez and Hernández 2022), reading Anzaldúa's work helped me feel adequate, closer to my culture, to the philosophers and theorists that spoke my language and embodied Brownness. I was able to see beyond my island of Puerto Rico, where I lived until the age of 21 and where I first encountered college courses. I was becoming part of Latin American thought, walking the roads forged by Anzaldúa—a lesbian, just like I am gay. Becoming a gay–Latinx–researcher is now possible since Anzaldúa showed me how to become one, how to transform myself and my writing while in-between spaces. That undoubtedly led me to becoming a Chicana feminist. Embodying being a man and a social worker, I could label my thoughts on issues of sex, race, ethnicity, class, gender, sexuality, and coloniality. I could think from the border, I could write from my center. Like performers on a stage, my writing and becoming is political—it pushes against boundaries of identities and embodiment (Muñoz 1999). It was with these thoughts in mind that I turned to the next assignment for the course.

5. Assignment #2: Interview Portfolio

Maureen asked students to conduct three interviews as an introduction to qualitative interviewing, data generation, and preliminary data analysis. These interviews built from their emerging research statement and ethnographic fieldwork, and students were encouraged to explore nontraditional methods.

5.1. The Doctoral Student: Reflections on the Interview

When I write it feels like I'm carving bone. It feels like I'm creating my own face, my own heart—a Nahuatl concept. My soul makes itself through the creative act. It is constantly remaking and giving birth to itself through my body. It is this learning to live *la Coatlicue* that transforms living in the Borderlands from a nightmare into a numinous experience. It is always a path/state to something else. (Anzaldúa 2012, p. 95) (*emphasis in original*)

The three Spanish-speaking *promotoras de salud* who participated in my study were Mexican immigrants, married, and mothers. Their ages ranged between 35 and 44 years, with most living in their communities for over a decade. All of them had been working for one year with the project. I gathered all three interviews in Spanish, and each interview lasted between 33 min and one hour. The interviews were conducted in a coffee shop, a participant's home, and while walking in a local park. This study was approved by the University of Georgia Institutional Review Board. The text that follows was part of my reflection after conducting all three of the interviews.

When writing the interview questions, I thought that the interviewees would struggle with answering the last question: "What does the future look like for you as a leader?" However, I was particularly surprised at how all three interviewees gave me a direct answer to this question. They all said that they see themselves continuing to do their work in the future. Their answers make me think of the interviewees' commitment to their roles as leaders and how not doing what they have been doing is not an option for them.

My interview with Flor, although technically a traditional interview, felt more ethnographic to me since I met her in her house, had breakfast with her and her family, and her husband was in the same room the interview was conducted. I noted on the transcript when her husband made comments during the interview. Outside of the interview recording, the interviewee and her husband talked to me about their breakfast routine when they first moved in together, among other things. These interactions inform how I understand the data in the interview, although they are not audio-recorded. As a social worker who has made many home visits, these dynamics seem common in my work. However, as a researcher, I should note more this interaction on my memos so as to not lose this nonrecorded data.

5.2. The Qualitative Instructor: Response to Interview

Great job on these interviews, Luis! I am listening to the audio of your first interview, and I am struck first by how fast she is talking and second, these long blocks of text with very little input from you. You can hear how excited she is to talk about this topic in her affect (there is one moment where she is talking so fast and then takes a big breath in—as though she was racing to the end of her sentence).

Looking over your transcription, I am stuck by the few pauses throughout here—later, you note a participant's husband speaking—so interesting! Was he there the whole time? I see where you note him above...and a few spaces below.... How did that affect the interview?

Nice job on your memos—a few things to think about going forward: You place a lot of emphasis on relationship building. How are your theories guiding you? Placing this type of relationship building over the extraction of data (e.g., Kuntz 2015) matters for the research you are doing. How do you decide what becomes data—is something only data when it is captured by the transcript? Think about reflexivity—who are you in relation to your participants? How does your identity entangle in this, how does the ways that you respond as an interviewer produce the interview? How does your positionality and identity come into play?

5.3. The Doctoral Student: Reflection on Feedback

My instructor asks me to understand the relationship between my participants and the theoretical underpinnings of Anzaldúa. To seemingly weave theoretical concepts with quotes from my participants. "This is easy," I say to myself. But then it isn't. I kept thinking about these connections and allowed myself to play with their weaving in the next assignment.

6. Assignment #3: Culminating Paper

Maureen asked students to more fully consider a qualitative study that could be used in their graduate work (i.e., a publishable article, a pilot study for their dissertation, etc.). This assignment again built from each of the previous assignments and attended to feedback provided by peers and the instructor throughout the semester to strengthen their research design. In this paper, students had the opportunity to flesh out more fully an analytic approach explored through the semester, and were welcome to approach this in a variety of manners, including experimenting with creative responses and forms.

6.1. The Doctoral Student: Approaching the Culminating Assignment

Like in the quote from Anzaldúa at the beginning of this manuscript, I was stuck, afraid of misconnecting, misunderstanding, misweaving. Academic writing is daunting and lonesome, so I decided to take on creative writing to have a conversation with theory and my data for this final paper. I have read Anzaldúa's work, and she makes no excuses for decolonizing academic writing by combining first-person accounts, poems, drawings, incomplete sentences. It is almost as if she is giving me permission to do the same. Perhaps my engagement in creative writing and poetical thinking allowed me to make sense of my theory and my data. I start to get unstuck, make some connections, and weave in theory and data through the use of creative writing and poetic exercises. In what follows, I offer two examples of these exercises.

Exercise One—A Conversation with Anzaldúa

This piece reflects how I, the doctoral student, put together the final research proposal when designing my qualitative study. During the process of writing my final proposal, I tried to connect theory, research questions, my subjectivity, and research design. I was feeling intimidated by needing to understand Anzaldúa's (2015) borderland theory. As a clinical social worker and a bilingual person, I thought, "What if I could speak with Anzaldúa and ask her questions? What would she tell me?" Following is what resulted from this creative writing inquiry. I did not edit this piece for the purpose of this paper—it may contain spelling and grammatical errors—to provide a raw example of the exercise.

The doctoral student and Anzaldúa:	Anzaldúa and I met on one of those days in which the wind comes by so passionately, that it takes you down to the US/México *frontera*, the border. Anzaldúa was sitting on top of the border, dangling her feet on the México side. I sat down next to her after I managed to fix my hair—it was a tumultuous landing. "Are you jumping to the other side?," I asked. Anzaldúa smiled, "I am always *en el otro lado*, on the other side," she replied. "I understand," I lied while trying to figure out what she was staring at. "Doña Anzaldúa, what are you looking at?"—I finally asked. She looked at me for the first time—"please don't call me doña, it makes me feel *vieja*, old." I felt embarrassed. "I am looking at the landscape. How the earth beneath us can be divided just on the surface, never deep enough," she said. I understood. She was really talking about herself—how she was *Mexicana, Chicana, Americana, Mestiza*, and *Latinoamericana* all at once, with no apparent divisions. "Yes, I am all and more. I am what I perceive myself to be, and what others perceive of me, my womanhood, my Brownhood, my lesbianhood," she said as if she had heard my thoughts. I ventured to ask her a question, "Would you consider yourself to be a leader?" She changed position, no longer dangling her feet but now sitting with her legs crossed, facing me. She was staring at me. I felt uncomfortable and intimidated; almost underserving of her attention. "What is a *líder*, a leader, to you?"—she said. I replied almost stuttering "A person who can stand in front of a group and command them." Anzaldúa started to challenge me, "Where did you hear that? Who are those leaders?" I knew I was in trouble and didn't dare to answer. She continued, "How we see leadership and leaders tend to be *desde el punto de vista colonizador y patriarcal*, from the colonizing and patriarchal point of view. Leadership is not something that only white men do. That politicians do. That Captain America does. A leader eats rice and beans, raises children, pays bills. Often, a leader is a woman with limitations with the language, who faces oppression, who fights back." I had to take a moment to process what she had just said. "So how can I find those leaders?"—I asked. Anzaldúa smiled and said, "Here is *mi consejo*, my advice to you. Listen carefully to the stories of others, to their *testimonios*. But also listen carefully to yourself when you hear these *testimonios*. *Testimonios* are co-constructed, and your insight will shape how others hear those *testimonios*." Oh, I had so many questions! And right when I was about to ask them, Anzaldúa was gone. She became the earth beneath me, the border where I was sitting, the wind that brought me to this place. I shifted the way in which I was sitting, and dangled my feet on the México side, staring at the landscape far away.

6.2. The Doctoral Student: Re-Worlding with Anzaldúa

Creative writing and poetical thinking have been linked to the process of qualitative research. Schulz (2006), for example, explored the role of creative writing from a hermeneutic phenomenology perspective. For Schulz, the process of writing involves creating and being. In this process, the writer is actively sense making, assigning meaning, thinking and feeling the experience of writing. Freeman (2016) also explored the process of poetical thinking as an experience of feeling and becoming. Freeman (2016) stated regarding poetical thinking that, "It is *felt* experience; the experience of *being* in the whirlpool of sensuous flow that we *are* as experiencing beings. This is a move away from an epistemological and representational form of knowing to an ontological one" (p. 72, emphasis in original). Likewise, Anzaldúa (2012) conceptualized being, becoming, and liberation as epistemological and ontological processes. Thinking with Anzaldúa provides me permission to get out of traditional writing practices and sedimented ways of knowing; she urges me to lean into our dreams, our memories, experiment with poetry and language and form. With Anzaldúa, writing is vulnerable, messy. Writing is felt, it is part of being and becoming with the world. This experience of the writing process and the data allowed me to engage in a process of becoming, not without moments of exasperation.

As I was attempting to make connections between my data and the theory, I often felt frustrated and defeated. How could I establish a connection between my participants and Anzaldúa? How could I, a non-Chicano cisgender man, truly understand Anzaldúa's words? How could I connect with the experiences of the *promotoras de salud*? Even more frightening, how could I make Anzaldúa and the *promotoras de salud* speak to each other through my academic writing? I would read Anzaldúa's work and feel inadequate—almost undeserving of understanding her words. We spoke the same languages, yet the words were becoming new and unexplored realities as I read them.

Exercise Two—Light in the Dark/Luz en lo Oscuro

A year later, when I returned to the data, I utilized Anzaldúa's (2015) book *Light in the Dark/Luz en lo Oscuro: Rewriting Identity, Spirituality, Reality* to engage in poetical thinking. I decided to overlap Anzaldúa's concept of the *nepantleras* with segments from my three interviews with the *promotoras*. After becoming familiar with my data and reading Anzaldúa's book, I thought of the connections between the work of the *promotoras* and the ways in which Anzaldúa described the *nepantleras*.

I first pulled segments from each interview in which the participants answered the questions: (1) How do you define leadership?, and (2) What is a leader to you? Then, I pulled the last sentences of the paragraphs from Anzaldúa's section "Las Nepantleras: Alternative Sense of Self," subsections "Lugares nepantleras—perspectives from the cracks" (pp. 81–83) and "The web of connection" (pp. 83–84). I kept the order of the sentences from Anzaldúa (in bold) and inserted the segments from the *promotoras* as if they were responding to Anzaldúa (in italics). I deleted symbols from the transcript, interruption of utterances, and things like "ums," etc. I decided to leave the segments from the interviews in Spanish in honor of Anzaldúa's way of writing. Underneath each quote is the English translation in brackets. Below is the result of this exercise:

Anzaldúa and the *promotoras de salud*:

We are forced (or we choose) to live in spaces/categories that defy gender, race, class, sexual, geographic, and spiritual locations.
Como fijar metas, por ejemplo en la familia o en las labores de la casa, por ejemplo. Como tener horarios, bueno como yo por ejemplo me dedico a la familia, verdad, a mis hijos, mi trabajo es relacionado en la casa.
[*Like setting goals, for example in the family or in house chores, for example. Like having a schedule, well like me for example I dedicate myself to family, right, to my children, my work is related to the house.*]

Nepantleras are not constrained by one culture or world but experience multiple realities.
La comunidad te hace líder.
[*The community makes you a leader.*]

Nepantleras use competing systems of knowledge and rewrite their identities.
Pero ahora, después de reconocer yo misma lo que hago, siento que tengo ese liderazgo conmigo.
[*But now, after recognizing myself what I do, I feel that I have that leadership with me.*]

Las nepantleras nurture psychological, social, and spiritual metamorphosis.
Y siento que es bueno porque haces sentir bien a la gente, la gente confía en ti.
[*And I feel it is good because you make people feel good, people trust you.*]
Pues para mí personalmente pues, líder hacia mí misma porque para hacer mejor las cosas.
[*Well, for me personally, well, leader towards myself because to do things better.*]

Las nepantleras are spiritual activists engaged in the struggle for social, economic, and political justice, while working on spiritual transformations of selfhoods.
Como saber guiar, como aprender para saber guiar, saber entender y analizar los puntos de cada persona sin juzgar ni- ¿judging es juzgar, no, es lo mismo?
[*Like knowing how to guide, like learning to know how to guide, knowing how to understand and analyze the points of view of each person without judging.*]

(Identities such as those of neo-Nazis and other hate groups with unethical behavior are not included).
Un líder yo supongo que es una persona que debe de saber guiar a un grupo de personas, aún sabiendo que cada persona piensa y analiza diferente.
[*A leader, I suppose that it is a person that should know how to guide a group of people, even knowing that every person thinks and analyzes differently.*]

6.3. The Qualitative Instructor: Sitting with Anzaldúa

As I read Luis's exercises, I take a breath. "This is beautiful," I write in the comments. "I wonder if you might add a few sentences to explain/expand/talk about what engaging with these exercises did. Particularly as this is a paper that you're framing as a "how to guide" so you might do a little more of this work given who you are speaking with." I sit a little longer, I sense the earth beneath me, the wind in my hair, Anzaldúa next to me. Then I write, "You could also resist this and not do it (Anzaldúa might agree with letting the reader dangle as she leaves you to figure it out as well…)." As I write back to Luis, I reflect on my teaching, the unexpected places it can lead. I sit a little longer on the border, grounded and grateful for these unexpected moments and places, murmuring my appreciation. As I return to my day, my week, the classroom, I keep thinking of the ways that refusal and resistance might take shape in other ways. How an artful and creative aesthetic might offer possibilities for resistance and refusal of traditional ways of doing research and imagining science.

7. An Afterword: The Doctoral Student and Reflections on Writing with Anzaldúa

In looking at this book that I'm almost finished writing, I see a mosaic pattern (Aztec-like) emerging, a weaving pattern, thin here, thick there. […] If I can get the bone structure right, then putting flesh on it proceeds without too many hitches. The problem is that the bones often do not exist prior to the flesh, but are shaped after a vague and broad shadow of its form is discerned or uncovered during beginning, middle and final stages of writing. (Anzaldúa 2012, p. 88)

I strived to connect, understand, and weave Anzaldúa's borderland and *nepantla* theories and my interviews in Spanish with three Mexican *promotoras de salud*, in which they discussed their experiences with leadership. However, I had not stopped to think about the actual process of writing. During the process of engaging in creative and poetic writing, I frequently felt curious, excited, adequate. Like other researchers (Prince 2022; Thomas 2021), creative and poetry writing led me to experience moments of becoming.

English is my second language, and academic jargon often seems like its own language at times. Hence, academic writing was a tedious and often cumbersome process. While engaging in nonacademic writing to understand my data and the theory, I felt a sense of becoming a writer. I was inhabiting a more familiar place—a place where the rules are not as rigid, and Spanish could be peppered into my analysis. This, in turn, made me feel a sense of accomplishment as I became a qualitative researcher—able to see lived experiences and follow the path to connections. These becomings, as a writer and a qualitative researcher, made me feel, somehow, like I was becoming more myself.

8. The Doctoral Student and Qualitative Instructor: Dear Reader

Writing produces anxiety. Looking inside myself and my experience, looking at my conflict, engenders anxiety in me. Being a writer feels very much like being a Chicana, or being queer—a lot of squirming, coming up against all sort of walls. Or its opposite: nothing defined or definite, a boundless, floating state of limbo where I kick my heels, brood, percolate, hibernate and wait for something to happen. (Anzaldúa 2012, p. 94)

The academic writing process can be daunting, especially for those of us who struggle to cement our thoughts in sterile style and composition. In Luis's experience, thinking with Anzaldúa, his theoretical proponent, offered an entry point to reimagine, interrogate, decolonize, and queer qualitative research design and data analysis. Writing with Anzaldúa offered a way to express a sense of authenticity and become in multiplicity. Telling a story through creative writing and poetic processes allows for vibrant epistemological and ontological spaces and opportunities. Theories are to be used to understand our experiences, not to make our experiences fit their molds. Qualitative data represent the constructed realities in which we live. Through using creative writing and poems to connect/understand/weave theory and data, Luis was able to feel more comfortable with the academic writing process. He allowed himself to feel and explore the process of becoming. Through this process, he encountered many worlds: the self, the cultural, the queer, the academic. At times, it seemed as if these worlds collided, creating a picture of bits and pieces of the self. Creative writing allowed him to weave in the pieces into a world of insight, belonging, resistance, and possibilities.

We both walked into the same classroom a few years ago. Today, from two different parts of the country, we enter and re-enter Zoom meetings to continue weaving our thoughts and experiences. Our worlds have changed, not only from the physical room to the virtual space, but from the point of view of our relationship. We re-examine our interactions in the past while continuing to weave what seems like a never-ending tapestry. We continue to learn from each other's worlds, sharing experiences in the classroom, with colleagues, with life. The boundaries of instructor and student have blurred through this re-worlding; we teach one another (we were always teaching one another, we see now). Our journey continues to ripple into critical connectedness.

To follow are some ideas for qualitative researchers, particularly doctoral students and those new to qualitative inquiry, to engage in as they sit with themselves, their theories, and their data. We offer these provocations as amplifications of the insights and contributions that emerged from our analysis and thinking together. We invite our readers to view these questions as further entry points to grapple with our discussions of refusal and resistance in writing and academic life. Thoughts from Luis are justified to the left, those from Maureen are justified are to the right, and provocations from us both are justified center. We conclude with a quote from Anzaldúa, bringing us and the reader full circle in our co-constructions.

Take time to understand your positionality as a person–researcher and engage in creative and critical reflexivity—Who am I? What do I bring to this study/participants/process? How do I show up in the data analysis process? What have I become? Who am I becoming? How is this study and writing personal to me? How is my voice showing up in my writing? (Harris 2016; Rodricks 2022)

Ask a lot of questions. Wonder, why this research topic and me?

Humanize theory—Who are the main theorists? What was the life of the theorists like, and what motivated them to develop this theory? How do the theorists show up in their own theory? How did the theory become theory?

Imagine your theorists at the kitchen table with you, looking over your shoulder as you write. How would they chime in? Where would they disagree? How would they interact with your participants?

Think of your methodology as a facilitator of a conversation—How can I have a conversation with my data and theory that would help me answer my research questions? What can I do to become an active listener–participant in the conversation?

Why this site and not another? Why this method and not another? (Marshall and Rossman 2015)

Have conversations with your data—What is not being said by my data? Where are the silences? What sticks out for me? What do I wish I could have said or asked of my participants, documents, or observations? What is my data becoming?

What does your data want? (Koro-Ljungberg 2015)

Have your data and theorist have a conversation with each other—What would the theorist tell me about my data? What would my data tell me about my theory? What would the theorist and data tell each other?

Ask: Who are we becoming as we engage in these conversations?

Sit on your border or join us in ours. Let's fearlessly dangle our feet together as we write, experience, and become.

For me, writing begins with the impulse to push boundaries, to shape ideas, images, and words that travel through the body and echo in the mind into something that has never existed. The writing process is the same mysterious process that we use to make the world. (Anzaldúa 2015, p. 5)

Author Contributions: Conceptualization, L.R.A.-H. and M.F.; methodology, L.R.A.-H. and M.F.; formal analysis, L.R.A.-H. and M.F.; investigation, L.R.A.-H.; data curation, L.R.A.-H. and M.F.; writing—original draft preparation, L.R.A.-H. and M.F.; writing—review and editing, L.R.A.-H. and M.F.; visualization, L.R.A.-H. and M.F. All authors have read and agreed to the published version of the manuscript.

Funding: This research received no external funding.

Institutional Review Board Statement: The study was conducted in accordance with the Declaration of Helsinki, and approved by the Institutional Review Board of The University of Georgia (MOD00006992 of STUDY00004909, 2019). for studies involving humans.

Informed Consent Statement: Informed consent was obtained from all subjects involved in the study.

Data Availability Statement: The data are confidential and under the custody of the first author.

Acknowledgments: We would like to acknowledge the *promotoras de salud* from *Lazos Hispanos* for sharing their leadership experiences with us. In addition, we express our appreciation for Brigette Adair Herron and Paul Eaton for their generous feedback on earlier drafts of this manuscript. We also want to acknowledge the Editors of this Special Issue, as their feedback added layers to our theoretical weaving.

Conflicts of Interest: The authors declare no conflict of interest.

References

Alexander, Dagmar, and Jonathan Wyatt. 2018. In(tra)Fusion: Kitchen Research Practices, Collaborative Writing, and Re-Conceptualising the Interview. *Qualitative Inquiry* 24: 101–8. [CrossRef]

Alvarez-Hernandez, L. R., and J. Maria Bermudez. forthcoming. Entre Madres y Comadres: Trans Latina Immigrants Empowering Women Beyond Marianismo. *Affilia*.

Anzaldúa, Gloria. 2012. *Borderlands/La Frontera: The New Mestiza*. San Francisco: Aunt Lute Books.

Anzaldúa, Gloria. 2015. *Light in the Dark/Luz En Lo Oscuro: Rewriting Identity, Spirituality, Reality*, Bilingual ed. Edited by AnaLouise Keating. Durham: Duke University Press Books.

Bhattacharya, Kakali. 2021. Rejecting Labels and Colonization: In Exile from Post-Qualitative Approaches. *Qualitative Inquiry* 27: 179–84. [CrossRef]

Bright, David. 2017. Becoming-City: Thinking and Writing Differently After Deleuze. *Qualitative Inquiry* 23: 416–22. [CrossRef]

Caine, Vera, and Pam Steeves. 2009. Imagining Playfulness in Narrative Inquiry. *International Journal of Education & the Arts* 10: 1–14. [CrossRef]

Cannon, Susan Ophelia, and Stephanie Behm Cross. 2020. Writing Excess: Theoretical Waste, Responsibility, and the Post Qualitative Inquiry. *Taboo: The Journal of Culture & Education* 19: 89–112.

Cisneros, Nora Alba. 2018. 'To My Relations': Writing and Refusal Toward an Indigenous Epistolary Methodology. *International Journal of Qualitative Studies in Education* 31: 188–96. [CrossRef]

Colyar, Julia. 2009. Becoming Writing, Becoming Writers. *Qualitative Inquiry* 15: 421–36. [CrossRef]

Denzin, Norman K. 2017. Critical Qualitative Inquiry. *Qualitative Inquiry* 23: 8–16. [CrossRef]

Evans-Winters, Venus E. 2019. *Black Feminism in Qualitative Inquiry: A Mosaic for Writing Our Daughter's Body*. New York: Abingdon, Oxon.

Evans-Winters, Venus E., and Jennifer Esposito. 2018. Researching the Bridge Called Our Backs: The Invisibility of 'Us' in Qualitative Communities. *International Journal of Qualitative Studies in Education* 31: 863–76. [CrossRef]

Foster, Susan. 2010. *Choreographing Empathy: Kinesthesia in Performance*. London and New York: Routledge.

Freeman, Melissa. 2016. *Modes of Thinking for Qualitative Data Analysis*. London: Routledge.

Gale, Ken, and Wyatt Jonathan. 2017. Working at the Wonder: Collaborative Writing as Method of Inquiry. *Qualitative Inquiry* 23: 355–64. [CrossRef]

Harris, Kate Lockwood. 2016. Reflexive Voicing: A Communicative Approach to Intersectional Writing. *Qualitative Research* 16: 111–27. [CrossRef]

Hein, Serge F. 2019. Deleuze, Immanence, and Immanent Writing in Qualitative Inquiry: Nonlinear Texts and Being a Traitor to Writing. *Qualitative Inquiry* 25: 83–90. [CrossRef]

Helin, Jenny. 2019. Dream Writing: Writing Through Vulnerability. *Qualitative Inquiry* 25: 95–99. [CrossRef]

Keating, AnaLouise. 2015. Re-Envisioning Coyolzauhqui, Decolonizing Reality: Anzaldúa's Twenty-First-Century Imperative. In *Light in the Dark/Luz En Lo Oscuro: Rewriting Identity, Spirituality, Reality*. Edited by AnaLouise Keating. Durham: Duke University Press, pp. ix–xxxvii.

Koro-Ljungberg, Mirka. 2015. *Reconceptualizing Qualitative Research: Methodologies Without Methodology*. Southend Oaks: SAGE Publications, Inc.

Kuntz, Aaron M. 2015. *The Responsible Methodologist: Inquiry, Truth-Telling, and Social Justice*. London: Routledge.

Marshall, Catherine, and Gretchen B. Rossman. 2015. *Designing Qualitative Research*, 6th ed. Southend Oaks: SAGE.

Mazzei, Lisa A., and Alecia Y. Jackson. 2013. In the Threshold: Writing Between-the-Two. *International Review of Qualitative Research* 5: 449–58. [CrossRef]

Mazzei, Lisa A., and Laura E. Smithers. 2020. Qualitative Inquiry in the Making: A Minor Pedagogy. *Qualitative Inquiry* 26: 99–108. [CrossRef]

McKnight, Lucinda, Owen Bullock, and Ruby Todd. 2017. Whiteout: Writing Collaborative Online Poetry as Inquiry. *Qualitative Inquiry* 23: 313–15. [CrossRef]

Moore, Amber. 2017. Eight Events for Entering a PhD: A Poetic Inquiry into Happiness, Humility, and Self-Care. *Qualitative Inquiry* 24: 107780041774510. [CrossRef]

Moraga, Cherríe, and Gloria Anzaldúa. 2021. *This Bridge Called My Back: Writings by Radical Women of Color*, Fortieth Anniversary ed. Albany: SUNY Press.

Muñoz, José Esteban. 1999. *Disidentifications: Queers of Color and the Performance of Politics*. Minneapolis: University of Minnesota Press.

Orpinas, Pamela, Rebecca Matthew, Luis R. Alvarez-Hernandez, Alejandra Calva, and J. Bermúdez María. 2021. Promotoras Voice Their Challenges in Fulfilling Their Role as Community Health Workers. *Health Promotion Practice* 22: 502–11. [CrossRef]

Orpinas, Pamela, Rebecca Matthew, María J. Bermúdez, Luis R. Alvarez-Hernandez, Alejandra Calva, and Darbisi Carolina. 2020. A Multistakeholder Evaluation of Lazos Hispanos: An Application of a Community-Based Participatory Research Conceptual Model. *Journal of Community Psychology* 48: 464–81. [CrossRef]

Prince, Cali. 2022. Experiments in Methodology: Sensory and Poetic Threads of Inquiry, Resistance, and Transformation. *Qualitative Inquiry* 28: 94–107. [CrossRef]

Richardson, Laurel, and Elizabeth Adams St. Pierre. 2005. Writing: A Method of Inquiry. In *The Sage Handbook of Qualitative Research*. Edited by Norman K. Denzin and S. Yvonna. Lincoln: SAGE Publications, pp. 959–78.

Rodricks, Dirk J. 2022. Theorizing Mishritata: A Queer Desi/South Asian Making Meaning of Multiple Minoritization in a Transnational Context. *Qualitative Inquiry* 28: 70–79. [CrossRef]

Sánchez, Nydia C., and Estee Hernández. 2022. Theorizing Home in The Academy: Chicana Doctoral Student Testimonios From the Borderlands. *Qualitative Inquiry* 28: 23–27. [CrossRef]

Schulz, Jennifer. 2006. Pointing the Way to Discovery: Using a Creative Writing Practice in Qualitative Research. *Journal of Phenomenological Psychology* 37: 217–39. [CrossRef]

St. Pierre, Elizabeth Adams. 1997. Circling the Text: Nomadic Writing Practices. *Qualitative Inquiry* 3: 403–18. [CrossRef]

Sword, Helen. 2017. *Air & Light & Time & Space: How Successful Academics Write*. Cambridge: Harvard University Press.

The Latina Feminist Group. 2001. *Telling to Live: Latina Feminist Testimonios*. Durham: Duke University Press.

Thomas, Rhianna. 2021. Poetic Juxtaposition, a Method for Connecting Data, Theory, and Every Day Texts. *Qualitative Inquiry* 27: 626–36. [CrossRef]

Tierney, William G., and Ronald E. Hallett. 2010. In Treatment: Writing Beneath the Surface. *Qualitative Inquiry* 16: 674–84. [CrossRef]

Ulmer, Jasmine Brooke. 2018. Composing Techniques: Choreographing a Post-qualitative Writing Practice. *Qualitative Inquiry* 24: 728–36. [CrossRef]

Ulmer, Jasmine, Susan Nordstrom, and Mark Tesar. 2017. Writing E/Scapes. *Reconceptualizing Educational Research Methodology* 8: 66–78. [CrossRef]

Yardley, A. 2008. Living stories: The role of the researcher in the narration of life. *Forum: Qualitative Social Research* 9. [CrossRef]

Zapata, Angie, Candace R. Kuby, and Jaye Johnson Thiel. 2018. Encounters with Writing: Becoming-with Posthumanist Ethics. *Journal of Literacy Research* 50: 478–501. [CrossRef]

Disclaimer/Publisher's Note: The statements, opinions and data contained in all publications are solely those of the individual author(s) and contributor(s) and not of MDPI and/or the editor(s). MDPI and/or the editor(s) disclaim responsibility for any injury to people or property resulting from any ideas, methods, instructions or products referred to in the content.

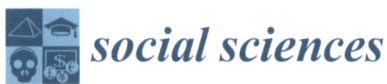

Article

Re-Making Clothing, Re-Making Worlds: On Crip Fashion Hacking

Ben Barry [1,2,*], Philippa Nesbitt [3], Alexis De Villa [4], Kristina McMullin [2] and Jonathan Dumitra [2]

1 Parsons School of Design, The New School, New York, NY 10011, USA
2 The Creative School, Toronto Metropolitan University, Toronto, ON M5B 2K3, Canada
3 Communication and Culture Program, Toronto Metropolitan University, Toronto, ON M5B 2K3, Canada
4 Human Ecology Department, University of Alberta, Edmonton, AB T6G 2R3, Canada
* Correspondence: barryb@newschool.edu

Abstract: This article explores how Disabled people's fashion hacking practices re-make worlds by expanding fashion design processes, fostering relationships, and welcoming-in desire for Disability. We share research from the second phase of our project, Cripping Masculinity, where we developed fashion hacking workshops with D/disabled, D/deaf and Mad men and masculine non-binary people. In these workshops, participants worked in collaboration with fashion researchers and students to alter, embellish, and recreate their existing garments to support their physical, emotional, and spiritual needs. We explore how our workshops heeded the principles of Disability Justice by centring flexibility of time, collective access, interdependence, and desire for intersectional Disabled embodiments. By exploring the relationships formed and clothing made in these workshops, we articulate a framework for crip fashion hacking that reclaims design from the values of the market-driven fashion industry and towards the principles of Disability Justice. This article is written as a dialogue between members of the research team, the conversational style highlights our relationship-making process and praxis. We invite educators, designers, and/or researchers to draw upon crip fashion hacking to re-make worlds by desiring with and for communities who are marginalized by dominant systems.

Keywords: crip technoscience; design; Disability; dress; intersectionality; pedagogy

Citation: Barry, Ben, Philippa Nesbitt, Alexis De Villa, Kristina McMullin, and Jonathan Dumitra. 2023. Re-Making Clothing, Re-Making Worlds: On Crip Fashion Hacking. *Social Sciences* 12: 500. https://doi.org/10.3390/socsci12090500

Academic Editors: Nadine Changfoot, Eliza Chandler and Carla Rice

Received: 21 December 2022
Revised: 12 February 2023
Accepted: 16 February 2023
Published: 6 September 2023

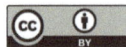

Copyright: © 2023 by the authors. Licensee MDPI, Basel, Switzerland. This article is an open access article distributed under the terms and conditions of the Creative Commons Attribution (CC BY) license (https://creativecommons.org/licenses/by/4.0/).

1. Cripping Fashion and Fashioning Design

I'm holding hands with my Disability
I have the other hand free
Could I hold the hand of someone who fights me?
Or I could hold the hand of someone who loves me?

It might seem that the dominant fashion industry is becoming more 'inclusive' of Disability.[1] There is a rise in the number of fashion products specifically designed for Disabled people from brands such as Tommy Hilfiger, Nike and IZ Adaptive. However, when Disabled people are 'invited' into the fashion industry, their participation primarily rests on the capitalist logics of assimilation, objectification, and depoliticization. During the design process, non-Disabled people are situated as the experts whose practices are focused on "designing *for* Disability rather than *with* or *by* Disabled people" (Hamraie and Fritsch 2019, p. 4). Disabled people are either excluded from the design of fashion, or restricted to the transactional roles of 'user' in an initial research phase or during the testing of prototypes (Critical Axis n.d.; Hamraie 2017). This relationship reduces Disabled people to being passive recipients of design, while it glorifies non-disabled people as the creators of design (Hamraie and Fritsch 2019). The clothing designed through this process often sanitizes Disability for non-Disabled audiences by concealing or normalizing boldly differences, erasing intersectional Disability experiences by centring white cis-heteronormative aesthetics, and pricing Disability-friendly fashion at amounts that ignore the financial barriers that many Disabled people experience due to ableism and other systems of oppression (Barry 2019; Cubacub 2019). As with other diversity gestures towards inclusion in the fashion industry, this engagement is no surprise because discourses of ableism 'laid the foundation, built the house, and are now opening the door (Mulholland 2019, p. 213).

This article analyzes our practice of crip fashion hacking as a process that reclaims design from the values of the market-driven fashion industry and towards a desire for intersectional crip experiences. We draw on Hamraie and Fritsch (2019) concept of crip technoscience and Otto von Busch's (2009) understanding of fashion hacking to ground our understanding of crip fashion hacking. Hamraie and Fritsch (2019) define crip technoscience as the use of scientific knowledge and technological-making by and with Disabled people in order to intervene into the exclusionary material world and systems that construct it. These anti-assimilationist "world-building and world-dismantling practices"—and fields of knowledge that emerge from them—-are grounded in the political reclamation of the word crip (Hamraie and Fritsch 2019, p. 4). Drawing on Disability studies scholars Robert McRuer (2006), Mitchell and Snyder (2015) and Kelly Fritsch (2016), crip refuses dominant narratives in which Disability is understood as an experience to be cured, fixed or eliminated, and instead recognizes it as generative, creative, and desirable. We understand fashion hacking as a design method that can apply the ethos of crip technoscience in the context of Disability and fashion. Following von Busch (2009), fashion hacking is a political and anti-capitalist practice in which communities who have been excluded from the dominant fashion system have open access to fashion knowledge. These communities are supported to use, modify and expand this knowledge to design garments that centre their needs, desires and imagination.

By bringing together crip technoscience and fashion hacking as design practices that intervene into dominant knowledge and remake existing material arrangements, we coin the term crip fashion hacking. We understand it as a "knowing-making" practice (Hamraie 2017) that shares, questions and overhauls dominant fashion knowledge to remake clothing by and with Disabled people in ways that centre access, aesthetics and desire for Disability. In this article, we draw upon this understanding to ask how crip fashion hacking might expand dominant fashion design practices and remake worlds that cultivate desire for Disability.

We draw on our project, Cripping Masculinity, which explores Disabled, D/deaf and Mad-identified men and masculine non-binary people's experiences with gender, fashion and Disability. We recruited participants—across a range of race, sexuality and other social locations—who have diverse experiences of Disability. We invited these participants to engage in the three project phases: wardrobe interviews to explore their relationships with clothing; fashion hacking workshops where they remake clothes to offer access for their bodyminds and reflect their desired intersectional identities; and fashion shows and exhibitions to showcase their clothing and expand public understanding about Disability experiences. For this article, we focus on phase two of the project: fashion hacking.

We had originally conceived that fashion hacking would take place through one-day, in-person workshops. However, due to the COVID-19 pandemic, we moved these workshops to a virtual format in which participants and research team would work in small groups over several months by communicating with each other online and mailing garments back-and-forth. One iteration of these virtual workshops, which we will focus on in this article, took place in an undergraduate elective course. The course aimed to honour and heed the principles of the Disability Justice "movement building framework" in the context of fashion design (Kafai 2021, p. 22). In 2005, Patty Berne and Leroy F. Moore Jr.—co-founders of the performance group Sins Invalid that centres queer and trans Disabled people of colour—developed Disability Justice with Mia Mingus, Stacey Milbern, Sebastain Margaret and Eli Claire (Kafai 2021). While we will discuss Disability Justice later in this article, we were mindful of the concerns that Disability Justice has been co-opted—especially by white academics—without crediting its Disabled, queer and trans of colour origins or enacting Disability Justice politics (Kafai 2021). The course was intentional about engaging with readings, films, podcasts, and art by its founders and other Disabled queer and trans people of colour as the guide, as well as to centre its principles in the context of fashion design. In the course, each student was paired with a research team member, whom we called the mentor, and a participant, whom we call the collaborator. They collaboratively hacked one of the collaborator's existing garments that did not, in its current form, work for their bodymind or aesthetically express their desired intersectional identities. Each design team, or what we refer to as design pod, altered, embellished, and recreated the garment to centre the collaborator's physical, emotional, and spiritual needs. By exploring the experiences of these workshops, we articulate a framework of crip fashion hacking. We position it as a political practice that educators, researchers and fashion professionals can draw on to re-make worlds by desiring with and for multiplying marginalized Disability communities.

2. Cripping Academic Writing

As we hold onto crip fashion hacking as a political practice to re-make worlds, we also hold onto *how* we tell the stories of these hacking processes to re-make how knowledge is generated and shared within academia. We selected a format for this article that falls outside of the typical style of scholarship. It is a mix of poetry and direct dialogue between us, the core members of the Cripping Masculinity research team. Our rationale for writing in this format is to honour the work of Indigenous, Black, Disability and feminist scholars who resist conventional approaches to academic writing, and to practice the politics on which our project is build.

Shawn Wilson (2008) observes that conversation is a more egalitarian format for sharing knowledge because it works against academic hierarchies that prioritize academic position. bell hooks (1994) highlights the value of dialogue by observing that it allows for a more intimate experience of sharing knowledge, allowing a reader to feel as though they are present for the conversations occurring. Hannah McGregor et al. (2020) understand this conversational format as a practice of feminist consciousness raising—explaining that it builds analysis not only by engaging with academic thought, but also by centring stories and lived experiences. Recognizing we each have "partial perspectives" based on our positionalities and lived experiences, Mel Y. Chen (2014, p. 172) observes that academic work should be developed by working together among people with diverse embodiments and cognitions, or as they note, differently "cognating beings". Moreover, interdependence—building relationships that support each other's needs—is a core tenant of practicing Disability Justice (Sins Invalid 2016). In this article, we therefore use dialogue to break down the hierarchies within our group and open-up desire for the unique offerings that each person brings to the research by generating ideas *together*. Our hope is that you can feel us as researchers working through challenges, sharing experiences, and playing with theory. We hope that you will find spaces to fit in and fill the gaps in our conversation. That way, we can start to build relationships so we can all move together.

Before we begin our conversation, it is important to note that publishing scholarship comes from a position of privilege, with power and with a responsibility to the communities about whom we are speaking. We recognize that academic publishing excludes many Disabled people, such as through inaccessible language and by restricting access to the capital that comes with writing in peer-reviewed spaces. As a group, we are still writing about shared experiences with the collaborators through our voices and we are receiving the value of authorship. Our choice to write this paper as a dialogue between us aimed to practice a process that we can use with collaborators in the future. By writing this here, we hope to stay accountable to that goal.

3. About the Authors

Our research team comprises a diverse group of people who come to the project from different positions, both within the hierarchical framework of academia and within our embodied ways of being in the world. To critically and collaboratively engage with one another and with collaborators, we have centred practices of reflexivity throughout the project. Key to reflexivity is maintaining transparency about our relationships with the various fields with which our research engages, the act of doing research, and the ways in which we produce knowledge (Haggerty 2003; Crooks et al. 2012). We share our positionalities to acknowledge that our identities influence how we interact with collaborators, as well as how we think about, experience, and reflect upon the project (England 1994). In sharing pieces about ourselves, we aim to position ourselves within the project through transparency and care.

Ben (he/him): I am a queer, Disabled person with low vision, and my relationship to clothing centres tactile experience. I am also a white, thin, middle-class, cisgender man, and my Disability is primarily invisible. My embodied privilege has granted me access to fashion; I can easily find clothing that fit my body, buy them, and express my being. As a fashion educator, designer and lead of this project, my own embodied experiences helped me to conceptualize this project while also recognizing the importance of bringing together a community of collaborators who do not have my embodied and social privileges.

Kristina (she/her): I am a white, visibility Disabled woman, a settler to the north part of Turtle Island in Tkaronto (colonially known as Toronto). My privilege to live and work in Tkaronto is due to the colour of my skin, the legacies of colonialism and white supremacy that have provided wealth and resources to my family. I share this information to contextualize how experiences of sexism and ableism exist within my identity. Alongside being an academic researcher, I am also a creative producer, arts administrator, and designer, rooting my practice in a drive to build spaces and experiences that make my community feel seen, desired, valued, and loved.

Alexis (they/them/sikato): I am a queer/non-binary, neurodivergent and mad-identified, second-generation Filipino and Pangasinan settler/migrant, community organizer, and textile artist. I share these parts of me as the intergenerational knowledge of those before me who have identified as such inform my understanding of the world and to whom I am accountable with the labor I put forth. My hopes within this project are to do the prescribed work, in the least violent way, to get materials, money, and resources to community members while I am in this space of privilege.

Jonathan (he/him): I am a gay/queer, Austrian-Romanian, neurodivergent fashion designer. Specializing in accessible fashion, I design queer-masculine lingerie, underwear, fetish, and intimate wear with the strong belief that all bodies deserve to feel sexy and erotic, without inherent negative fetishization. With the understanding that my fit, cis, white man's body has a classically "model-esque" figure, my work decentres people who look like me from the fashion narrative to create a more holistic and accurate representation of the bodies on the planet.

Philippa (she/her): I am a white, cisgender, and neurodivergent settler currently pursuing my Ph.D. with a focus on fashion and disabilities. I approach my work with a recognition that I hold privileges that have facilitated easier access to academic spaces and fostered a positive personal relationship with fashion, and an understanding that my own personal embodiment limits my understanding of the lived experiences of others. I strongly value the way collective knowledge generation can develop a more holistic view of the world and foster greater social change.

4. Fashion Hacking and Disability Justice

Holding is loving, caring
To hold hands is for someone to hold it back
given and received at our own pace
given and received willingly and eagerly.
To hold with mutual desire

Ben: von Busch (2009) observes that the word "hacking" originates from the early programming culture in the 1960s, as a do-it-yourself practice of intervention into closed online networks. When applied to fashion, hacking redistributes power from the elite fashion system to previously excluded consumers. The practice transfers knowledge about the creation of fashion to them, and it supports them to modify it for themselves (von Busch 2009). Alice Payne (2021) notes that "fashion hacking" is a method within the larger fashion design strategy of "rewilding". According to Payne (2021), rewilding aims to "seize back fashion as cultural expression from its continual commodification by industry. Rewilding actions are those that make wild spaces for fashion practices to flourish beyond the dictates of the dominant fashion system" (p. 160).

Philippa: Why do you think that fashion hacking worked well for a project on Disability?

Ben: To survive in an ableist world as Disabled people, we have long engaged in "making, hacking, and tinkering with existing material arrangements" in order to produce forms of access unavailable or economically inaccessible for us (Hamraie and Fritsch (2019, p. 4). These design interventions—what Hamraie and Fritsch (2019) call the field and practice of crip technoscience—are generated from knowing what works best for us, as well as from the shared expertise developed within Disability communities. For example, Bess Williamson (2019) details how Disabled people in postwar America have drawn on their Disability experiences to hack assistive equipment and everyday household tools to offer access for their bodyminds. These hacking practices recognize that Disabled people "are not merely formed or acted on by the world—we are engaged agents of remaking" (Hamraie and Fritsch 2019, p. 7). The knowledge and material arrangements that result from these hacking practices centre what Leah Lakshmi Piepzna-Samarasinha (2018) refers to as "crip science": the skills, wisdom and resources that Disabled people have uniquely developed to navigate inaccessible worlds. Our experiences of "misfitting" into environments that do not sustain our bodyminds have therefore helped us generate the knowledge that we can use to dismantle and remake them (Garland Thomson 2011).

Following this approach, our crip fashion hacking workshops focused on re-making clothing that were owned by collaborators but that did not support their bodyminds or express their desired identities. Our objective was to explore alternatives to profit-driven fashion design that enable crip communities to affirm their embodied selves. Engaging in fashion hacking through a crip technoscience framework centred the knowledge and creativity that comes from Disability experiences, as well as an understanding that fashion hacking makes access through friction. According to Hamraie and Fritsch (2019), crip technoscience challenges the dominant assumption that accessibility is about the inclusion and assimilation of Disabled people into non-Disabled environments. It draws on Kelly Fritsch's (2016) understanding of access as a site of friction and contestation. In this way, fashion hacking in a crip context intentionally pushes beyond assimilationist-based approaches to access in fashion design. Rather than aiming to hide or eliminate Disability through accessible clothing features, fashion is redesigned to be accessible through the lens of "non-compliance and protest" (Hamraie and Fritsch 2019, p. 10).

Philippa: The hacking workshops focused on small group experiences, where participants worked with one or two research team members via Zoom to hack their garments. Ben, you also created an elective course as a branch of Cripping Masculinity. What was this course about?

Ben: The course aimed to cultivate a deeper understanding and practice of social justice in the context of Disability and fashion design. For the first half of the course, students learned about the Disability Justice movement, crip fashion and fashion hacking. They watched Sins Invalid's *Crip Bits* video series, read their *Skin, Tooth and Bone: A Disability Justice Primer* (2016), and engaged with works by Disabled queer of colour scholars, activists and designers such as Shayda Kafai, Mia Mingus and Sky Cubacub. For the second half of the course, each student-designer worked in a virtual 'pod' with a mentor (research team member) and a collaborator (research participant) in order to hack one of the collaborator's garments. The pod was led by the collaborator's experiences and desires, and the student supported the redesign of the collaborator's garment. A mentor facilitated the collaboration, supported the knowledge exchange, and provided care for the student and collaborator throughout the process.

Philippa: The aspect of exclusivity in fashion that Ben spoke about is also something that is foundational to academic spaces. To me, it is amazing to witness both fashion students and scholars work against this and, by doing so, work against harmful, ableist systems built out of capitalist frameworks. This is something that's key to Disability Justice.

Kristina: Disability Justice, at its core, is a movement led by Disabled people of colour. It aimed to expand upon the Disability Rights Movement that sought equal rights for Disabled folks within the legal system. One of the most well-known examples of the Disability Rights Movement's activism was the passing of the Americans with Disabilities Act (ADA) in 1990. The ADA granted legal protections based on Disability status in the United States, and it has been a framework for similar legislation around the world. Disability Justice was developed to respond to gaps in the Disability Rights Movement that focused on whiteness, maleness, heteronormativity and mobility as the default Disability experience (Kafai 2021). Disabled activists of colour and who are queer and trans were rarely reflected in the Disability Rights movement; it was primarily led by white, cis heterosexual Disabled people who discussed Disability as a single and isolated issue. Disability Justice aimed to centre leadership of Disabled people of colour and to cultivate community with them. It underscores how ableism, white supremacy, racism, sexism, colonialism, patriarchy, cis-heteronormativity and other forms of oppression work together to oppress people whose bodyminds do not conform to dominant understandings of normalcy, intelligence and behaviour (Sins Invalid 2016; Lewis 2022).

As we discussed in the introduction, the performance group Sins Invalid has been invaluable to Disability Justice. They outline ten core principles of the movement: intersectionality; leadership of those most impacted; an anti-capitalist politic; a commitment to cross-movement organizing; recognizing wholeness; sustainability; a commitment to cross-Disability solidarity; interdependence; collective access; and collective liberation (Sins Invalid 2016). The definition of Disability Justice that I relate to most on both an emotional and physical level is Mia Mingus' (2018) declaration that Disability Justice is just another term for love. To practice Disability Justice is to love Disability, and to love it *publicly*. A crip and loving approach to time and pace is one aspect that J has said he personally connected with in Cripping Masculinity.

5. Cripping Time While Hacking Fashion

Jonathan: I came to form an intimate relationship with crip time throughout the development of the project. Crip time is a concept and a practice developed by Disability scholars and activists (e.g., Kafer 2013; Price 2011; Samuels 2017), and it is one that we have been utilizing for our project to reject capitalist ideals about productivity, creation, and collaboration. Crip time reimagines temporality through a recognition that current expectations of productivity and time have been based upon ableist frameworks (Kafer 2013, p. 27). It creates new temporalities that attend to the needs of our bodyminds, allowing us to take breaks and refuse to push through when the dictates of capitalist expectations tell us to continue (Samuels 2017). Throughout the hacking workshops in the course—as well as in the earlier iterations of them—crip time has been central to our design practice and relationships. We encouraged every group to organize their schedules in ways that centred their needs and created a space to reimagine what productivity could look like for them. One pairing between the student-designer Julie and the collaborator AJ really highlighted crip time throughout their process of collaboration. Julie often felt the pressures of university time and felt overwhelmed during the process. They didn't complete the garment by the end of the course, and it's still a work in progress, but this is actually something we encouraged. We wanted Julie to experience the practice of crip time by being supported to question and reimagine the pace that she was taught to expect of herself in a university course. AJ reinforced these ideas using comforting words and plenty of encouragement. To many members of crip and Mad communities, crip time is not just a theory, but an active force in their life. It is a reality of survival in a world with ableist barriers, and a way of respecting the changing capacity of each bodymind, even when the constraints of capitalism work against it.

Jonathan: Although we wanted to encourage crip time and support an anti-capitalist, Disability-centred approach to time and pace in our workshops, there was another 'time signature' with which we had to grapple: university time. University time follows a capitalist-based system of time that requires progressive and consistent work, with set due dates and expectations. It often leaves little room for adaptation because results are based on scores or grades rather than experiences. Unfortunately, no matter how much we wanted to encourage crip time, we still had to work within the constraints of university time. Just as in music, it is next to impossible for a song to exist within two different time signatures simultaneously—this was the dissonance we felt while undertaking fashion hacking through the structure of a university class. When practicing crip time in the workshops, the greatest success we found has been when it was not just our dominant time signature, but our *only* time signature. By stripping down the capitalist timeframes, crip time can flourish and cultivate crip fashion hacking.

Ben: I have been reflecting on the differences of embedding crip time into the university compared to the fashion industry. Plural understandings of fashion and fashion design have historically existed since time immemorial and continue to operate geographically today. However, a singular white European definition of fashion has become hegemonic and it associates fashion with capitalist production and consumption, as well as with clothing of the moment. This definition was developed during the European modernist period, and it prioritizes novelty, constant change, and speed (Payne 2021). We can therefore coin 'fashion industry time' that requires a fast pace for fashion design to support the demand of constant change. In the fashion industry, this timestamp is practiced by the expectation that designers produce at least four distinct collections per calendar year—fall/winter, spring/summer, pre-fall and resort—and showcase these collections at four scheduled industry events (Wong 2013). In the university, there are specific timestamps for courses, semesters and academic years, yet the university also provides the material conditions that can make space for crip time. Individual faculty—particularly those with more security and seniority—have agency over their courses, and they can intentionally bend their pacing and deadlines toward crip time. Students and faculty can also request and receive formal 'accommodation' through their university in order to develop a schedule and deadlines that better supports their pace. While the fashion industry does not offer these same conditions, fashion design in the university can offer more flexible timestamps to support the pace of the design collaborators. While our hacking workshops provided this flexibility, I wonder about the extent to which this affirmation of participants' intersectional crip embodiments moved beyond our design spaces and into their everyday lives.

Philippa: The collaborator Birdie really comes up for me. Her student-designer, Aris, helped her to create a new bra that worked for her body (Figure 1). For context, Birdie had top surgery years ago, but during the workshop, she was de-transitioning and identifying as female again. It was important for Birdie to find a bra for her flat chest, which didn't seem to exist in the world. Even though it wasn't something that was necessarily seen by other people, a bra was something that created a sense of gender euphoria and validation in her own embodiment. Under Birdie's guidance, Aris ensured that none of the alterations to the bra were permanent, should Birdie want to take it apart so it returns to its original cup size. Aris also created a document of how to do similar alterations to other pieces (Figure 2). This provided a format for Birdie to follow if she wanted to alter other pieces. In our closing meeting, Birdie talked about how important that document was going to be for her future. For example, she had a wedding coming up and had nothing to wear but had a lot of dresses that held potential. She would use that document to fix the chest and be able to wear the dresses again, helping to give her the confidence and validation to be in the world. I know that didn't necessarily happen in all the groups, but this was one case that did show a deep impact on Birdie's intersectional crip embodiment in their everyday life.

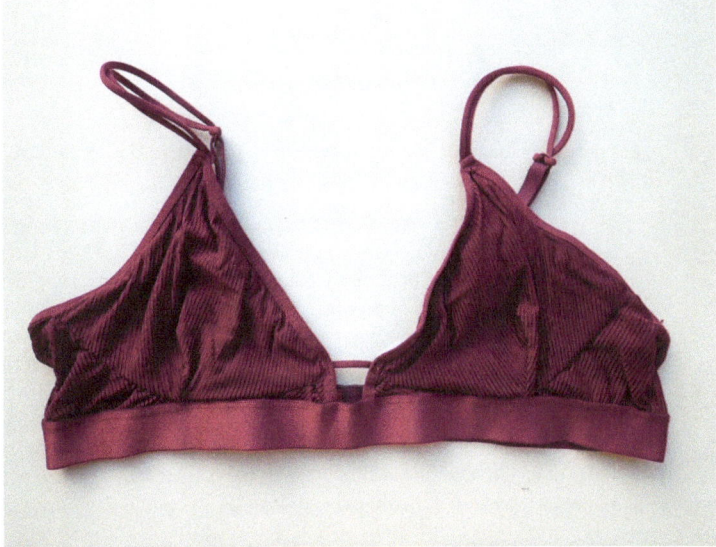

Figure 1. Birdie's finished garment. The image shows a maroon bralette lying flat on a white background. The fabric is ribbed, with an iridescent band on the bottom.

1) Pin the area of your garment you'll be working on to the tabletop. Then, fold up the area you'll be sewing to flatten it (in this case, I used a v-shaped "cut" along the original dart) and pin that down in as many places as needed. Try to have some places that anchor into the bottom band or binding on the edge of the cups so that there's some extra stability holding the shape in place once you let all the pins loose. When pinning your fold, keep in mind how the rest of the cup looks too; you might have to keep it a little looser so that both the folded area and the fabric around it aren't pulled too tight. I took some time to play with the balance on both sides to create a look I felt was natural.

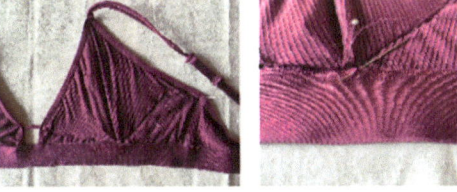
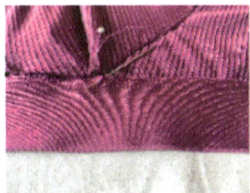
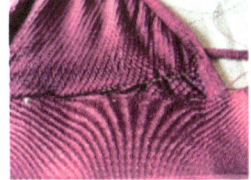

fg. 1 pinned bralette   fg. 2 anchoring in binding   fg. 3 ladder stitch

Figure 2. A sample of the hacking document created for Birdie by Aris. The image shows a screenshot of black text that reads "(1) Pin the area of your garment you'll be working on to the tabletop. Then, fold up the area you'll be sewing to flatten it (in this case, I used a V-shaped "cut" along the original dart) and pin that down in as many places as needed. Try to have some places that anchor into the bottom band or binding on the edge of the cups so that there's some extra stability holding the shape in place once you let all the pins loose. When pinning your fold, keep in mind how the rest of the cup looks too; you might have to keep it a little looser so that both the folded area and the fabric around it aren't pulled too tight. I took some time to play with the balance on both sides to create a look I felt was natural". Below the text are three photographs: the first, labeled "fg. 1 pinned bralette", shows one side of a maroon ribbed bralette with pins, flat against a white linen textile; the second, labeled "fg. 2 anchoring in binding" shows a bra cup and band that have been pinned together; the third, labeled "fg. 3 ladder stitch" shows the bralette's band with visible stitching.

6. Honouring Collective Access

Holding hands in all the ways we can
The form taking different shapes
with all the fingers or none of the fingers
All of the glorious ways our genders, races and sexualities
meet our stutters, disassociations and aches

Philippa: Another tenant of Disability Justice we explore through the project is a major shift away from that singular Disability rights-based framework Kristina spoke about toward Disability Justice. That really comes through when thinking about different understandings of access.

Ben: It does. From a Disability Rights perspective, access is focused on supporting Disabled people solely based on their Disability experiences. In contrast, access from a Disability Justice lens understands Disabled people as whole people rather than siloing their Disability from their other social positions. In our fashion hacking workshops, we aimed to incorporate this latter understanding of access through every encounter—from how we remade clothing to how we communicated with collaborators. We recognized that each encounter would not always be accessible, but we would do our best with small-scale actions to bring about access. As Lakshmi Piepzna-Samarasinha (2021) has observed about Disabled mutual aid, "We were maybe not going to save the world, but we were going to save each other" (n.p.).

Philippa: There are so many examples of encounters with access needs that happened in tandem with much larger, perhaps more obvious access needs. I think one great example is in the way the student-designer Eesha worked with the collaborator Cam.

Ben: Yes! Cam wanted their garment to support their experiences as an East Asian, trans masculine, fat-identified, Lolita-loving Disabled person. Their original pre-hacked garment was a long vest that did not care for their intersectional experiences (Figure 3). It was too tight. The lining caused sores on their sensitive skin, while its floral pattern didn't reflect their trans masculinity. The silhouette also did not have the volume they desired for their Lolita aesthetic. Cam and student-designer Eesha hacked the vest to centre an intersectional understanding of access and care for all the parts of Cam's identities (Figure 4). The vest was made larger; the lining was changed to an ultra-soft blue textile; and a removable bustle skirt was added. This latter hack especially brought about care for Cam as a racialized, trans, Disabled person by recognizing that the exaggerated volume might get tangled in Cam's crutch when they moved about their city, and its hyper visibility might put Cam in danger in particular social contexts. The removable design offered Cam the agency to detach the bustle and easily store it in their backpack when they traveled from one location to another, and to then reattach it when they arrived at the destination where they felt safe to wear their voluminous piece.

Philippa: We also see this in the experience between the collaborator Rowan and the student-designer Lisa. What really came through here was what Jonathan spoke about— navigating time and capacity within deeply-entrenched, capitalist systems of productivity.

Alexis: One small but significant practice where Rowan and Lisa's needs were navigated was in how this collaboration actually took shape rather than how we as a research team planned for it. Originally, these hacking workshops and virtual meetings were to take place during the class, using that time to build relationships and hack the clothing. However, it was still under the misguided assumption that when the meetings were set, folks' capacity would remain the same and each person would have the emotional, physical and mental energy readily available. In order to meaningfully address access barriers, we had to first recognize that it would be impossible for each group to stick to the format that we had intended. We had to recognize that our first draft of this process was essentially flawed. That opened up discussions about alternative ways to maintain communication and build relationships. We talked about how we could support this process, get Rowan the sweater they desired, honour Lisa's schedule and labour, and honor my capacity. We created a Google drive that allowed each of us to input design inspirations and concepts while sharing personal interests and tidbits of who we are, as we might in a virtual or in-person conversation. All of these small interactions looked to collective access to care for each persons' needs.

Philippa: It's interesting how personal interests came up in some of the collaborations, which was fostered by these dialogues between the collaborators and student-designers.

Alexis: Talking about personal interests created a pathway for more tender and intimate collaboration. For example, Lisa and Rowan had a common interest in Gangnam, which influenced what their collaborative design looked like. Furthermore, meeting up became easier because there was an eagerness to come to a meeting, knowing that we were all desired as full humans, rather than just meeting up to complete a goal.

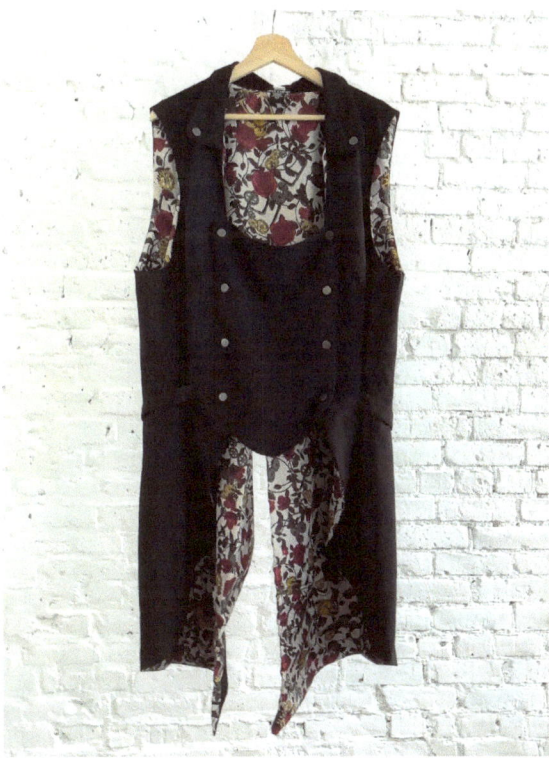

Figure 3. Cam's original garment. The image shows a long, black vest hanging on a wooden hanger against a white painted brick background. The vest has brushed silver buttons along each side, fastening a front panel together. The interior of the vest is visible. It is white with a pattern of dark red and yellow roses with green stems, leaves, and thorns.

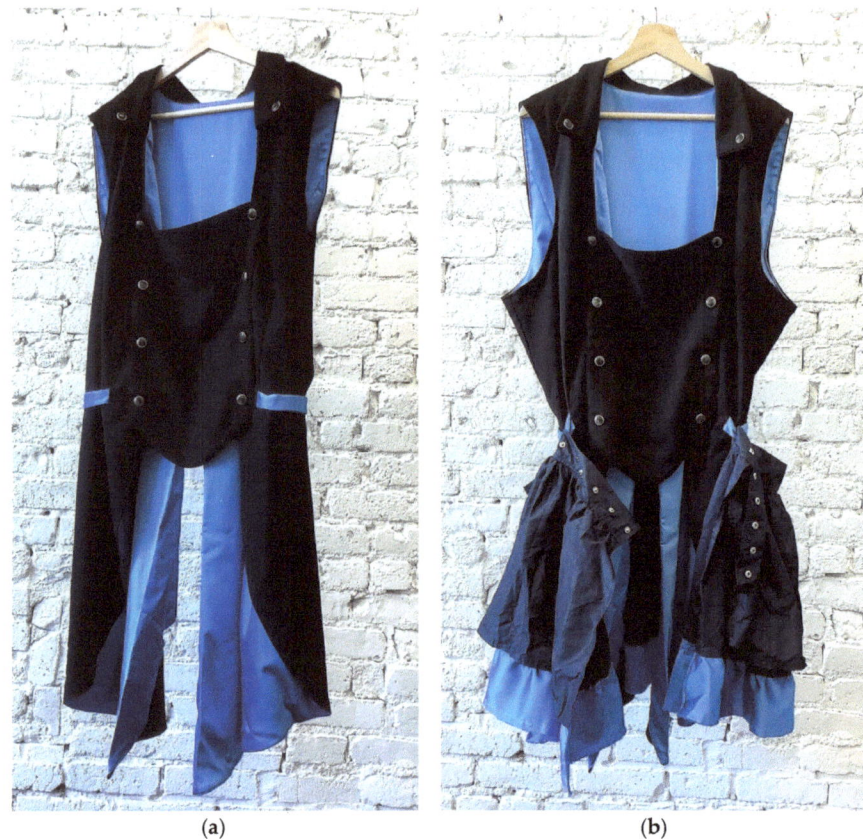

Figure 4. (**a**) Cam's hacked garment without bustle. The image shows a long black vest with a blue interior on a wooden hanger against a painted white brick background. The vest has silver buttons on each side and a narrow blue belt at the waist that matches the vest's interior. (**b**) Cam's hacked garment with removable bustle attached. The image shows a long black vest with a blue interior on a wooden hanger against a painted white brick background. Attached at the waist is a bustle that resembles a skirt, with a blue bottom layer and a black top layer. It is left open with silver snaps showing.

7. Interdependence through Fashion Hacking

I'm holding hands with my Disability
I'm holding hands with my clothes
I have the other hand free
Could I use that hand to throw it away?
Or could I use that hand to mend it?

Philippa: Interdependence is a core principle of Disability Justice (Sins Invalid 2016). I wonder if we could discuss a little bit more about how this practice played out in our workshops.

Kristina: Mingus (2017) explains that "Interdependence moves us away from the myth of independence, and towards relationships where we are all valued and have things to offer" (n.p.). Counter to dominant ableist logics, in interdependence there is no 'lack' to remedy, but an abundance of 'have', to share and to share willingly and eagerly. However, much like access intimacy (Mingus 2011), interdependence cannot be artificially created; it grows naturally in loving and care-filled environments. In the workshops, we attempted to create interdependent hacking pods, in some cases pairing two students with less fashion experience with one collaborator and an experienced mentor. We didn't always experience our desire for interdependence between the two student-designers. In fact, the opposite occurred—it ended up being more challenging to build interdependent relationships within the time constraints of the course when an additional person was integrated. While the integration of an additional student-designer was intended to lessen the labour of the hacking itself, it disproportionately increased the amount of labour and time it took to foster relationships within the set meeting times. On a strictly logistical level, it takes four people more time to introduce themselves than it takes three. On a more nuanced level, it takes more labour to understand two people's desires, intentions, politics, and capacities than to understand the same facets of one person. The meetings were filled with greetings, pleasantries, and technical updates, but there simply was no time to discuss hobbies, interests, or creative endeavours, essentially developing relationships. As Jonathan mentioned, we were working within the time constraints of a university, an institution built from the roots of capitalism and not always hospitable to interdependent relationships.

A friend of mine, Jenna Reid (2022) once said: "It's a beautiful thing to *learn* how to *receive* love". Through this project our team is not only learning how to receive love within our work, but how to foster interdependence within our hacking pods. This learning, like all forms of love, takes time, intention, and freedom to develop. Although we saw deep relationships form in some pods, there were others that were disconnected. We could not control the time of the course, or the emotional intentions of our student-designers or collaborators. We will continue to desire the cultivation of interdependence within this project, and we will continue to fail in relationships that are not given the time, intention and love that we have developed as a team.

Alexis: A question that arises for me when thinking about interdependence is: How can fashion build interdependent relationships by being both a relational medium—like a mutual friend that two people can share conversation about and find connection through—and an active community member? The hacking workshops could not unfold without textiles and garments. Garments became a support system that offered care to collaborators because these materials connected how they presented their intersectional identities in an embodied way. Furthermore, through the process of fashion hacking, we further developed emotional and tactile relationships with garments—we made sure that these unused garments are getting used again. To me, this is rooted in Indigenous worldview and practices. Wilson (2008), Rebecca Sockbeson (2009), Manu Meyer (2008) are some people who come to mind that explore this connection.

Philippa: You worked closely with the collaborator Keith and the student-designer Melanie. They had a deeply interdependent relationship that was built on a lot of what you are discussing.

Alexis: Although this is my interpretation from being in the same space as them, I witnessed Keith and Melanie's relationship develop through their transcultural shared experiences, Keith being Métis and Melanie Native Hawaiian. The three of us talked about how we viewed the inclusion of more-than-humans and Land as community and how the Land can offer such generous insights. Halfway through our conversation, it felt like our shoulders relaxed, to use the words of Mingus (2017). Our friendship felt so immediate and special. I want to share something Keith offered during our last conversation: "I think Melanie and I, our connection, which is a weirdly amazing, intergenerational, transcultural . . . I don't know, I can't even describe it. But I just feel like we connected right away, and our ideas flowed together in a really good way. And then [the hacked shirt] that came out of it is the most beautiful transformation of something that used to hold some negative connotations. And it's been transformed into this beautiful, powerful symbol of solidarity between nations". There was a meaningful relationship between all of us and a shifted relationship with the shirt Keith and Melanie hacked.

Philippa: Keith's words and summary of their relationship with Melanie is just so perfect. What were those negative connotations embedded in Keith's original, unhacked piece—a rodeo shirt?

Alexis: When Keith, Melanie and I all first discussed the shirt they wanted to hack, Keith talked about the idea of rodeo and how in Alberta, where Keith lived, there was and continues to be violence against Indigenous communities at rodeos. However, Keith shared that the elements of rodeo are rooted in many Métis traditions and shares roots in other Indigenous communities. Melanie immediately chimed in about how her mom goes to the rodeo every year in Hawaii and how rodeo is popular amongst Native Hawaiians. What came from this was a collective choice to use traditional beading and embroidery knowledge to adorn flowers along this rodeo "western shirt". The hacking served a reclamation of Indigenous relationships to the rodeo, and symbolized a rebuilt relationship with the rodeo through the design process and final shirt. When the hacking plan was decided, Keith offered to give Melanie the beads to make it possible. I was able to go to Keith's place to pick up these beads, and Keith gifted me a pin that said "babies against colonialism" because they had found out that I was pregnant. I mention these small parts that may not seem related because these practices nurtured our embodied, interdependent relationships in material ways that included more-than-human entities.

8. Desire for Disability as a Design Principle

Palms touching

Holding all of it

All of our bodies-minds-spirits

All of the kinships and fabrics that embrace them, embrace us

Philippa: Sins Invalid (2016) shares, "A Disability Justice framework understands that: All bodies are unique and essential; All bodies have strengths and needs that must be met; We are powerful, not despite the complexities of our bodies, but because of them; All bodies are confined by ability, race, gender, sexuality, class, nation state, religion, and more, and we cannot separate them" (p. 19). In this project, this ethos of Disability Justice was not only experienced through the relationships that were formed, but in the design process too. Ben, how did you, the student-designers and the collaborators engage with these principles in the design process?

Ben: When fashion design includes Disabled people, the design approach is often that of adaptive fashion. Here clothing originally designed for non-Disabled people is modified for Disabled wearers. This practice centres non-Disabled bodies as the starting place in the fashion design process, and then adapts these designs for Disabled bodies. While these adaptive features recognize the needs of Disabled bodies, these elements are often visually concealed in the overall design of garments and, as such, sanitize Disabled bodies for non-Disabled people. For example, the Tommy Hilfiger adaptive polo is designed with magnets along the front to open and close in the same way as a button-down shirt. This design feature supports ease of dress for people with limited mobility and dexterity. However, rather than making these closures visible, using this access feature as an aesthetic feature and celebrating Disability, the magnets are hidden inside the shirt and disguise the fact that the shirt is designed for Disabled people. Adaptive fashion design therefore does not embrace desire for Disability but instead views Disability as a problem that fashion design can conquer, solve, hide, and normalize. In contrast, Disabled designer Liz Jackson explains their crip approach to design, "Usually in design when people consider Disability, typically the goal is to smooth things out or to fix a thing. But for me, it's really about honoring the friction of Disability. Really thinking about what sort of creative opportunity Disability has to bring to design". (in Fonder 2019, n.p.). Our approach heeded Jackson's understanding by honouring the beauty and imagination of Disability experiences, and inviting desire for what Disability disrupts and generates into the design process and outcome.

Philippa: This crip approach was exemplified by our student-designer, Brigit, in the workshop with you, Kristina, and the collaborator Adam.[2]

Kristina: Absolutely, it was. It's important to note that when participating in this project, it's not the first time some of our collaborators have worked in a proudly crip space, specifically the visibly Disabled community members who cannot hide or camouflage their bodies through clothing or other means. For Adam, as for other visibly Disabled participants, the Disabled body has been the entry point to community. For them, to desire Disability is not a political act, but rather a tool for survival. To quote trans and Disabled scholar Syrus Marcus Ware (2017), "the desire for our Disabled kin is desire". For Adam, a power chair user working as an artist, desire was the centre of the hacking workshops. Adam wanted to make a worn-out jacket of Adam's favourite NHL hockey wearable again. Adam loved wearing this jacket out in public, as people would speak to Adam about the most recent game or even ask about the score if a game was happening. But the jacket was no longer wearable for Adam. Adam works with care attendants to dress each day, a practice that puts unexpected stress on the fabric and seams of the jacket's shoulders and arms. To be able to wear the jacket again would be an act of love, for Adam's team and body.

Adam worked with Brigit who had a keen interest in technology but had never worked with, or even engaged with, someone who looks like Adam, who moves through space like Adam. In our first meeting, Adam's Disabled body was proudly on display: Adam's face was close to the screen, the joystick of Adam's wheelchair obscuring a corner of the camera, and Adam's speech was non-normative in both sound and pace. Adam spoke about the way care attendants help dress Adam each day, mobility limitations, and Adam's favourite hockey team with the same type of pride. For Brigit, this was a jarring experience, highlighting that unless we are entrenched in the crip community, we rarely see crip pride. But Adam's pride is not unique. As Disability scholar Catherine Frazee notes, "Before we can begin to push back against injustice and indignity, before we can rise up from the swirl of rate and despair, before we can speak back to a script and that casts us as tragic victims and bitter villains, we must have pride" (Roman and Frazee 2014, p. 5). As Brigit moved through the design process, she designed to represent and desire Adam's pride in Adam's body and favourite hockey team. She removed the leather sleeves, replacing them with sleeves of a down filled bomber jacket and making them adjustable from underneath the arm, facilitating easier dressing. Brigit moved the team's logo from the back of the jacket to the front so it would not be obscured by Adam's chair, and then added other logos and symbols that Adam selected. Brigit integrated a micro-LED pixel thread that outlines the logos and lights up via a Bluetooth connection controlled by Adam's iPad. This is a jacket that demands to be seen, demands to be admired and desired. In wearing it, there is no hiding Adam's body, nor Adam's love for Adam's favourite hockey team —There is only to celebrate, to enshrine with love, to desire with pride.

Philippa: A very different example of this desire for Disability through fashion hacking was with the collaborator Sean and the student-designer Diego Ortega. The garment that these two created was one that reflects sort of a 'capital F fashion' aesthetic, something that feels rather avant-garde, and also celebrates the physicality of Sean's body. Ben, you worked with this pod.

Ben: It was an incredible hacking experience. Sean is a queer, East Asian visibly Disabled art curator with a very experimental fashion aesthetic. His hacked garment was a pair of voluminous jersey black pants that he never wore because the length did not work for his short, asymmetrical body. Sean's access needs require the garment to not constrain or constrict his body, but instead allow for an ease of mobility and an offering of comfort. Diego deconstructed the pants and draped the fabric into a top. The design did not force Sean's body into a particular shape or structure but allowed the garment to take the shape of his body. Moreover, the top has six possible openings for Sean's arms and head. It also has five yards of detachable chiffon that can go through these openings and can be shortened by buttoning it to a custom wristband (Figure 5). This modular design gives Sean agency to style the garment in a multitude of ways, create novel silhouettes, and centre comfort and mobility.

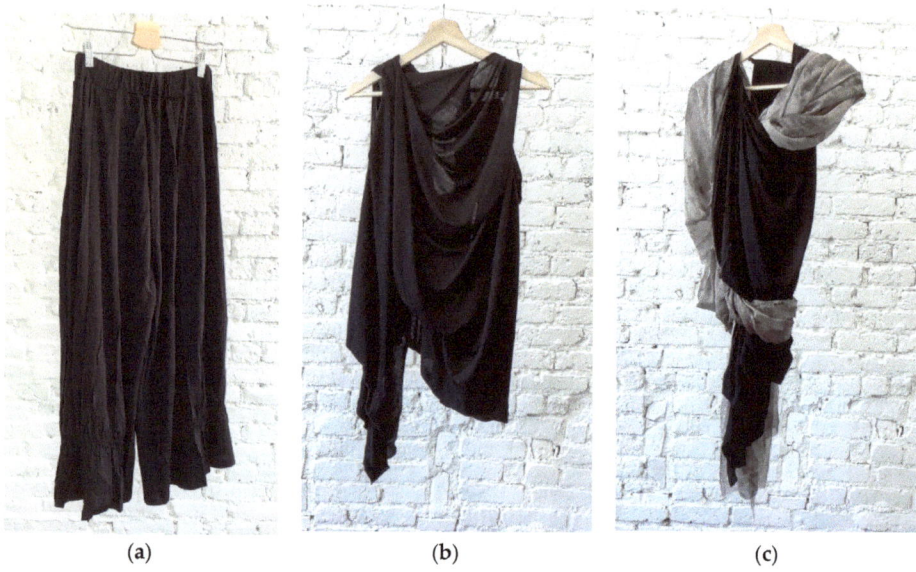

Figure 5. (**a**) Sean's original garment. The image shows a pair of black, wide-leg pants with an elastic waist on a metal clip hanger against a white painted brick wall. (**b**) Sean's hacked garment. The images shows a black, slightly sheer sleeveless top on a wooden hanger against a white brick wall. The top is drapey with a cowl neck. (**c**) A different styling option for Sean's hacked garment. The image shows a sleeveless garment on a wooden hanger against a white painted brick background. Grey material is woven into the right arm of a black sleeveless top, coming through the left arm and attaching at the bottom of the garment.

Ben: An important moment in this hacking exchange was when Sean shared his measurements with Diego. Diego originally sent Sean an illustration of a non-Disabled cis man's body that a tailor would use to collect measurements to make a suit. However, the illustration and requested measurements didn't reflect Sean's short and asymmetrical proportions. Sean redrew the illustration to mirror his body and sent it back to Diego (Figure 6). This intervention allowed the design process to honour Sean's body as the starting point in the design, desiring for the ways in which Sean's body would direct the garment.

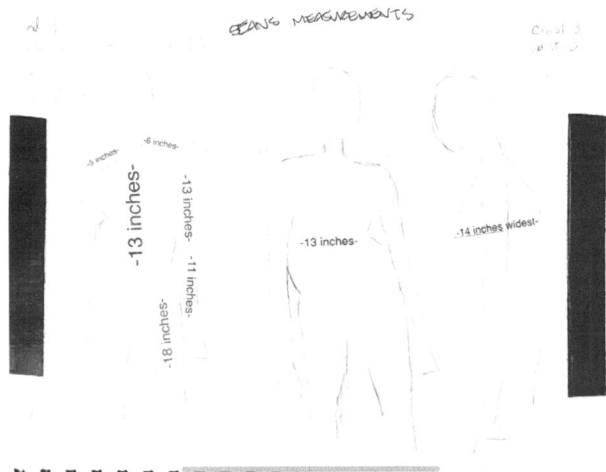

Figure 6. Sean's drawing of their body with measurements. At the top of the sketch reads "Sean's Measurements", with the measurements handwritten on either side of the text. The sketch shows three views of a body: a front view, a back view and a side view, with the relative measurements listed on top of the drawings.

9. Reflections on the Fashion Hacking Workshops

Kristina: One of the biggest challenges in these workshops was the balance of how much time there was to teach the students in the classroom through texts about Disability Justice and Disability Studies. We understood these texts to be formative to creating a space for our student-designer to be informed and collaborators to feel safe. This learning took space, and reduced how much time student-designers and collaborators had to work together, to develop relationships, share embodied knowledge through conversation, and ultimately hack garments.

As much as academic knowledge can be a tool of teaching, there are only so many readings you can give someone in the first six weeks of a course, and we can only hope that reading these works will shift everyone's perspective. There needed to be time dedicated to this, time for the students to understand what they were going into, as that knowledge generation does feed into the relationship building and the creation of the actual garments. While the time for hacking itself was limited by university time, it was also limited by the research teams' conception of what knowledge was necessary to foster interdependent relationships. University time became a problem because so much needed to be done in such a short amount of time. In a utopian world, the students would have met the collaborators earlier and had a longer time to develop relationships and make the garments. There was a consistent and paradoxical struggle between time to develop knowledge about theory and to develop relationships that require both an understanding of theory and a removal of time constraints to be generative and comfortable.

Jonathan: To build on that, groups that faced the most challenges were the ones where there was less of a connection, and so it didn't necessarily come down to the academic content that they were learning at the beginning of the course. While that content shared important knowledge, it was more so the connection of their lived experiences, or the desire to learn about these lived experiences and apply them in the context of the hacking workshops. As Mingus (2011) explains, access intimacy doesn't always come down to a person's political understanding of Disability or access— it's an elusive sense of someone "getting" your access needs. Those connections are what made both the collaborator and the student-designers want to go above and beyond, because there was an interpersonal value beyond the class grade.

Philippa: That's something I was thinking about as well, getting out of this mindset of this being just a class, which is a really hard thing to ask of students who are *in a class* and working for a grade. And Ben, as much as you fostered an environment that does work against those structures, it's hard for a student to get outside of that. It speaks not only to the academic system, but also to the fashion industry. These are students who are working toward a particular industry that is grounded on a restrictive ideal of time, or in 'fashion industry time' as you called it. Even though we had good relationships develop, it was hard to get some of the students out of that designer-client mindset rather than these interpersonal relationships; it was hard to get them to understand that part of making garments with their collaborators was getting to know them and their whole selves. Sins Invalid (2016) includes "recognizing wholeness" as one of their ten principles of Disability Justice. They explain, "Each person is full of history and life experience. Each person has an internal experience composed of our own thoughts, sensations, emotions, sexual fantasies, perceptions, and quirks. Disabled people are whole people" (Sins Invalid 2016, p. 24). To recognize the wholeness of the collaborators, we need time and space to work closely with them. This was possible in the first workshops that we had outside of the course, but less possible within the structure of the course and the university timeline of an academic term.

Ben: Going back to the experience of Aris and Birdie is important because our hacking workshops spanned different formats. Aris and Birdie worked with the same timeline as the course, but Aris wasn't a student in the course, so they had more flexibility. I think that understanding the differences of what we could do, what we couldn't do and how these different contexts changed relationships is valuable. Beyond that, I'm thinking a lot about this "versus" mindset you mention, Philippa. In the context of a course in a fashion design program, there is a critical perspective as well as an industry focus. There was this idea of designing for a client in the course, even though we tried to move away from it, but isn't there also value in that? I'm cautious to dismiss it as inherently negative. For example, I remember one student-designer sharing with me that they've never designed with or for an actual person in school – talking to them, learning about them and creating for them. It's valuable to gain experience designing for living, breathing humans with lived experiences and bodies who navigate the social world in different ways. Students were also not designing for people who have an idealized fashion body or who are wealthy and can afford custom clothing. There is value in learning about those experiences, designing with those experiences, and bringing those experiences with you in your future courses and career. Designing with and for Disabled people disrupts how design pedagogy typically operates in fashion school—The human body is absent, or if a human body is present, they are an idealized model who does not share their perspectives.

Philippa: I think this is something that happens so much in fashion for people who don't fit within that idealized fashion body. If you're outside of that ideal, it's considered peripheral or sub-cultural by the fashion industry. The fashion needs of people with embodied differences are met mostly in DIY spaces, or through movements that fall outside of the mainstream fashion industry. These are incredibly valuable spaces of resistance and community, and that shouldn't be diminished. But it's something that frustrates me with the ways that fashion is talked about, especially for Disabled bodies, where embodied differences are defined only as resistant. It is valuable to treat Disabled people as couture clients and offer access to custom fashion, having garments made specifically for bodyminds that are not always valued in the mainstream industry. There is value in showing students this reality as an industry practice. Some of the collaborators are people who want customized fashion in the same ways as those who are non-Disabled.

This came through with Max Q and Audrey Chou—their meetings were short, usually only ten minutes, even though we would put aside an hour. I tried to facilitate a deeper relationship between them, but they didn't seem to connect in a more personal way. Nonetheless, Audrey created this couture feeling piece for Max that reflected Max's identity (Figure 7). In the garment, Audrey included aspects of art that Max made, reflecting his work in the colours, textures and techniques that were part of the design. Audrey also included aspects of comfort that were essential to Max without foregoing the couture feeling of the piece. The relationship perhaps felt transactional in the beginning, but it resulted in this beautiful hacked piece. To me, their relationship and the final garment perfectly illustrated access intimacy where even in short meetings, Audrey got what Max's needs were and built that directly into the garment. This highlights that transactional relationships can, too, be cripped. While we encouraged deeper relationships between the student-designers and collaborators, these couldn't be forced, and in a case like Audrey and Max, it didn't seem to be necessary. Carrying with them lessons from Disability Justice activists, Disability studies scholarship, and the experiences of those with whom they collaborated, students can move forward in their work with an understanding of the need to centre Disability in their design practice, even in transactional relationships. It is important to distinguish that a lot of Disabled people don't want to participate in that fashion system, but there are also Disabled people who *do* want to participate but aren't welcome. It is important to show students that Disabled people can and should be part of the fashion industry.

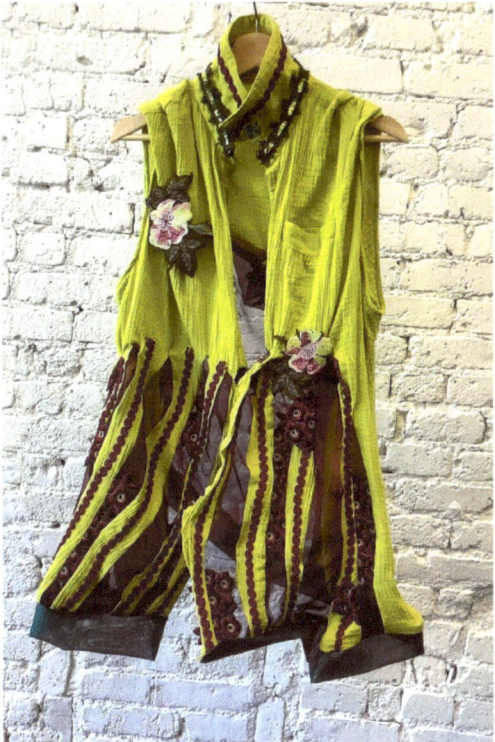

Figure 7. Max Q's finished garment. The image shows a bright green, long, sleeveless vest with a high neck on a wooden hanger against a painted white brick background. The neck is embellished with burgundy piping alongside silver and green piping that resembles a vine. The body of the vest is embellished with two white and pink textile flowers. The bottom half of the vest is a dark, sheer fabric overlaid with green textile and burgundy piping and embellished with clusters of small burgundy flowers.

Ben: I have been thinking about this Philippa—the impact of fashion hacking on students-designers and collaborators, and the bigger shifts that might come from them in the future. Collaborators have shared with us that they valued creating a garment that honours their bodyminds and through a process in which their intersectional Disability experiences were desired. That might not systemically transform the fashion industry or culture-at-large, but it impacts individuals. Collaborators emotionally carry and physically wear this experience with them in their everyday lives, and they can share these experiences with their communities.

As you shared Philippa, the students who participated in the course might bring the knowledge and practices that they learned into their other courses, and eventually into the fashion industry during their internships and when they finish school. I don't want to be too utopian about the changes that students might enact solely because of taking this course, but the fact that they will enter other fashion spaces opens up possibilities. For example, students might draw upon crip theory to centre the beauty of crip embodiments rather than assume non-Disabled embodiments as the standard when they design. They might recognize the fashion knowledge that comes from Disability experiences and subsequently intentionally heed and hire Disabled people when they work on projects about design and Disability. Students might introduce crip time into their design processes in order to slow-down tight scheduling, and they might engage with Disability Justice principles to expand one-dimensional understandings of Disability. Bringing these concepts—and others from this class—into their other university courses and workplaces can start to reduce stigma and cultivate new understandings among peers, faculty and colleagues and, eventually and slowly, transform practices in fashion education and the fashion industry.

Alexis: There are a lot of challenges that come with having classes like this—classes that offer different ways of knowing and then experiment with putting that into practice. These ways of knowing were in tension with other courses that the students were taking. Despite telling some students that they did not have to finish the project and to honour their bodymind's cues, they still told me they stayed up all night working and lost sleep. It is a slow build to break down dominant practices, but the fact that some practices, such as drawing on crip time and desiring Disability, actually manifested within this space, no matter how small, should be recognized.

Kristina: Another challenge was the disconnect that sometimes happened as a result of the project taking place virtually. I know it was impossible to all come together during a pandemic and while working in different locations, but there is a lot of embodied knowledge in actually sharing a physical space and sharing a material environment.

Ben: We were facilitating a material and embodied process virtually, but this format provided access for some collaborators who wouldn't have been able to visit campus. This opened up participation to take part in a fashion design that is typically an in-person experience.

Philippa: It would have also been so much easier for the student-designers and collaborators to do fittings on the body if they were together in the same space, as you talked about Kristina. At the same time, the virtual space was a site of so much possibility that we didn't foresee. For example, the virtual spaces allowed collaborators and student-designers to communicate and collaborate through the flexible and frequent scheduling of meetings, the intimacy of each person being in their own homes, the mitigation of safety and anxiety that may have come from traveling to and from an in-person space. I think it's difficult to say whether in-person or virtual or hybrid would be best in the future, but I do think the virtual format was both a benefit and a challenge.

Alexis: Further to that, there's no choice in the vulnerability that you hold when you're in a body. In a society embedded with white supremacy, I will always come into a space and be a racialized body. In a society entangled with ableism, Kristina will always come in with a visible, physical Disability. And that's something that can't be hidden at any time. Therefore, entering any new space means the possibility of subjecting oneself to harm, leaving one vulnerable. This isn't to say that online is better than in-person, but having the choice to be online can help some people navigate how vulnerable they want to be with themselves and their embodied experience. For example, I could choose to keep my camera off, and Kristina can meet from wherever she chooses to be. In a lot of ways, being online and being in the pandemic has allowed us to take on this space that a lot of Disability communities have always been occupying (Kafai 2021).

10. Conclusions

This article has articulated the practice of crip fashion hacking that fosters relational ways of designing fashion to centre intersectional crip experiences and decentre ableist logics. As explored in our dialogue, crip fashion hacking creates the conditions that foster flexibility of cripping time, collective access, interdependence, and desire for intersectional Disabled embodiments. More importantly, crip fashion hacking offers the possibility of fostering social justice beyond one's singular engagement in its practice. We recognize that not all collaborators and student-designers in our hacking workshops finished with the experiences, resources or desire to implement their crip fashion learnings. However, we are hopeful that some collaborators might carry out future alterations of their garments and share their learnings with their communities, and some student-designers might centre intersectional crip embodiments in their future fashion design practices. As adrienne maree brown (2017) observes, "What we practice at the small scale sets the patterns for the whole system" (p. 53). In this way, the learnings and skills developed in our workshops can be practiced in spaces in the future, re-making fashion paradigms and re-making worlds. We invite educators, researchers, and fashion professionals to explore using crip fashion hacking by desiring with and for communities who are marginalized by the dominant systems.

For those who wish to try out crip fashion hacking, we encourage reflection about the benefits of different workshop formats. Prior to developing the course, we conducted one-on-one virtual workshops between a small number of participants and research team members. These workshops did not have the time restraints of a university course, and therefore provided the space and pace for collaborators and research team members to develop relationships by working slowly on alterations together on Zoom over a few months. Strong, intimate and interdependent relationships were formed—some of which lasted beyond the scope of the project. These relationships took on aspects of collective access, or what many Disability Justice activists refer to as care webs: these complex webs and small exchanges that resist concepts of charity and favour care (Lakshmi Piepzna-Samarasinha 2018). Beyond sharing skills and hacking clothing, the participants and research team members shared images and memes over social media that brought them joy, and they exchanged physical notes and handmade items unrelated to the project. They were also conscious of each other's time and changing capacity. As we implemented the hacking workshops within a university course, we intended to continue the focus on fostering relationships through the facilitation of virtual meetings, check-ins and other exchanges. However, we quickly learned that interdependent, intimate relationships are impossible to manufacture. We could not insist that student-designers and collaborators engage with each other in a particular way, or expect that they would fully engage in collective access and interdependence. While some groups developed meaningful relationships during the course, other groups did not. It was difficult for this not to feel like a failure, as we had seen it work well in past workshops. However, we observed that less intimate relationships in our fashion hacking workshops still cripped transactional relationships that typically occur during adaptive fashion design because our workshops centred intersectional crip embodiments. Our hacking workshops led to the creation of custom garments that were accessible, fashionable and desirable—pieces that reflected the embodiments of collaborators but that were created in conditions that we initially wanted to resist. We learned that the intimacy that we were perhaps trying to force was not always necessary to honour intersectional crip experiences with fashion design.

Conducting our fashion hacking workshops virtually led to both benefits and challenges. Disabled people have long engaged in online communities in order to resist the loneliness and isolation that comes from living in an ableist world. Many virtual spaces have fostered Disabled queer-of-colour activism and Disability Justice practices (Kafai 2021; Lakshmi Piepzna-Samarasinha 2021). The virtual fashion hacking spaces illuminated the creativity of our Disabled collaborators, who came up with imaginative ways to share inspiration, workarounds for sharing custom measurements and alternative ways of collaborating when Zoom fatigue set-in. However, we also recognize the beauty and vitality that can come from coming together in a physical space, and the opportunities that in-person workshops may have had for building communities of Disabled people with shared interest in fashion and fashion design. Perhaps the embodied knowledge that arises from a material environment was lost in the virtual space. We look forward to exploring what we can differently experience through crip fashion hacking during the next iteration of shorter, in-person workshops.

The start of each section of this article has begun with pieces of a poem. As we shared in the introduction, one objective of this article is to think through our learnings from crip fashion hacking through dialogue—a format that might creatively re-make how we do academic analysis and writing. We endeavored to experiment with format not only by using dialogue but also by crafting a poem. Our poem was inspired by our wardrobe interview with the collaborator Cam who shared: "Picking out clothes is a spiritual process for me. It's touching the clothing and saying hi to it and being like, do you work? . . . It's like holding hands with someone. I'm holding hands with my Disability and have this other free hand. Could I hold the hand of someone who's barking angrily at the other person? Or I could hold the hand of someone who's loving towards them". Grounded in Cam's words, we have collectively written this poem as a research team to share how we have experienced the ways in which crip fashion hacking re-makes worlds that centre desire for intersectional crip embodiments and resist ableist logics of the fashion industry.

I'm Holding Hands with my Disability

I'm holding hands with my Disability
I have the other hand free
Could I hold the hand of someone who fights me?
Or I could hold the hand of someone who loves me?
Holding is loving, caring
To hold hands is for someone to hold it back
given and received at our own pace
given and received willingly and eagerly.
To hold with mutual desire

Holding hands in all the ways we can
The form taking different shapes
with all the fingers or none of the fingers
All of the glorious ways our genders, races and sexualities
meet our stutters, disassociations and aches

I'm holding hands with my Disability
I'm holding hands with my clothes
I have the other hand free
Could I use that hand to throw it away?
Or could I use that hand to mend it?

Palms touching
Holding all of it
All of our bodies-minds-spirits
All of the kinships and fabrics that embrace them, embrace us

Thank you for holding my hand.

Author Contributions: Conceptualization, B.B., A.D.V., J.D., K.M. and P.N.; formal analysis, B.B., A.D.V., J.D., K.M. and P.N.; writing—original draft preparation, B.B., A.D.V., J.D., K.M. and P.N.; writing—review and editing, B.B. and P.N.; supervision, B.B.; project administration, P.N.; funding acquisition, B.B. and Megan Strickfaden. All authors have read and agreed to the published version of the manuscript.

Funding: This research was funded by The Social Science and Humanities Research Council of Canada (SSHRC) Insight Grant #435-2019-1231, The SSHRC Partnership Sub-Grant #895-2016-1024, The New School General Research Funds, and The New School Student Assistant Research Fund.

Institutional Review Board Statement: This research project was approved by the Research Ethics Board of Toronto Metropolitan University (REB# 2019-406), the Research Ethics Board of the University of Alberta (REB# Pro00097341), and The New School (BRANY File #23-063-1244).

Informed Consent Statement: All participants in this research project have given their informed consent for inclusion prior to their participation in the project.

Acknowledgments: We are grateful to the participants who collaborated in the project by sharing their experiences, wisdom, and creativity, and for collaborating with us on these garments. We thank the fashion hacking design support team, Aris Cinti, Madison Hollamon, Diego Ortega, Alex Piefer and Kishan Tehara, and all the students who participated in hacking these garments. We also thank co-investigator Megan Strickfaden for her support in project.

Conflicts of Interest: The authors declare no conflict of interest.

Notes

[1] In the article, we intentionally capitalize D in Disability and Disabled as political acts that proudly centre these terms as a culture and identity respectively. Similarly, we capitalize the first letters of Disability Justice to honour the labour, work and impact of the Disability Justice movement and the Black, Indigenous and People of Colour Disabled activists who founded it.

[2] Adam uses Adam as pronouns. Adam's decision intends to resist the de-humanization that Disabled people experience.

References

Barry, Ben. 2019. Fabulous Masculinities: Refashioning the Fat and Disabled Male Body. *Fashion Theory* 23: 275–307. [CrossRef]
brown, adrienne maree. 2017. *Emergent Strategy: Shaping Change, Changing Culture*. Chico: AK Press.
Chen, Mel Y. 2014. Brain fog: The Race for Cripistemology. *Journal of Literary & Cultural Disability Studies* 8: 171–84.
Critical Axis. n.d. World's First Adaptive Deodorant. Available online: https://www.criticalaxis.org/critique/worlds-first-adaptive-deodorant/ (accessed on 19 July 2022).
Crooks, Valorie A., Michelle Owen, and Sharon-Dale Stone. 2012. Creating a (More) Reflexive Canadian Disability Studies. *Canadian Journal of Disability Studies* 1: 45–65. [CrossRef]
Cubacub, Sky. 2019. Radical Visibility: A QueerCrip Dress Reform Movement Manifesto (Abridged). *Radical Visibility Zine*. Available online: http://rebirthgarments.com/radical-visibility-zine (accessed on 19 July 2022).
England, Kim V. L. 1994. Getting personal: Reflexivity, Positionality, and Feminist Research. *The Professional Geographer* 46: 80–89. [CrossRef]
Fonder, Alison. 2019. Liz Jackson Doesn't Want 'Design for Disability'—She Wants Disabled People to Be Part of Designing Better Products. Core77. August 1. Available online: https://www.core77.com/posts/89571/Liz-Jackson-Doesnt-Want-Design-for-Disability---She-Wants-Disabled-People-to-Be-Part-of-Designing-Better-Products (accessed on 12 July 2022).
Fritsch, Kelly. 2016. Accessible. In *Keywords for Radicals: The Contested Vocabulary of Late Capitalist Struggle*. Edited by Kelly Fritsch, Clare O'Connor and AK Thompson. Chico: AK Press, pp. 23–28.
Garland Thomson, Rosemarie. 2011. Misfits: A Feminist Materialist Disability Concept. *Hypatia: A Journal of Feminist Philosophy* 26: 591–609. [CrossRef]
Haggerty, Kevin D. 2003. Review essay: Ruminations on Reflexivity. *Current Sociology* 51: 153–62. [CrossRef]
Hamraie, Aimi. 2017. *Building Access: Universal Design and the Politics of Disability*. Minneapolis: University of Minnesota Press.
Hamraie, Aimi, and Kelly Fritsch. 2019. Crip Technoscience Manifesto. *Catalyst: Feminism, Theory, Technoscience* 5: 1–34. [CrossRef]
hooks, bell. 1994. *Teaching to Transgress*. New York: Routledge.
Kafai, Shayda. 2021. *Crip Kinship: The Disability Justice and Art Activism of Sins Invalid*. Vancouver: Arsenal Pulp Press.
Kafer, Alison. 2013. *Feminist, Queer, Crip*. Bloomington: Indiana University Press.
Lakshmi Piepzna-Samarasinha, Leah. 2018. *Care Work: Dreaming Disability Justice*. Vancouver: Arsenal Pulp Press.
Lakshmi Piepzna-Samarasinha, Leah. 2021. How Disabled Mutual Aid Is Different than Abled Mutual Aid. Disability Visibility Project. Available online: https://Disabilityvisibilityproject.com/2021/10/03/how-Disabled-mutual-aid-is-different-than-abled-mutual-aid/ (accessed on 1 July 2022).

Lewis, Talia A. 2022. Working Definition of Ableism—January 2022 Update. Tu[r]ning into Self. Available online: http://www.talilalewis.com/1/post/2022/01/working-definition-of-ableism-january-2022-update.html (accessed on 15 July 2022).

McGregor, Hannah, Cheryl Ball, and Carla Rice. 2020. Bonus Episode: Season 3 Peer Review of Secret Feminist Agenda. Secret Feminist Agenda. Podcast Audio. Available online: https://secretfeministagenda.com/2020/04/07/bonus-episode-season-3-peer-review-of-secret-feminist-agenda/ (accessed on 15 July 2022).

McRuer, Robert. 2006. *Crip theory: Cultural Signs of Queerness and Disability*. New York: NYU Press.

Meyer, Manu. 2008. Indigenous and authentic: Hawaiian epistemology and the triangulation of meaning. In *Handbook of Critical and Indigenous Methodologies*. Edited by Norman K. Denzin, Yvonna S. Lincoln and Linda Tuhiwai Smith. London: Sage, pp. 217–232.

Mingus, Mia. 2011. Access Intimacy: The Missing Link. Leaving Evidence. Available online: https://leavingevidence.wordpress.com/2011/05/05/access-intimacy-the-missing-link/ (accessed on 18 June 2022).

Mingus, Mia. 2017. Access Intimacy, Interdependence and Disability Justice. Leaving Evidence. Available online: https://leavingevidence.wordpress.com/2017/04/12/access-intimacy-interdependence-and-Disability-justice/ (accessed on 18 June 2022).

Mingus, Mia. 2018. 'Disability Justice' Is Simply Another Term for Love. Leaving Evidence. Available online: https://leavingevidence.wordpress.com/2018/11/03/Disability-justice-is-simply-another-term-for-love/ (accessed on 29 July 2022).

Mitchell, David, and Sharon Snyder. 2015. *The Biopolitics of Disability: Neoliberalism, Ablenationalism and Peripheral Embodiment*. Ann Arbor: University of Michigan Press.

Mulholland, Monique. 2019. Sexy and Sovereign? Aboriginal Models Hit the "Multicultural Mainstream". *Cultural Studies* 33: 198–222. [CrossRef]

Payne, Alice. 2021. *Designing Fashion's Future: Present Practice and Tactics for Sustainable Change*. London: Bloomsbury.

Price, Margaret. 2011. *Mad at School: Rhetorics of Mental Disability and Academic Life*. Ann Arbor: University of Michigan Press.

Reid, Jenna. 2022. Crip Times Episode 9: The Jenna Reid Episode. Crip Times. Podcast audio. Available online: https://bodiesintranslation.ca/crip-times-episode-9-the-jenna-reid-episode/ (accessed on 24 July 2022).

Roman, Leslie G., and Catherine Frazee. 2014. Launch of The Unruly Salon Series at the University of British Columbia Green College. *Review of Disability Studies* 5: 1–7.

Samuels, Ellen. 2017. Six Ways of Looking at Crip Time. *Disability Studies Quarterly* 5. [CrossRef]

Sins Invalid. 2016. *Skin, Tooth and Bone—The Basis of Movement is Our people: A Disability Justice Primer*. San Francisco: Sins Invalid.

Sockbeson, Rebecca. 2009. Waponahki Intellectual Tradition of Weaving Educational Policy. *Alberta Journal of Educational Research* 55: 351–64.

von Busch, Otto. 2009. *Becoming Fashionable: Hacktivism and Engaged Fashion Design*. Philadelphia: Camino.

Ware, Syrus Marcus. 2017. Sit With the Discomfort. Filmed May 31, 2013 at The Walrus Talks National Tour: We Desire a Better Country, Toronto, ON. Video, 9:17. Available online: https://www.youtube.com/watch?v=DhMosU68N68 (accessed on 22 June 2022).

Williamson, Bess. 2019. *Accessible America: A History of Disability and Design*. New York: NYU Press.

Wilson, Shawn. 2008. *Research Is Ceremony: Indigenous Research Methods*. Halifax: Fernwood Publishing.

Wong, Zara. 2013. What Is Resort and Why Is It Important—Pre-Collections Explained. *Vogue*. Available online: https://www.vogue.com.au/fashion/news/what-is-resort-and-why-is-it-important-precollections-explained/news-story/2cfc8b69a857a5a1776ae44e5075950f (accessed on 1 July 2022).

Disclaimer/Publisher's Note: The statements, opinions and data contained in all publications are solely those of the individual author(s) and contributor(s) and not of MDPI and/or the editor(s). MDPI and/or the editor(s) disclaim responsibility for any injury to people or property resulting from any ideas, methods, instructions or products referred to in the content.

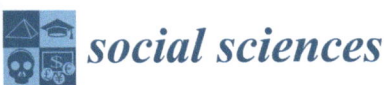

Article

Performing Fat Liberation: Pretty Porky and Pissed Off's Affective Politics and Archive

Allison Taylor [1,*], Allyson Mitchell [2] and Carla Rice [1]

1. Re•Vision: The Centre for Art and Social Justice, University of Guelph, Guelph, ON N1G 2W1, Canada
2. School of Gender, Sexuality and Women's Studies, York University, Toronto, NE M3J 1P3, Canada
* Correspondence: ataylo60@uoguelph.ca

Abstract: This article uses collaborative auto/ethnography to explore the circulation and potentiality of affect in the live performances and archive of Pretty Porky and Pissed Off (PPPOd), a Toronto-based queer fat activist performance art collective active during the late 1990s and mid-2000s. Drawing on video and audio recordings of five PPPOd performances alongside other performance ephemera and a series of conversations relating to these archival objects among the article's three authors, we identify and theorize our affective responses to and situated recollections of these performances, both in their current form as archival objects and as historical live events. We argue that PPPOd's archival objects/live performances disrupt the constellation of affects that constitute fat hate (e.g., fear, loathing, shame) and set in motion more affirmative affects (e.g., playfulness, pride, desire, love) that contribute to micro-worldings and prefigurative fat politics, as ephemeral as these might be. In capturing these fleeting moments of radical possibility, PPPOd's activism and archive offer opportunities for touching and feeling a future where fat lives are more livable.

Keywords: fat; archive; art; fat activism; affect; Pretty Porky and Pissed Off; performance art; queer; world-making; fat hatred

1. Introduction

This article engages with the artful politics of Pretty Porky and Pissed Off (PPPOd), a Toronto-based queer fat activist performance art collective that was active from the late 1990s to the mid-2000s. We use a carnal methodology focused on bodily experiences and sensations such as feeling and touching, explored via collaborative auto/ethnographic insights from live performances and affective analyses of the collective's archive, to get closer to the affects circulating during PPPOd performances and their effects on performers and audiences, emphasizing the potential of fat performance art to disrupt and transform sensory (e.g., felt, tactile, kinesthetic) experiences of fat. Drawing on video and audio recordings of five PPPOd performances alongside other performance ephemera[1] and conversations relating to these archival objects among the three authors of this article, we theorize our affective responses to and situated recollections of these performances, both in their current form as archival objects and as historical live events. Teasing out the affects produced by these archival objects/live performances, we meditate on the force of affect in determining the transformative potential of fat performance art to activate new and vibrant sensory fields surrounding fatness. Rather than offering grand claims about all fat performance, we remain tangibly focused on the artifacts from five performances by PPPOd, getting close to, touching, and feeling these archival objects and moments in time. Our investigation into the force of PPPOd's fat performance activism finds that the archival objects/live performances disrupt the constellation of affects that constitute fat hate (e.g., fear, loathing, shame) and set in motion more affirmative affects (e.g., playfulness, pride, desire) that contribute to micro-worldings and prefigurative fat politics, as ephemeral as these might be.

Citation: Taylor, Allison, Allyson Mitchell, and Carla Rice. 2023. Performing Fat Liberation: Pretty Porky and Pissed Off's Affective Politics and Archive. *Social Sciences* 12: 270. https://doi.org/10.3390/socsci12050270

Academic Editor: Nigel Parton

Received: 16 November 2022
Revised: 29 March 2023
Accepted: 30 March 2023
Published: 2 May 2023

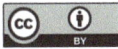

Copyright: © 2023 by the authors. Licensee MDPI, Basel, Switzerland. This article is an open access article distributed under the terms and conditions of the Creative Commons Attribution (CC BY) license (https://creativecommons.org/licenses/by/4.0/).

2. Context

From the late 1990s to the early 2000s, Pretty Porky and Pissed Off (PPPOd) a fat activist and performance art collective, based in Toronto, Canada, aimed to set its audiences on fire—to incite a "queen sized revolt." PPPOd consisted of core members Allyson Mitchell, Tracy Tidgwell, Zoe Whittall, Lisa Ayuso, Joanne Huffa, Abi Slone, and Mariko Tamaki with contributions from many others, including Gillian Bell and Ruby Rowan. From producing and performing shows centered on fat dance and drag across southwestern Ontario, to direct actions and teach-ins where they passed out flyers and treats to highlight the issues of fat hate and their effects on those who embody fatness; to developing zines, writing articles, and engaging in other cultural production to resist fat hatred; to hosting fat girl clothing swaps; to lecturing and leading workshops on size acceptance, PPPOd sought to bring fat people together in politicized, fat-affirmative spaces and offered fat people and their experiences greater visibility and "new possibilities for imagining fat" (Cooper 2016, p. 69). Within the fat studies literature, PPPOd has often been celebrated as a germinal example of Euro-Western queer fat feminist activism (Cooper 2016; Ellison 2020; Johnson and Taylor 2008; Rice 2014, 2015; Tidgwell et al. 2018).

The *Archiving the Ephemeral History of Pretty Porky and Pissed Off* (*Archiving PPPOd*) research project preserves PPPOd's legacy. Led by Allyson Mitchell, with the support of Allison Taylor, the project sources a range of materials—including audio and video recordings of events, interviews, and meetings; print materials such as posters, meeting notes, and creative writing; and objects such as visual art, crafts, swag, and costumes—from group members and affiliated community members and partners. These materials are largely unconventional, informal, and personal, and many of the items capture the ephemeral. The materials have been digitized, and Taylor and Mitchell are currently working towards making them publicly accessible via an online archive. With funding through the SSHRC Partnership Grant, *Bodies in Translation, Activist Art, Technology, and Access to Life* (BIT), this archival project takes interest in the potential of activist arts to provoke social, cultural, and political transformation—or world-making. With the support of grant co-directors Carla Rice and Eliza Chandler and research associates, in particular former PPPOd member Tracy Tidgwell, at the *Re•Vision Centre for Art and Social Justice* (University of Guelph), the *Archiving PPPOd* project offers a rare glimpse at the possibilities engendered by archives created *by* and *for* fat activists and scholars.

The *Archiving PPPOd* project finds theoretical footholds in Ann Cvetkovich's (2003) work on the gay and lesbian archive, which conceives of how the archive might exceed "conventional forms of documentation, representation, and commemoration" (7), because fat people, like queers, have struggled to preserve our histories "in the face of institutional neglect" (8). Because "symbolic annihilation" largely characterizes the representations of fat people in mainstream archives, assembling unconventional, informal, personal, and ephemeral materials on fat activists and activisms into a "fat community archive" safeguards against the systemic erasure of fat resistance from the historical record (Pratt 2018, p. 236). A fat activist archive also makes it possible to map out how, in different times and places, fat people "conceive of our collective past, how we understand and record our present, and how we imagine our futures" (Pratt 2018, p. 236). While Pratt's (2018) work is a jumping off point for us in framing this article, it is important to note that there are exciting fat activist materials available in Canadian archives such as the Toronto ArQuives, Library and Archives Canada, and the Canadian Women's Movement Archive in Ottawa. Fat activist materials are also held in U.S. archives, including the Schlesinger Library at Harvard, the Mazer Archives in Hollywood, the Lesbian Herstory Archives in Brooklyn, and the John J. Wilcox Archives in Philadelphia, to name a few. Each of these repositories makes it possible to trace fragments of past fat activism. However, not all of the named archives digitize their materials or make them available online and some of these archives exist in institutions of higher education with complex infrastructures that may make access intimidating or off-putting to those who are not attached to universities.

The collection of objects in the PPPOd archive includes many of the historical and root texts influencing this group, as well as the objects and texts that they themselves created (e.g., zines and a special guest edited issue of the magazine *Fireweed*). Further, the archive contains the process-based ephemera that the group used to conceptualize as well as reflect on the art they were making, and the direct action and teaching that they were undertaking. For example, the archive contains performance documentation, brainstorming notes, video documentation in change rooms before performances, and recorded conversations after performances. The archival documentation also includes video, audio, and photographic recordings of meetings that may help future researchers to understand more deeply (and affectively, as we argue) the intentions, failings, triumphs, day-to-day administrivia, and even drudgery, of art and activist processes. Adding another layer, the archive also contains documentation of television spotlights and radio interviews that indicate how PPPOd's work was being represented in popular media at the time. This complex gathering of materials offers multiple entry points and perspectives into PPPOd's history and allows for complex insights in analysis.

In our affect-suffused encounters with the PPPOd artifacts, we acknowledge that archival objects "represent far more than the literal value of the objects themselves" (Cvetkovich 2003, p. 268), because they produce a range of emotive experiences, from melancholy, nostalgia, and indignation, to comradery, disappointment, and fantasy. As we demonstrate in this article, these affects are central to the world-making potential of the PPPOd archive. We theorize the flows of affects coursing through our bodies as we interact with PPPOd archival materials by drawing on Sara Ahmed's (2004a) socio-political exploration of the work of affect in creating, sustaining, subverting, and resisting cultural economies, both hegemonic and counter cultural. Rather than orienting to emotions as internal psychic states—as perceptions and sensations originating from and contained within bodies—Ahmed (2008) understands emotions as "sociable" if nebulous forces that arise from and circulate through our embodied relations in the world, which move us to feel with, for, and against others. Here emotion indivisibly entangles with cognition for, as Ahmed notes "to hate or to fear is to have a judgment about a thing as it approaches" (Schmitz and Ahmed 2014, p. 99); and the judgment-tinged affects generated in cultural encounters across power and difference help to establish the sensory boundaries and relationalities of bodies and collectivities. Emotions thus circulate between individual and social bodies, binding certain people together and casting others out of the body politic; and emotions are powerful in mediating knowledge, influencing what knowledge gets produced and which claims to truth are accepted, greeted with ambivalence, or denied/opposed (Ahmed 2004b; see also Rice et al. 2022b). Ahmed's monist understanding of affective economies as entangled emotive-cognitive forces that are socially shaped and acquire intensity as they circulate helps to explain why fat (and non-fat) peoples become attached to hegemonic and oppressive knowledge; and it also explains why, given their corporeality, emotions stigmatizing fatness are difficult to cast off. As we narrate our carnal (i.e., embodied and felt) encounters with archival objects, we invite readers to feel the clashing affects surrounding fatness that PPPOd performances set in motion, and vicariously experience how the group artfully received and remade these affects through performer-audience encounters (see Hoang (2018) for further discussion of carnal methods).

3. Methodology

We engaged with five recordings (four video and one audio) from the PPPOd archive that document moments of live PPPOd performances. Each of us watched and listened to these independently, and then we met together over Zoom four times to discuss our layered responses. The discussions centered on our intimate contact with each object, generating visceral descriptions ripe with the feelings, sensations, and memories that we collectively analyzed. After stewing in the affects the artifacts stirred up, we reflected on our different positions in relation to the archive materials and the collective as a whole, and how these positionalities affected our engagements with the archival objects: Mitchell as a producer-artist creating and participating in the performances, Carla Rice as a fangirl and audience member at performances, and Taylor as a next-generation researcher viewing the recorded performances a number of years later. We recorded and transcribed our discussions and analyzed the transcripts using thematic analysis (Braun and Clarke 2006). Threaded throughout our discussion are insights derived from "performance autoethnography" (Chalklin 2016a), by which we mean Mitchell's critically reflexive recollections of "the affective, intersubjective and corporeal levels of experience" (Chalklin 2012, p. 110) generated whilst viewing the PPPOd performances. This is layered with Rice's felt memories of participating in the performances as a fat activist and PPPOd follower, and Taylor's emotive experiences of watching these historical performances in the present moment. To better reflect our weaving together of both audience and performer recollections, we refer to this aspect of our method as a *collaborative* performance auto/ethnography. What follows is an experimental attempt to describe and theorize our carnal encounters—emphasizing the felt, visceral, and material—with the selected artifacts from the PPPOd archive. By attending closely to our affective encounters with these ephemeral, digital objects, we aim to enhance, nuance, and deepen our embodied readings of the archive, and provide readers with a different mode of engagement with artifacts than that which is typically offered in archival research.

4. The Artifacts

4.1. Blubber

Blubber was a body positive cabaret put together by PPPOd, sponsored by the Wellington Dufferin-Guelph Eating Disorders Coalition and performed at the River Run Centre in Guelph, Ontario in February 2001. The video documentation[2] starts with emcee Roy Mitchell provoking and rousing the audience members with promises of boundary-pushing performances by PPPOd, locally-known performance artists, writers, musicians and poets, a fan-favorite drag king troupe, and the musicians Queen Size Shag. What unfolds on the footage is an hour-long show featuring a dozen or so performers and over 100 fans shouting, laughing, hooting, and dancing to a curated playlist, films, songs, jokes, choreographed performances, poems, stories, and live drawing projections, alongside a craft sale of items made specifically for the event. PPPOd named the show *Blubber* to pay homage to and reclaim the young adult novel of the same title by Judy Blume which was popular in the 1970s, when the troupe members were growing up. PPPOd prefaces the show by contextualizing how the book was one of the only representations of fat (white) girls in popular culture that several members of the group could relate to with its bittersweet representation of othering, bullying, and self-realization.

4.2. Big Judy

PPPOd mounted *Big Judy*, another cabaret-style show at George Brown College in Toronto, Ontario on 23 and 24 March 2004.[3] Arts curator Anna Camellari, working for the Mayworks Festival of Working People, invited PPPOd to develop and present this show for several Toronto venues, including George Brown College, York University, and Buddies in Bad Times Theatre, the self-proclaimed largest and longest-running queer theatre in the world. A grant from the Canada Council for the Arts supported the show's development and presentation. PPPOd members borrowed the title, *Big Judy*, from the name given to the "plus size" mannequins used for fashion design at the time. As a performance, *Big Judy* takes shape as a composite of the mostly white collective's most translatable and dramatic coming-of-age experiences, and as a character, Big Judy comes alive as a singular fat girl whose life experiences the collective knits together from relatable or affecting autobiographical vignettes. The scenarios follow a chronological order of fat experiences, such as bullying in the schoolyard, fat shaming by a mother in a change room, visions of pop star fame, and dreams of fulfilling careers, friendships, and queer love affairs. The live performance consists of accumulative storytelling through soliloquies by each troupe member which are stitched together with choreographed dances using props such as mannequins, skipping ropes, music, and slides. Kaleb Robertson choreographed the dances and co-shot the video documentation with Lukas Blakk.

4.3. Double Double

PPPOd originally performed the show *Double Double* at Toronto's Buddies in Bad Times Theatre on 9 November 2002, following this up with another performance at the MIX underground film festival in New York City on 23 November 2002 as part of the *Baby Got Back* fat film program. Christina Zeidler shot the video documentation.[4] As we discuss the artifact's contents, Rice recalls attending the show when it was staged at Buddies Theatre, the archival video telescoping her back to being a spectator, whooping, whistling, laughing, clapping, and stamping in sync with the raucous crowd whose collective energy to dislodge and defeat fat hate seemed boundless on that riotous night. Dwelling in the affect-tinged recollection that still sends shivers down her spine, she realizes that this was one of the first shows to introduce her to the affective power of fat performance.

4.4. NOLOSE

The archive also contains video documentation[5] of PPPOd and King Size performance troupe members as they journey to perform at the National Organization for Lesbians of Size Everywhere (NOLOSE). Originating as an organization exclusively for lesbians of size, NOLOSE had expanded into a community of fat queer and trans people seeking to end fat oppression when they invited PPPOd to perform at their semi-annual conference in Chery Hill, New Jersey from 7–11 July 2004. Archival documentation of the event includes unscripted footage of the road trip to NOLOSE punctuated by singing, dancing, eating, flirting, and crosstalk in the two-car queer convoy travelling from Toronto to New Jersey and back, with dance sequence rehearsals in gas stations and picnics at various pit stops along the way. The footage also captures the PPPOd NOLOSE live performance, which they titled *Slim Down Road Show*, with members Tracy Tidgwell, Allyson Mitchell, and Kaleb Robertson, as well as performances by King Size. Gigi Basanta documented the performance. The performance video stitches together choreographed dance pieces and lip sync performances and features a special collaborative tap dance number choreographed by Keith Cole and performed by PPPOd and King Size to Eminem's *Lose Yourself*. The video also contains footage of various conference events and moments of unscripted conversations, where a mic carrying PPPOd member cheekily interviews random conference attendees about their thoughts and impressions on PPPOd's and King Size's performances. The comments from the pumped-up attendees echo Rice's affective experiences of PPPOd performances: attendees not only delight in PPPOd's commitment to their craft, but they also revel in PPPOd's commitment to shattering the false and limiting assumptions about what a fat body can be and do. The footage ends with documentation of the road trip returning to Toronto, culminating in a picnic in a field off the highway as the sun sets and the travelers' snack, feed each other suggestively, mug for the camera, and hang out.

4.5. Sudbury Super-Size Sunday Night

Also part of the archive are audio recordings[6] of PPPOd members processing their performance of *Sudbury Super-Size Sunday Night* at Thornloe University Theatre at Laurentian University in Sudbury, Ontario on 30 November 2003; their workshop *Using Your Body to Make Social Change* for the *Myths and Mirrors* Youth Theatre Group also held in Sudbury on that date; and their invited guest lecture for an undergraduate Women's Studies course sponsored by Professor Suzanne Luhmann and the Department of Women's Studies at Laurentian on 1 December 2003. During the recording, the crew eats lunch with Dr. Luhmann and two students from the undergraduate class they spoke to. The guests and hosts discuss the PPPOd members' experiences of publicly performing to a lukewarm audience the night before and then presenting to a more warmed-up class of undergraduate students the next day. They banter about the food they eat and their experiences in the classroom and theatre.

This artifact is especially intriguing given that it is accompanied by two other objects: email exchanges between dissatisfied audience members and PPPOd after the performance.

5. Analysis

5.1. Fat Hatred

Rinaldi et al. (2020) argue that "fat hatred circulates as an affective economy ... it flows across, attaches to, and comes to define or value different bodies" (37). While fat hatred is nefarious and omnipresent, it can be difficult to pinpoint or identify. In most documentation of PPPOd performances the audience is seemingly on board and supportive. Mitchell recalls audience responses ranging from loud applause and laughter in the right places to uproarious screaming and whooping. Rice remembers being in those audiences and participating in performances with wild abandon. However, Mitchell also recalls moments when audiences were not on side. Amongst rowdy crowds some attendees engaged in back talk and made snide remarks expressing distaste. Most frequently these moments happened when PPPOd performed for captive audiences in spaces such as classrooms, where attendees could not always choose to opt out without consequence. Mitchell describes how these audiences at times met PPPOd performances with confusion and discomfort that morphed into disgust and dismissal. She recalls one classroom performance of *Big Judy* that felt like the young people were thinking something along the lines of "what the fuck? This is stupid, this is gross, who are these old ladies?"

It is in the archive's artifacts that the fat hatred circulating in PPPOd's activism becomes especially clear. In the audio documentation of PPPOd members debriefing the *Sudbury Super-Size Sunday Night* event with the co-sponsoring professor and students, we hear performers and hosts wonder about the audience's coldness, which seemed to form an invisible wall of sullenness in response to the performance. And, shortly after the performance, PPPOd members received emails from two disgruntled audience members. The critiques issued by both were that the dances were unprofessional, the performers failed to memorize their lines, and that they, as theatre patrons, did not "get" the message of the performance. One writes in their email that PPPOd's performance was not "celebratory" or educational enough, stating, "I left [the performance] feeling like I witnessed a group telling us they are angry and there was no sense of closure ... They are pissed off [and] just another activist group." In agreement, the other critic writes, "To think that our tax dollars are funding this ... It's time to stop telling the story and get on with it, how long are you going to be angry and stay wrapped up in content?".

This negative feedback "landed with a thud" for PPPOd members, as Mariko Tamaki wrote in her response to one of the emails. When we, co-authors of this article, gathered years later to review the archival artifacts, we concluded that while correct in many senses, particularly when one considers the relational and reciprocal nature of the audience–performer dynamic—when a performance falls flat for an audience, it falls flat—much of this critique could still be attributed to fat hatred (and even activist disdain). We understand the feedback as surfacing affects constitutive (at least in part) of fat hatred (e.g., loathing, disgust, hostility, distain, fear) woven throughout the dominant discourse about fat circulating at the time that still have a stronghold in normative culture, including discourses upholding hegemonic standards of health, productivity, ability, and desirability. When enough people with enough authority carrying enough of these affects come together, their force amasses and unleashes, taking the joy and pleasure out of PPPOd's work. This entangled cognitive-affective response from audiences, rooted in fat fear and hatred, has a political function: to absorb PPPOd's prefigurative political praxis—its enactment of livable fat life now and otherwise—back into the bounds of neoliberal self-responsibilization narratives, thus thinning out PPPOd's thick potential. Rather than sitting with the affective-cognitive complexities of the performance, the spectators quoted above insist that PPPOd deliver a neat lesson on fat discrimination: they presume that there is a right way to identify and deconstruct fat discrimination (i.e., ignore it, get on with it) and to exist as a fat person—as a "good fatty" (Gibson 2022), a fat person who, despite not losing weight (or gaining and losing it and gaining it again), dutifully subjects their body to food deprivation and other restrictive dictates in order to perform as a well-adjusted, self-accepting, "healthy" fat person, as someone who otherwise adheres to all possible social norms.

Our carnal reading of the PPPOd archival ephemera suggests that the visceral materiality of fat played, and in our intimate encounters with the objects, continues to play a significant role in mapping the circulation of affects in PPPOd's performances. The PPPOd members put their fleshy bodies on display in ways that directly contradict popular messaging about how fat bodies should be seen, sensed, and known. This elicits constellations of both abjecting and desiring emotions, and a comingling of the two, creating an affective atmosphere that is perceptible in audiences and can tip in different directions, towards audience joy and pleasure, and/or discomfort with and resistance to PPPOd's performances. These conflicted affective responses surface in the viewers' e-mails where they hold PPPOd's performers to the standards of professional actors and artists, and to conventional white middle-class notions of what constitutes well-staged storytelling (DeMars and Tait 2019); in doing so, the attendees dismiss the jarring affects and ideas stirred up by the performance rather than sit with the discomforting feelings it generates.

We understand the patrons' discomforting affects as socio-politically produced in the confrontation between hegemonic expectations about what a "good" or "healthy" (fat) body is and fat people's thick desires for something otherwise and yet-to-be, sensed in the PPPOd performers' staging of their unresolved, resistant, pleasurable, and prideful embodiments and experiences. The critics, desiring closure, could not receive or accept the message sent by the visceral storywork—that the force of fat oppression, in discursively and viscerally casting unwanted bodies out of the body politic, far exceeds individual-level efforts to overcome or defeat it. This seems to shake up the two attendees enough to protest the radical space and generative possibilities for fat life that PPPOd puts on offer. Indeed, PPPOd strongly resisted the homogenized, hyper-individualized, and medicalized understandings of the good fatty, and the associated "it gets better" narratives (Berlant 2011) circulating at the time in favor of a queer politics of contradiction, anti-assimilation, and non-closure. Their performances centered less on celebrating fatness than on working through the intense emotions arising from difficult experiences at the nexus of fatness, queerness, and other axes of oppression. Rather than staging progress narratives about "overcoming" trauma or enacting a social justice vision of utopia, Mitchell describes how PPPOd used performance "to work through feeling bad most of the time", drawing on dance, personal narrative, spoken word, visual props, singing, and storytelling to convey experiences of ambivalence, pain, and defiance. The performances staged experiences of shame, loathing, and anger, but also emphasized joy and pleasure in fat embodiment, and, ultimately, the political importance of holding complexity. PPPOd's happiness was "happiness in alterity"—a happiness that did not deny or push away the harm caused by the imposition of a certain standard of the human body as part of a system of corporeal supremacy, but rather the joy, love, and desire that performers channeled, felt, and embodied when they loosed their smart, incisive, absurd critique carnally onto the sensory fields of spectators (Chandler and Rice 2013). We thus understand the two e-mail exchanges as representative of some audience members' decisions to retreat from, rather than embrace, the potential of fat performance art and collective activism to "undo" us (i.e., our sense of ourselves, our culture's normative standards). Jennifer Nash (2019), drawing on Judith Butler, theorizes this undoing as willful or intentional vulnerability, as "the experience of 'coming up against' the bodies of others, [the] practice of intimate proximity to others ... [that] requires us to embrace the fact that we can be—and often are—'undone' by each other" an undoing that can take the form of "grief and mourning, desire and ecstasy, solidarity and empathy, and mutual regard". Nash (2019) points to the possibilities and limits of counter-cultural world-making through the type of performance that we next discuss: performance-based worldmaking in spaces of alterity that asks the spectators to become actors who both receive and contribute to the affects that the performance sets in motion. If enough spectators and performers do not open up to their own undoing, the collective shuts down the potential to experience alternative fat existences. It is "the decision to embrace rather than retreat from the possibility of our potential undoing" (Nash 2019) that enables liberatory politics and possibilities for social transformation.

5.2. World-Making

Despite having to contend with audience discomfort and hostility, for Mitchell this deflating reception also "reinforce[d] that we were doing what we needed to do." The goal of public performance was not to elicit affirmative responses (though those were life-giving), rather it was to bust a seam to allow more breathing space for fat bodies. When PPPOd formed in the mid-to-late 1990s, prior to widespread internet availability, few people had access to alternative representations of fatness, so the work of changing representational fields and carving out a fat-desiring space in a bid to change fat peoples' lives was a key group aim. Like the disability arts (Rice et al. 2017), fat-activist art finds power in taking back the spectacle-making of the fat body, taking hold of the spectacle, turning tropes of fatness on their head, setting prohibited or forbidden affects in motion (desire, love, joy), and keeping under question fat oppression (rather than the fat body) through subversively staging the absurdities, contradictions, problematics, and clashing world-senses in a play to open space for something new or otherwise. PPPOd saw their engagements as opportunities to intervene in local cultures and reach people situated wherein who were open to different ways of thinking and feeling, with an overarching aim to transform normative spaces into spaces of radical potential. Indeed, PPPOd's performances took place, at times, in conservative spaces saturated with fat fear, shame, and distaste, including public health spaces, university-based, industry-driven fashion programs, and outpatient and inpatient eating disorder treatment centers. For Mitchell, the possibility that PPPOd performances might create a paradigm shift for those present made the riskiness of exposing herself to fat hatred in order to set in motion fat desire/pleasure to advance fat-affirmative politics worth it. For Rice, PPPOd's dramatization of the contradictory affects swirling around fatness contributed to dislodging/displacing the affective edges of stereotyping which offered spectators new subject positions, and with these new ways of being fat and of being in the fat community. For Taylor, in the footage lie glimpses of alternative affective possibilities for fat bodies to those of (self-) loathing and isolation that she so often feels in the present; the performances make her feel hope, joy, and connection to a past and potential future legacy of radical fat embodiment.

Through our carnal engagements with the PPPOd fat archive, we found that in staging fat agency and desire, and in taking those energies to new places and people, PPPOd performances created occasions for world-making, for experimenting with previously unconsidered ways of being in a fat body as a prefigurative fat liberation politics. By staging the undiscovered possibilities of fat embodiment, PPPOd engaged and implicated the audience in micro-acts of worlding with an impassioned commitment to cultivating livable fat lives. Fat studies scholars such as Chalklin (2016a) and Hernandez (2020) demonstrate the world-making potential of fat performances using the late queer theorist José Esteban Muñoz's (2009) notion of a queer utopia. Muñoz queers utopia to push against fantasies of the "future perfect"—the hegemonic vision of utopia that white masculinist philosophers have built based on the tenets of sameness, order, and reason, and that has depended on the elimination or assimilation of all bodies, individual and social, that exceed or transgress its hard-edged orderly bounds (Rice et al. 2017, p. 217). We understand PPPOd performers as intervening in this thinned-out utopia in order to thicken the narratives and affects of fatness and, by extension, to thicken spaces and futures for fat people, even if fleetingly, as part of a political commitment to fat queer liberation. We also take our conceptualization of world-making, in part, from the dance scholars Klein and Noeth (2011) who argue that the "world" is neither fixed nor given but in a constant process of creation, "made when actions and language bring forth [new] meanings". World-making, they assert, does not refer to "one world"; rather, "different way[s] of worldmaking provoke different, interlocking worlds" (Klein and Noeth 2011, p. 8). In this account, performers and audiences come together to make and re-make worlds over the span of a performance, joining in co-creating micro-worlds in which the participants and audiences want to live (Rice et al. 2022a). As Hernandez (2020) writes in her performance autoethnography of a fat women of color burlesque troupe, "the cowitnessing of fat flesh onstage makes it possible to be hopeful about a fat future in which [audiences] too can engage in a fat-liberating present/future" (109).

The world-making generated via PPPOd's performances occurred through the coming together of many different forces and energies, human and nonhuman. For instance, the assemblage of music, lights, and other visual and sound elements woven into the performances sometimes worked in conjunction with the energy and exhilaration radiating from the PPPOd performers' bodies to create a perceptual-affective wall of caring, loving resistance that shielded the troupe members from potential audience or off-stage hostility. At other times, audiences, opening to the affective, kinesthetic experiences that PPPOd members set in motion, also contributed to growing those affective experiences in ways that thickened the space for fatness, if only for the duration of the performance. For example, audience members felt the performers' excitement and euphoria, and often began moving in their seats and wheelchairs, on makeshift dance floors, cracking jokes, telling vulnerable stories, and flouting bodies, and parts of bodies, that those present knew the wider world reviled. Rice recalls feeling the intensity of this euphoria, its bursts and exuberances, and how it dissipated over time. In moments of euphoria, she felt the affective wall that protected PPPOd from the harmful affects begin to dissolve as audience members warmed up, and the performers' carnal energy would take over the space, bringing audiences into a sensuously fat bubble with them. There was a clear chemistry between performers and audiences, comprised of all the different elements of the performance, resulting in spurts and sprees of world-making.

Kinship played a central role in PPPOd's artful world-making. Mitchell describes how the group met regularly to process their experiences of fat oppression and to reflect on the personal and political impacts of their performance activism. Whether on car rides back from performance venues, or in regular meetings, or at clothing swaps, PPPOd members centralized the sharing of space, feelings, and experiences as critical to their wellbeing and activist artistic practice. The kinship that members felt relates to the intimacy created when fat (or otherwise marginalized) people come together, find comfort and familiarity in sharing experiences of embodied being, and exchange stories of surviving in a world that imposes a supremacist body standard that utterly fails to welcome difference (Chandler and Rice 2013). This kinship can further forge what Mitchell calls a "protective critical mass" where "you create this atmosphere by moving together in your bubble of kin, protecting each other from taking those gazes in, sardonically, satirically, saying 'fuck you' to the fat despising world." The affective kinship ties that PPPOd members enacted on stage did shut out some harmful hegemonic affects circulating around fatness during performances. Yet the group did not bond to each other or to audience members solely, or even primarily, through affect-laden experiences of injury and alienation. Desire figures prominently in PPPOd's interactions with spectators and each other, as seen in the NOLOSE footage, which oozes with flirtatious energy and carnal cravings, and the "full-on fat crushes" that members felt for each other. From the up-close shots of members giving each other sexy and loving looks, to the micro movements of hands stroking faces or fixing hair, to the sensuous consumption of sweet, salty, sticky, and acidic foods, desire is free-floating. Everybody feels it: desire for each other's fat, desire for queer bodies, desire for each other's arm rolls, desire for food, desire for love, desire for care, desire for freedom.

Viewers can likewise access the worlds created by PPPOd's performances via the archival footage. The recordings include group members walking through the back halls of venues like Buddies in Bad Times Theatre, spending time in dressing rooms, flirting, joking, planning, and pep talking. Other clips capture the group nervously exchanging energy in a classroom at Sheridan College before the students enter; they rehearse, joke around, flirt with each other and camera operators, and while the tech is being sorted, they plan and plot in palpable excitement. In moments when the camera focuses on their performances you can hear the audience screaming, hooting, and clapping, and sometimes even drowning out the actual performance dialogue. Viewers of the video recordings may not have been present originally, but they gain entry into background moments, such as the preparatory moments before the members step on stage and moments when they come on stage that capture the intensity of the initial audience response. For instance, Taylor, not present at the live event, in watching this footage years later, feels an intense desire to have been in the bubble. As the performance euphoria envelops her, she feels a sense of carnal kinship with fat-activist histories, and pride in being fat. Taylor feels that it is impossible for her *not* to be infected and affected by the joy emanating from the screen, as she was transported via video from today to that moment in time. As Cooper (2016) writes of finding fat activist materials in an archive, for us, the PPPOd archive "put [us] in touch with past lives, people [we] knew vaguely, and past instances of [our] own activism . . . [we felt] part of something bigger than [ourselves], and this enabled [us] to think of . . . fat feminism and fat activism as entities that travel and shift over time and space" (as cited in Pratt 2018, p. 236).

Relatedly, Mitchell, in relaying how she had goosebumps just viewing and talking about the footage, and Rice, in reliving the spine-tingling moments of participating in a PPPOd performance, demonstrate how past moments can touch us in the present and future. Affects from those moments not only stick to the object, they also stay in the body: the body remembers and becomes an archive in and of itself. In this way, we can think about goosebumps or tingles as the body's testimony, as testifying to its history and the history of other unwanted bodies, as testifying to what they know, what they carry, what they want. Goosebumps and tingles bring us back in time to those spaces and moments of queer fat world-making and re-ignite feelings of longing and hope in the present for alternative futures and worlds.

Ultimately, PPPOd's performances facilitate an emotional intensity, both celebratory and anguish-infused, that encourages the release of pain and, with it, the possibility for catharsis amongst audiences. This "cocktail of contradictory and ambiguous affect in which joy, delight, excitement, misery, anger, and indignation [can] co-exist . . . is exactly where [fat performance art's] queer potential lies" (Chalklin 2016a, p. 93). PPPOd's performances thus liberate queer fat desires by dramatizing the systemic trauma that fat people experience and flipping it to create access to the desires denied to those same people: desires for connection, visibility, and (other ways of existing in) fat bodies.

5.3. Feeling Bad

Performing the undoing of fat hatred in front of live audiences had its repercussions for PPPOd members. Mitchell remembers needing to withdraw and retreat after the exhausting emotional and physical output of a performance. At other times, PPPOd members might have absorbed the negative feelings emanating from audiences or perhaps even projected those feelings onto audiences by, for example, automatically attributing an audience member's lack of enthusiasm for the performance to fat disdain or hatred. For PPPOd members, as for audiences, fat activism could be scary; it took guts. PPPOd had to "feel" their way to understanding when, how, and with whom their performances produced the desired effects—creating social change by broadcasting their messaging to various groups of people and demonstrating alternate ways of embodying fatness.

Like the troupe members, supporters, allies, and audiences also experienced the affects of fear, anxiety, (self-)hatred, and exhaustion circulating around PPPOd's performance activism. As an early active supporter of PPPOd, Rice recalls feeling intense anxiety in response to invitations from Mitchell to join PPPOd's artful street activism (which involved approaching strangers to hand out DIY "queen-sized revolt" stickers or asking them provoking questions, such as, "Do you think I'm fat?") when the group was first forming in the 1990s. From a working-class community where she was schooled in the respectability politics embraced by heteronormative families such as her own, Rice responded to the invitation to join in PPPOd's boundary-crossing street activism with anxiety, fear, and even dread of the threat it posed to her aspirations to middle-class professionalism. In one conversation, Rice spoke candidly about how, at the time of the invitation, she was striving to embody the figure of the middle-class white professional, given that the dominant image of the professional reflected (and continues to reflect) a hard-edged "expert" mode of embodiment (Rice et al. Forthcoming). She "couldn't imagine doing a PPPOd demonstration because it was violating everything that I was trying to become". PPPOd's leaky and self-described embarrassing tactics posed a direct challenge to Rice's embodiment of professionalism and, more broadly, to white, middle-class notions of respectability (Lind 2020).

Archival objects carry these feelings through to the present moment. For example, Mitchell discloses feeling swells of shame and vulnerability in digitizing the archive, at once excited to preserve PPPOd materials so that future scholars and activists can engage with the work and fearful of the judgments that can come from opening access to the material—especially a collection of objects that no one foresaw would be frozen in a capsule to be accessed, slowed down, analyzed, and disseminated. Mitchell imagines that when activist-artists are debriefing a performance-intervention, they don't imagine (or at least she didn't) that one day, 20 years later, documentation of their performances and their preparation for and debriefs of these stagings would be digitized, shared in an open access library, and made available to the public, allowing for the kind of scrutiny which the original creators had never intended. The limitations and opacities of any movement's politics often only become clear in hindsight, leading Mitchell to experience "that feeling of shame attached to the thought that this is self-indulgent, this is a bunch of white middle-class women working through very 'first world' issues". Vulnerability and self-doubt re-insert themselves through her posing reflexive questions, such as: Does this work count? Did it make a difference? What kind of difference did it make? Did we waste our energy? As the co-authors listened, we began to pose other, more theoretical and methodological questions of activist-oriented art and the archive: How do you translate complex moments, thick with affect and ideas, into an inventory list in an archive? How do you measure/record/interpret/understand the affects and effects of an activist artistic intervention? For creators? For audiences? How do you quantify the impacts of PPPOd's and others' fat activist art? These questions reflect the deep anxieties and insecurities about the relevance, purpose, and effectiveness of fat art and activism, as well as an awareness of the forces of intersecting oppressions shaping fat embodiment and expression, including fat hate, classism, ableism, and racism.

Mitchell also worked through feelings of resistance to revisiting the PPPOd materials as they became digitized, knowing that revisiting objects might elicit strong and unpredictable emotions. She worried about feeling mournful, nostalgic, sad, and humiliated. One object might make her recall a beautiful moment of friendship, and another rip the rug out from under her. Mitchell watched the NOLOSE footage, for instance, with a heavy heart, feeling grief and remembering people, like beloved fat-community member Luscious, who traveled to NOLOSE with PPPOd members and later passed away. Like PPPOd's fat performance art, the PPPOd archive conjures complex, conflicting, and not always "positive" or "easy" feelings, gesturing towards the importance of taking seriously so-called "negative" affects such as fear, anxiety, fatigue, and grief in theorizing the meaning, potential, and impact of fat performance art and archives.

5.4. Limitations and Future Directions

In this analysis, we have highlighted the liberatory, life-affirming and life-giving potential of Pretty Porky and Pissed Off's activism, and the affects its live performances set in motion, that, we have argued, remain attached to its archival artifacts. We hold strongly that interventions such as those staged and archived by PPPOd remain urgent and necessary in a world saturated with anti-fat affects and discourses (e.g., anti-fat science). However, we do not mean to suggest that PPPOd's activism constitutes the right, best, or only way to challenge the pervasive, insidious, and entrenched fat hate operating as a forceful agent of corporal supremacy. In many ways, the PPPOd troupe members resemble "The Rad Fatty", a figure described by Chalklin (2016b) as someone who "uncompromisingly rejects fat stigma from a position of critical knowingness usually gained through involvement in fat activism or an academic understanding of sizeism" (122). Chalkin stresses that to become "Rad Fatties", performers and audiences need to gain access to and accept certain counter-cultural knowledge and practices and acquire the kind of (counter) cultural capital and the "psychological resilience" needed to embolden those involved "to face [the] destruction of norms without being 'undone'" (Chalklin 2016b, p. 122). Indeed, reflecting on PPPOd's activism, Mitchell feels that, in many ways, it was quite tame in its methods of direct action and had its limits, such that PPPOd could be considered fierce but certainly was not radical according to many definitions of the term. In fact, Mitchell suggests that the truly radical aspects of PPPOd's activism may lie in its queer performance roots. Chalklin's (2016b) analysis raises important questions about the audience, limits, and accessibility of PPPOd's activism.

One critique of PPPOd's performances and the affects circulating around them that we consider here is PPPOd's limited engagement with the structures of racism and white supremacy as these intersected, and continue to intersect, with fat oppression. PPPOd organized their first street performances in the mid-to-late 1990s, a time when paradigm-shifting scholarship on the intersectional nature of oppression was first being published by Black feminist scholars such as Kimberlé Crenshaw (1989). Theoretical insights into the ways that fat oppression fuels anti-Black and anti-Indigenous racism were largely missing from the scholarly literature in (white) feminist studies, critical race studies, (white) queer studies, and the related critical fields that were then emerging; and many white feminist scholars and white cis activists were only beginning to grapple with feminism's power problem, its centering of privileged white women's issues, and its failure to center the intersecting-equity concerns of multiple marginalized wholly-or-partially-identifying-as-woman subjects. In this climate, fat studies and fat activism materialized as predominantly white spaces centrally concerned with interrogating fat oppression, with social actors extending this analytic frame mainly when considering gender and sexuality and sometimes, ability and class (Friedman et al. 2019). Across the conventional disciplines and within the fields of health and education, fat-destroying discourses had gained a stranglehold over almost all the funded research on fatness throughout the period of PPPOd's activism, intensifying and proliferating biomedical perspectives and thinning out and weakening social, political, and material inquiries into fat as a phenomenon (e.g., following the rise of the obesity epidemic discourse, see (Gard and Wright 2005)). This meant that knowledge-makers and -users fed into a hegemonic knowledge system that reproduced the epistemic ignorance about fatness by disfavoring knowledge claims about the oppression of fat people as an aggrieved group deserving of justice, and favoring the expertise that emphasized fat's pathology and pressed for its elimination. In this climate, few white fat studies scholars or activists could think through how fat oppression might function to uphold white supremacy, or how the empirical research informed by white supremacist knowledge systems might code fatness as a carnal sign of (familial, psychological) dysfunction that required correction to meet the standards and values of white abled middle-class life. For all of these reasons, PPPOd members mostly did not stage embodied experiences of fatness as those experientially entangled with race and coloniality.

Additionally, we recognize that our analysis highlights the celebratory and joyful affects engendered by PPPOd's activism; in fact, it was difficult for us to find negative or even lukewarm responses to PPPOd shows in the archived recordings of performances. The e-mails we discussed earlier evidence the existence of hurtful affects amongst audiences; and whilst our analysis could be critiqued for emphasizing the positive or for setting up an apparent binary between so-called "positive" and "negative" emotions that PPPOd performer–audience intra-actions set off, we also orient these as constellations of emotions or as affective atmospheres created by and through the specific dynamics of each audience–performer dance. We further suggest that the cognitive-affective ambiguity generated in the liminal space between creators and perceivers is part of the experience of any cultural production, and this is especially true of live performance. However, we believe that PPPOd accomplished the cognitive-affective work of creating space for fat joy and desire (and counter discourses oriented to the vitality of fatness) precisely through staging fat hate in ways that poked holes in it, that viscerally challenged its very premises, and that through exposing and upending its illogic, created potent spaces for unleashing queer, feminist, and fat desires. In the recordings, applause, laughter, and hoots from enthusiastic audience members drown out any ambivalent responses. We three authors, those at NOLOSE featured in the recorded interviews, the audience responses captured in other video recordings, and the published scholarly analyses of PPPOd performances, all align insofar as each source experiences PPPOd's activisms as intense, affect-infused, and highly energetic exchanges. Other than the examples given, discomfort in the audience responses to the messages that PPPOd created and disseminated through their street activism, media interviews, and performances, be these in the form of a grumbling theatre patron or an offended community member, is not glaringly obvious to us.

6. Conclusions

Touching and feeling Pretty Porky and Pissed Off's artful politics, embodied in past live performances and remembered through objects in an archive, reveals the power of affect in fat performance art and activism to move subjectivities and world senses. In our lingering over the objects and recordings examined in our collaborative performance auto/ethnography and thematic analysis, we have aimed to illuminate the significant role that affect plays in how PPPOd's fat performance art and activism created the conditions of possibility for the radical transformation of fat, both in meaning and materiality. Overall, we argue that PPPOd's performances, as live events and archival objects, elicit the constellation of affects constituting fat hatred and, simultaneously, disrupt and flip (or cast off) those affects by generating alternate feelings of hope, playfulness, pride, desire, love, and euphoria that contribute to ephemeral micro-worldings.

We hope that by centering others' and our own sensory and affect-laden experiences of fat bodies and counter-cultural activism we offer pathways for fat people to collectively hang onto, extend, and rework our histories spatially and temporally, making them legible and relevant both here and elsewhere, and now and into the future. For this article, we offer a snapshot of the responses from three different academics[7], who have made different contributions to fat activism, working intensively at different times over the last four decades of the fat liberation movement in Canada, and engaging with fat studies from discrete methodological angles and theoretical vantage points. We orient to the field itself as a form of activism that seeks to transform a fat-debasing world. The effectiveness of our activism is difficult to assess. The metrics are unclear and depend on the hope and desire of those who continue the work with faith that their contribution will engage, inspire, shelter, and embolden successive generations.

As they engage with the PPPOd archive, we urge readers to consider the pleasures and trepidations of picking up an object, pressing play on a digital video file, or clicking on a photo; to become mindful of what that object is, what it might have meant to its creators, subjects, and stewards, and what it brings to and might mean for the current moment. We recognize that this beginning analysis can only "scratch the surface" of the experience of creating an archive for the *archived*—for groups or individuals whose work finds its way to an archive while they are still living and participating in the activities archived. So often an artist's or activist's work is archived after their death. The archives of living people allow for deeply subjective and feeling-infused narrations of the objects and recordings. This adds weight to social movement histories. Ultimately, the PPPOd archive provides an alternate history and legacy for fat people by capturing ephemeral moments of radical possibility and, consequently, it offers unique and important opportunities for *feeling* our way to other, more livable fat lives in the present and future.

Author Contributions: Conceptualization, A.T., A.M. and C.R.; methodology, A.T., A.M. and C.R.; formal analysis, A.T. and C.R.; investigation, A.T., A.M. and C.R.; resources, A.M. and C.R.; data curation, A.T.; writing—original draft preparation, A.T., A.M. and C.R.; writing—review and editing, C.R., A.T. and A.M.; visualization, A.T., A.M. and C.R.; supervision, A.M. and C.R.; project administration, A.M. and C.R.; funding acquisition, C.R. All authors have read and agreed to the published version of the manuscript.

Funding: This research was funded by SSHRC Partnership Grant *Bodies in Translation, Activist Art Technology and Access to Life* (BIT), a project of Re•Vision: The Centre for Art and Social Justice at the University of Guelph.

Institutional Review Board Statement: Not applicable.

Informed Consent Statement: Not applicable.

Data Availability Statement: The data presented in this study are available at https://revisioncentre.ca/performing-fat-liberation using the password: performing (29 March 2023).

Conflicts of Interest: The authors declare no conflict of interest.

Notes

[1] These archival materials are available for viewing here: https://revisioncentre.ca/performing-fat-liberation. Password: performing (29 March 2023).

[2] This video documentation was created by the Wellington-Dufferin-Guelph Eating Disorders Coalition and a copy was shared with PPPOd. It was preserved in the personal archive of PPPOd co-founder Allyson Mitchell. This artifact is a VHS tape titled "Blubber Show—Raw Footage" (length: 1:54:55).

[3] This documentation is provided on a mini DV tape titled "PPPO-BJ-Casaloma Campus—25 March 2004" (length 1:04:26) and includes footage of set-up, rehearsal, and banter before the show at George Brown College's School of Labour and a question-and-answer period after the show. It was preserved in the personal archive of PPPOd co-founder Allyson Mitchell.

[4] This artifact originated as a VHS tape titled "PPPO'd at Buddies—November 2002" (length 32:14). It was preserved in the personal archive of PPPOd co-founder Allyson Mitchell.

[5] This artifact includes two separate mini DV tapes. The first tape is titled "No Lose 2004: Performance and Roadtrip" (length 1:03:32). The second tape is titled "No Lose 2004: Interviews and Picnic" (length 44:04). It was preserved in the personal archive of PPPOd co-founder Allyson Mitchell.

[6] This artifact includes one audio cassette with recordings on both sides titled "PPPO'd Women's Studies Sudbury Workshop/1 December 2003" (length: 47:55 side A and 46:28 side B). The audio cassette was preserved in the personal archive of PPPOd co-founder Allyson Mitchell and the emails were saved by PPPOd member Tracy Tidgwell.

[7] Who, because of our research interests and political orientations and embodied experiences, are indeed the enabling audience for this activism and archive.

References

Ahmed, Sara. 2004a. Affective Economies. *Social Text* 22: 117–39.
Ahmed, Sara. 2004b. *The Cultural Politics of Emotion*. Abingdon: Routledge.
Ahmed, Sara. 2008. The Politics of Good Feeling. *Australian Critical Race and Whiteness Studies Association* 4: 1–18.
Berlant, Lauren. 2011. *Cruel Optimism*. Durham: Duke University Press.
Braun, Virginia, and Victoria Clarke. 2006. Using Thematic Analysis in Psychology. *Qualitative Research in Psychology* 3: 77–101. [CrossRef]
Chalklin, Vikki. 2012. Performing Queer Selves: Embodied Subjectivity and Affect in Queer Performance Spaces Duckie, Bird Club and Wotever World. Ph.D. dissertation, Goldsmiths, University of London, London, UK.
Chalklin, Vikki. 2016a. All Hail the Fierce Fat Femmes. In *Fat Sex: New Directions in Theory and Activism*. Edited by Helen Hester and Caroline Walters. Farnham: Ashgate, pp. 85–100.
Chalklin, Vikki. 2016b. Obstinate Fatties: Fat Activism, Queer Negativity, and the Celebration of 'Obesity'. *Subjectivity* 9: 107–25. [CrossRef]
Chandler, Eliza, and Carla Rice. 2013. Alterity in/of Happiness: Reflecting on the Radical Possibilities of Unruly Bodies. *Health, Culture, and Society* 5: 230–248. [CrossRef]
Cooper, Charlotte. 2016. *Fat Activism: A Radical Social Movement*. Bristol: HammerOn Press.
Crenshaw, Kimberlé. 1989. Demarginalizing the Intersection of Race and Sex: A Black Feminist Critique of Antidiscrimination Doctrine, Feminist Theory and Antiracist Politics. *University of Chicago Legal Forum* 140: 139–67.
Cvetkovich, Ann. 2003. *An Archive of Feelings: Trauma, Sexuality, and Lesbian Public Cultures*. Durham: Duke University Press.

DeMars, Tony R., and Gabriel B. Tait, eds. 2019. *Narratives of Storytelling Across Cultures: The Complexities of Intercultural Communication.* London: Lexington Books.

Ellison, Jenny. 2020. *Being Fat: Women, Weight, and Feminist Activism in Canada.* Toronto: University of Toronto Press.

Friedman, May, Carla Rice, and Jen Rinaldi, eds. 2019. *Thickening Fat: Fat Bodies, Intersectionality and Social Justice.* New York: Routledge Press.

Gard, Michael, and Jan Wright. 2005. *The Obesity Epidemic: Science, Morality and Ideology.* Abingdon: Routledge.

Gibson, Gemma. 2022. Health(ism) At Every Size: The Duties of the 'Good Fatty'. *Fat Studies: An Interdisciplinary Journal of Body Weight and Society* 11: 22–35. [CrossRef]

Hernandez, Yessica Garcia. 2020. Longing for Fat Futures: Creating Fat Utopian Performatives in Burlesque. *Frontiers* 41: 107–29. [CrossRef]

Hoang, Kimberly Kay. 2018. Gendering Carnal Ethnography: A Queer Reception. In *Other, Please Specify: Queer Methods in Sociology.* Edited by D'Lane R. Compton, Tey Meadow and Kristen Schilt. Berkeley: University of California Press, pp. 230–48.

Johnson, Josée, and Judith Taylor. 2008. Feminist Consumerism and Fat Activists: A Comparative Study of Grassroots Activism and the Dove Real Beauty Campaign. *Signs: Journal of Women in Culture and Society* 33: 941–66. [CrossRef]

Klein, Gabriele, and Sandra Noeth, eds. 2011. *Emerging Bodies: The Performance of Worldmaking in Dance and Choreography.* Bielefeld: Transcript.

Lind, Emily R. M. 2020. Queering Fat Activism: A Study in Whiteness. In *Thickening Fat: Fat Bodies, Intersectionality, and Social Justice.* Edited by May Friedman, Carla Rice and Jen Rinaldi. Abingdon: Routledge, pp. 183–94.

Muñoz, José Esteban. 2009. *Cruising Utopia: The Then and There of Queer Futurity.* New York: New York University Press.

Nash, Jennifer C. 2019. *Black Feminism Reimagined: After Intersectionality.* Durham: Duke University Press.

Pratt, Laura. 2018. The (Fat) Body and the Archive: Toward the Creation of a Fat Community Archive. *Fat Studies: An Interdisciplinary Journal of Body Weight and Society* 7: 227–39. [CrossRef]

Rice, Carla, Chelsea Temple Jones, and Ingrid Mündel. 2022a. Slow Story-Making in Urgent Times. *Cultural Studies, Critical Methodologies* 22: 245–54. [CrossRef]

Rice, Carla, Eliza Chandler, Jen Rinaldi, Nadine Changfoot, Kristy Liddiard, Roxanne Mykitiuk, and Ingrid Mündel. 2017. Imagining Disability Futurities. *Hypatia* 32: 213–29. [CrossRef]

Rice, Carla, Meredith Bessey, Andrea Kirkham, and Kaley Roosen. Forthcoming. Transgressing Professional Boundaries through Fat and Disabled Embodiments. *Canadian Woman Studies.*

Rice, Carla, Susan D. Dion, Hannah Fowlie, and Andrea Breen. 2022b. Identifying and Working Through Settler Ignorance. *Critical Studies in Education* 63: 15–30. [CrossRef]

Rice, Carla. 2014. *Becoming Women: The Embodied Self in Image Culture.* Toronto: University of Toronto Press.

Rice, Carla. 2015. Rethinking Fat: From Bio- to Body-Becoming Pedagogies. *Cultural Studies, Critical Methodologies* 15: 387–97. [CrossRef]

Rinaldi, Jen, Carla Rice, Crystal Kotow, and Emma Lind. 2020. Mapping the Circulation of Fat Hatred. *Fat Studies: An Interdisciplinary Journal of Body Weight and Society* 9: 37–50. [CrossRef]

Schmitz, Sigrid, and Sara Ahmed. 2014. Affect/Emotion: Orientation Matters. A Conversation Between Sigrid Schmitz and Sara Ahmed. *FZG* 20: 97–108. [CrossRef]

Tidgwell, Tracy, May Friedman, Jen Rinaldi, Crystal Kotow, and Emily R. M. Lind. 2018. Introduction to the Special Issue: Fatness and Temporality. *Fat Studies: An Interdisciplinary Journal of Body Weight and Society* 7: 115–23. [CrossRef]

Disclaimer/Publisher's Note: The statements, opinions and data contained in all publications are solely those of the individual author(s) and contributor(s) and not of MDPI and/or the editor(s). MDPI and/or the editor(s) disclaim responsibility for any injury to people or property resulting from any ideas, methods, instructions or products referred to in the content.

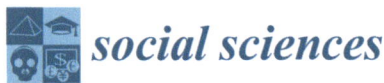

Article

Revisioning Fitness through a Relational Community of Practice: Conditions of Possibility for Access Intimacies and Body-Becoming Pedagogies through Art Making

Meredith Bessey [1,*], K. Aly Bailey [2], Kayla Besse [3], Carla Rice [1,4], Salima Punjani [5] and Tara-Leigh F. McHugh [6]

1. Department of Family Relations and Applied Nutrition, University of Guelph, Guelph, ON N1G 2W1, Canada
2. Department of Health, Aging & Society, McMaster University, Hamilton, ON L8S 4L8, Canada
3. Stratford Festival, Stratford, ON N5A 6V2, Canada
4. Re•Vision: The Centre for Art and Social Justice, University of Guelph, Guelph, ON N1G 2W1, Canada
5. Independent Self-Employed Artist and Curator, Montreal, QC H3N 1T7, Canada
6. Faculty of Physical Education & Recreation, University of Alberta, Edmonton, AB T6G 2R3, Canada
* Correspondence: besseym@uoguelph.ca

Abstract: *ReVisioning Fitness* is a research project and community of practice (CoP) working to reconceptualize "fitness" through a radical embrace of difference (e.g., trans, non-binary, queer, Black, people of colour, disabled, and/or fat, thick/thicc, curvy, plus sized), and a careful theorising of inclusion and access. Our collaborative and arts-based work mounts collective resistance against the dominant power relations that preclude bodymind differences within so-called "fitness" spaces. In this work, we build queer, crip, and thick/thicc alliances by centring relational and difference-affirming approaches to fitness, fostering a radical CoP that supports dissent to be voiced, access intimacies to form, and capacitating effects of body-becoming pedagogies to be set in motion. In this article, we consider how conditions of possibility both co-created and inherited by researchers, collaborators, and the research context itself contributed to what unfolded in our project and art making (multimedia storytelling). By a radical CoP, we mean that we mobilise a more relational and difference-affirming notion of CoP than others have described, which often has involved the reification of sameness and the stabilisation of hierarchies. Further, we call on leaders in fitness organisations to open conditions of possibility in their spaces to allow for alternative futures of fitness that centre difference.

Keywords: participatory research; fitness; communities of practice; disability arts; access intimacy; body-becoming

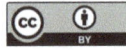

1. Introduction

Art and fitness in the western world may seem disparate, but they have at least one thing in common: both are known for precluding certain types of bodies—fat, raced, gendered, and impoverished—from accessing and enjoying recreation, leisure, physical activity, and cultural spaces (e.g., Chandler et al. 2018, forthcoming; Rinaldi et al. 2020). *ReVisioning Fitness* is a participatory arts-based research project, collective, and community of practice (CoP) made up of people with varied lived experience and expert knowledge, working together to reconceptualise "fitness" and movement practices with accessibility and inclusion in front of mind. This project brought together individuals from groups imagined as non-vital within the dominant culture (Bodies in Translation n.d.) to create a generative alliance of artists, activists, and thinkers invested in envisioning alternative futures for fitness. Our collaborative project undertaken across the northern part of Turtle Island (Canada) enacts collective resistance against eugenic and colonial forces that preclude difference within so-called fitness spaces. In this, we build on the existing efforts of queer, fat, racialised, and disabled leaders in the fitness sphere who have already undertaken the hard work of developing and teaching non-oppressive fitness and movement practices. These community-committed organisers include Free to Move in Canada, Decolonizing Fitness based out of North Carolina, GOODBODYFEEL located in Ontario, Dianne Bondy Yoga in Canada, Fringe(ish) Fat Positive Yoga based in Toronto, and Black Girl Fitness operating out of Nova Scotia. We believe in the movement-making and -reinvigorating potential of non-normative arts and cultures to help create necessary change and disrupt ableist, racist, fatphobic, heteronormative, and cis-sexist structures (e.g., Chandler et al. 2018, forthcoming; Rice et al. 2021) that dominate gyms, yoga studios, and other spaces intended for physical activity, leisure, and culture sharing. As disability scholars Eales and Peers (2016) note, researchers have seldom explored the transformative potential of the disability and non-normative arts and culture movements to disrupt the inaccessible praxis that dominates contemporary fitness and physical activity spaces. We thus engage with and across theories of coalition building, CoPs, access intimacies, body-becoming pedagogies, and capacity/debility to understand the potential of working together with disability and non-normative communities to reimagine fitness.

Our *ReVisioning Fitness* collective has a working definition of fitness that we intentionally leave open. So far, our alternative understanding of fitness hinges on a radical embrace and celebration of different ways of moving, sensing, and perceiving our bodies that invite joy, pleasure, and connection to ourselves, each other, and the land. In this reimagining of traditional notions of fitness, we urge relational understandings of access that create open-ended and supportive possibilities for movement and embodiment and that refuse neoliberal capitalist approaches to inclusion.

Building from our working definition of fitness, in this article we consider how conditions of possibility, both co-created and inherited (e.g., through the ongoing interactions between bodies and worlds that co-constitute both) by researchers and the research context itself have contributed to our revisioning of fitness and of what is typically understood as a CoP through the lens of access intimacy (Mingus 2011). Mia Mingus (2011) understands access intimacy conceptually as "that elusive, hard to describe feeling when someone else 'gets' your access needs" (para. 4). She describes access intimacy not as acting charitably or dutifully toward disabled "others" but rather as engaging relationally across nondominant differences through building and deepening interdependent connections: "Sometimes access intimacy doesn't even mean that everything is 100% accessible... Sometimes it is someone just sitting and holding your hand while you both stare back at an inaccessible world" (para. 9). Inspired by the possibilities of access intimacies, we mobilise a more relational conceptualisation of a CoP than what has been previously described (e.g., Cox 2005). Formulated in the early 1990s to explain processes of co-learning in group contexts (Lave and Wenger 1991), CoPs have since been taken up in management research and used as a tool to foster workplace innovation (e.g., Roberts 2006). Wenger (1998) argues that three key characteristics define a CoP: instructors' and learners' mutual engagement, a joint enterprise, and a shared repertoire, all of which can contribute to sameness or homogeneity in such communities. Being engaged in a CoP often involves absorbing the habits and values of the group, which may serve to stabilise hierarchical ideas of expertise and hegemonic power relations (e.g., Cox 2005). While a few researchers have reported on CoPs that subvert norms and centre difference, conflict, and challenge (e.g., Limatius 2019), many studies have found that praxis communities tend to stabilise power and aim for consensus and uniformity, and thus unintentionally reproduce dominant ideologies and normative standards of being and doing (e.g., Contu and Willmott 2003; Curnow 2013). This has led to critiques of CoPs as lacking attention to power and social marginalisation.

Based on their tendencies towards the normative, we believe both fitness and CoPs are ripe for reimagining. We have begun to reconceptualise the idea of CoP through our collective work and our engagement with the idea of *ReVisioning Fitness* as a generative coalition. We argue that enacting a relational orientation to collaboratively politicized praxis serves as fertile ground for power-attuned CoPs and access intimacies to form in difference-affirming spaces. We see this work as an example of micro-activist affordances (Dokumaci

2019), the "ongoing and (often) ephemeral acts of world-building" that transform the daily lives of disabled, queer, fat, thicc, gendered, and racialised people in ways "that the built social and material world fails to readily provide" (p. 493). Our work centres bodies of difference in order to (re)build the fitness world via micro-activist affordances in queer, crip, and thicc ways. To inform our use of this reclaimed terminology, we draw on crip and queer theories and fat studies: similar to the liberatory reclamation of the word queer, the term crip[1] recuperates cripple, calling into question "compulsory able-bodiedness" (McRuer 2016, p. 301) with its re-inscription of a singular (able-bodied, white, hetero, male) mind-body norm (Garland-Thomson 2017; Kafer 2013; Piepzna-Samarasinha 2021; Rice et al. 2018; Viscardis et al. 2019). We also thicken fitness by actively resisting the normativity that has crept into fat studies by drawing on intersectionality (e.g., Friedman et al. 2020). Thus, we take up the alternative spelling "thicc" in this article to resist the cooptation of the term and to gesture to its roots in celebrating Black bodies that were made invisibilised, hypersexualised, or stereotyped via the forces of sexism, fatphobia, and racism (Cooper 2021; Griffin et al. 2022).

In what follows, we describe and theorise our ways of working together as a CoP with one caveat: we do not consider the iterative approaches that we introduce as a playbook for how this sort of research *should* be done. Rather, we highlight forces acting on and within the research apparatus that have allowed for new insights to surface within the time-space of our project, and we also develop a case for relational and difference-affirming CoPs wherein access intimacies and body-becoming pedagogies *may* thrive in capacitating ways. In our writing and theorising, we draw on content from our group meetings, individual interviews, and multimedia creations (digital stories) and provide author reflections on the research process.

2. Framework and Conditions of Possibility

In what follows, we describe the elements or forces that have acted on us, constituted the project from the fore, and opened (and likely foreclosed) possibilities for what could be created. We call these elements conditions of possibility, which include who we are as a team, our engagement with disability art making, our work of building a community of care, our collective reimagining of CoPs in the online space, and our expansive approach to coalition building, including welcoming dissent.

2.1. Who We Are as a Team

The *ReVisioning Fitness* team began as five white mostly cis women co-investigators, Drs. Aly Bailey, Carla Rice, Evadne Kelly, and Tara-Leigh McHugh, and research assistant Meredith Bessey, working within the disciplines of kinesiology, dance studies, feminist studies, and critical dietetics, and straddling various normative and non-normative embodiments, with some of us identifying as queer, femme, fat, disabled, mad, and/or neurodivergent, and as having (or having had) eating/dieting/exercise/general body-related distress. To actively resist fitness imperatives to fit into a compulsory heteronormative, ableist, fat-hating world, the original research team recruited six additional participant co-researchers from our personal and professional networks, seeley quest, Skylar Sookpaiboon, Kayla Besse, Bongi Dube, Paul Tshuma, and Salima Punjani, who brought expert knowledge (e.g., community activism, disability arts, accessibility consulting, and academia) and lived/living and embodied experiences (e.g., trans, non-binary, queer, Black, people of colour, disabled, and/or fat, thicc, curvy, plus sized) to the project.

We intentionally blur the line between so-called "academics" and "non-academics" to challenge and flatten hierarchies of power in the academy, which is also why we use everyone's first name throughout this paper. We recognise that participatory research can, at times, be problematic, inequitable, and extractive (e.g., Williams et al. 2020). Acknowledging this history, the grant principal investigator (PI, Aly) and co-investigators (Carla, Evadne, Tara) decided to pay co-researchers an hourly rate (aligned with our host institution's graduate-level research assistant pay scale) for their participation in all project activities and for most of the writing that took place afterwards. Co-researchers also describe receiving non-monetary benefits, including camaraderie, new friendships (for some), opportunities for social connection during an isolating time, and a chance to reframe fitness in their/our lives. Regardless of these strategies, we recognize how systemic challenges always constrain efforts to mitigate hierarchies, which for us included bureaucratic hurdles and delays in paying participant co-researchers, harsh academic deadlines, time constraints when publishing, and more (see Williams et al. 2020 for more examples). Since this project intentionally intervenes at the vital edges of normative culture and outside existing fitness systems, we realize that structural-level impact is unlikely at this stage, but this is our intended goal for the future. Additionally, we orient to this CoP as fluid and ever-evolving, whereby we each resonate with or connect to this research in different ways at different times and where the connections in the group ebb and flow. Thus, the benefits and challenges of this project are likely not felt equally across the group or across time.

Beginning in early 2021, we met biweekly as a team in a curated online space (designed to meet and surpass the highest standards of accessibility) through Zoom, a total of eight times. These meetings involved sharing our own (positive and negative) experiences in fitness spaces, learning about the eugenic history of fitness, and discussing our ideas for how fitness's future could shift in difference-affirming ways. In her role as PI, Aly conducted one-on-one interviews with each participant co-researcher to gather individual perspectives on the topics. We also met online as a group in late summer 2021 for a co-analysis meeting. Our group continues to communicate regularly about ongoing writing projects and other knowledge-sharing opportunities (e.g., film screenings with fitness stakeholders). This praxis community had three main aims: to share and analyze our experiences of fitness; to question and subvert dominant meanings of fitness; and to imagine alternative futures for fitness through engagement with disability arts via a multimedia storytelling workshop.

2.2. Disability Art Making

In addition to the elements of our project outlined above, we engaged in a four-week virtual multimedia storytelling workshop in June 2021, supported by the Re•Vision Centre for Art and Social Justice at the University of Guelph (Evans et al. 2022). In this workshop, all six participant co-researchers and three of five co-investigators created multimedia stories—or short videos paired with audio recordings of first-person narratives, images, and other soundscapes. These digital stories can be a powerful way to speak back to dominant discourses and norms, challenge the stories that are told *about* people with bodymind differences, and be a powerful pedagogical tool in helping to shift cultural narratives (LaMarre and Rice 2016; Rice et al. 2015). We intend to use the stories in film screenings with various stakeholders to help disrupt conventional ideas of fitness. Story-making included an in-depth framing of the themes and issues that brought us as storytellers together (e.g., questioning fitness), and each storyteller also had support to develop whatever story was most important for them to tell in the moment. The workshop included a story circle to share initial ideas; writing exercises to develop scripts; tutorials about the use of online editing software; and access to technical, writing, and conceptual support throughout the process. To conclude the workshop, we voluntarily shared our stories in a screening, and everyone left the workshop as the creator and owner of their video. This means that the creators have autonomy in how and when their videos are published or shared (for further details on methodology, see Rice and Mündel 2018, 2019; Rice 2020). Then, in post-production, Re•Vision Centre facilitators supported creators in learning closed, open, or creative captioning[2] as a disability cultural practice.

Our centring of disability arts and culture contributed to makers going to the edges of, and making meaning from, their unique embodied needs, interests, and desires within movement practices. These conditions of possibility stemming from disability cultural practices were present in the workshop and in the broader research activities we engaged in; and notably they laid the foundation for what emerged as art making allowed us to imagine alternative futures of fitness through centring and celebrating difference.

2.3. Building a Community of Care

A disability cultural practice that helped establish our terms of being together entailed group consideration of the politics of "no." The capacity to say no is often stripped from disabled people via structural forces (e.g., substitute decision makers, medical ableism; e.g., Rice et al. 2022a), and in fitness spaces where non-disabled practitioners often make assumptions about what disabled bodies can and cannot (or should not) do (Saxton 2018). At an early meeting, we discussed what it meant for us to feel our no, both in our work together and in fitness spaces, where "no pain, no gain" and "don't stop" mentalities often dominate and saying no feels impossible (see Richardson/Kianewesquao and Reynolds 2014 for more about safety and saying no). We also considered how saying no may not be accessible to everyone and that power dynamics influence people's ability to refuse something—shaping when, how, and with whom we, as people who are differently embedded in uneven power, can say no. Yet, we wanted to create an open space where people could honour each other's limits and engage in capacitating and fulfilling ways rather than depleting or debilitating ones. For example, while we could financially compensate participant co-researchers for most of the work, we could not pay everyone for all writing (due to a budgeting oversight), so we instead ensured that folx could say no to this unpaid work, which some did. We draw on the concepts of capacity and debility, whereby within westernized neoliberalized democracies, certain bodies are seen as capable of being productive or of living, while others are seen as debilitated or targeted for slow death (Puar 2012). We subvert neoliberal notions of capacitating by considering how this work fulfilled and satiated us in ways beyond the market's expectations of productivity and progress, in line with Puar (2012), whereby we supported each other's "no" in resisting neoliberal academic pressures that threaten to debilitate us. We return to an exploration of what capacitated each of us near the end of this paper.

During one of our early group meetings, one participant co-researcher, Salima, named an important condition of possibility for doing good work together: "being part of a community of practice... *ReVisioning Fitness* really feeds into that, because it feels like I can still be part of a community that is centred around care." She further elaborated that "when we come together and think about accessibility, even in an online space, and care and connection is thought about throughout the whole process, that in itself is a motivating reason to be part of *ReVisioning Fitness*." Her invitation for us to become a CoP centring on care and connection struck us as especially significant given the COVID-19 lockdown conditions we were then confronting. The phrase stuck, shaping what we have accomplished in revisioning fitness and how we now orient to our work together.

2.4. Online Nature of Our Work

The sudden shift to the online space in the face of the COVID-19 emergency surfaced as another powerful force acting on our research. Zoom, WeVideo, Mentimeter, and other technologies opened pathways for us to think, feel, perceive, and create together in a virtual space. We consider the pandemic coupled with these online affordances as both enabling and constraining forces in our work.

One enabling component involved intentionally creating a relaxed space that we co-constituted by enacting a disability cultural practice called "relaxed performance" (e.g., Collins et al. 2022; Jones et al. 2022). Relaxed performance has emerged in the last few decades from a growing recognition of the contributions of disability, d/Deaf, mad, ageing, and fat activist-artists to disability rights and justice movements and the need to educate the mainstream about non-normative cultural practices to improve access to art (LaMarre et al. 2021). As a cultural practice, relaxed performance aims to make art and cultural spaces more accessible through technical modifications, such as dimmed lights, warnings about and/or reductions in loud noises and pyrotechnics, the choice to move freely in and out of the space, and the creation of a "chill-out space" where people can relax, and more (LaMarre et al. 2021; Collins et al. 2022). Within *ReVisioning Fitness*, we enacted this practice by encouraging people to engage in the ways that worked for them, including turning their cameras on or off as needed, situating themselves anywhere that made them feel comfortable (e.g., their bed), and inviting freedom to eat/drink, take breaks, and flow in and out of the online meeting space as desired. In addition, because we met online, team members could join from British Columbia, Alberta, Ontario, Quebec, and Nova Scotia, allowing us to connect across provinces in ways that would not have happened otherwise. However, we recognise that online research also required everyone to have access to a computer or phone and a stable internet connection, which may have excluded some from participating. We also acknowledge that our relaxed approach to working online (e.g., the option to turn cameras off) made perceiving dissent or someone's "no" more challenging since reading the body language or facial expressions of others was not always possible.

Another constraint of the online space surfaced in our inability to explore movement in embodied ways as we had planned to in person. For example, in the original project proposal, we planned to spend two meetings exploring body movement, which was not something we could ethically enact in the online space. While not viscerally sensing or directly engaging with our own and each other's bodies limited some activities, this ostensible constraint created a certain amount of freedom, allowing us to escape the friendly but exposing gaze of others in our explorations of fitness. For example, at our second group meeting, co-investigator Evadne described how the gaze of others interferes with her ability to feel pleasure in fitness and impedes her internal perceptual-sensory experience of movement:

> a barrier to pleasure is sometimes when I feel the gaze of others and feel that I can't fit into what their—what their idea of fitness is, and yeah, so mirrors and, you know, that's one of those things that creates that feeling of being watched as opposed to an internal experience for me...

While Evadne was not specifically speaking to the experience of online fitness, her words feel apt in demonstrating why the relaxed nature of *ReVisioning Fitness* became so important in cultivating a space where we could explore freely and subvert the gaze.

2.5. Our Expansive Approach to Coalition Building

Our intentional creation of a coalition across bodymind differences (Price 2015)—queer, trans, non-binary, Black, racialised, disabled, mad, neurodivergent, fat, thick/thicc, and plus sized—comprised another condition of possibility for revisioning fitness. Although some of us knew each other prior to joining the project, many of us were strangers. Despite this, and the fact that many of us have only engaged with one another online, we felt a sense of relationality and community almost immediately. In her theorising on coalition building, Alison Kafer cites Catriona Sandilands on the power of coalitional rhetoric to forge connections across seemingly incommensurate differences. Sandilands writes: "A vital moment in coalitional political rhetoric is its ability to construct connections among struggles that may be not only diverse but opposed to one another in many respects" (as quoted in Kafer 2013, p. 149). We argue that effective coalition building across embodied differences must embrace disagreement and the possibility of dissent in its goal-making. Our team came together with the common goal of refusing the damaging "fit" and "unfit" dichotomy that continues to be tethered to eugenic notions of worthy/unworthy bodies (e.g., Kelly et al. 2021). At the same time, we push against sameness, taking up a politics of coalition that embraces dissent (Lorde 1997; Samantrai 2002) rather than suppressing it.

We recognise that the benefits of coalition politics are also bound up with the difficulties of such politics (Kafer 2013). It was not always easy, but we invited disagreements, tensions, and frictions in the group because otherwise we risk not recognising our own biases, assumptions, or exclusionary habits (Kafer 2013), particularly amongst the white, cis, thin, and straight and straight-passing academics on the team. These practices included disagreements being welcomed verbally by Aly as the group meeting facilitator, embracing "no" and supporting each other in our no throughout the project (e.g., choosing not to make a video, not to share a video in publication, or not being an author on a publication), giving space for people to hold opposing views, and offering opportunities to question the research process. For example, one participant co-researcher, Paul, contacted Aly to inquire whether participants would be compensated fairly for their time outside of the storytelling workshops when working independently on their videos. This is an example of Paul's refusal to be exploited in his art making; even though he was paid for all art making hours, exploitation of his video in the future is still a risk, which is why he declined to include his story in other academic articles we have written.

An openness to refusal sits in sharp contrast with the conventional nature of the fitness industry and traditional conceptualisations of a CoP, both of which seem to value normativity and consensus (e.g., Wenger 1998). Co-investigator Tara-Leigh, in reflexive writing for this paper, spoke to the uniqueness of *ReVisioning Fitness* and the power that came from learning together through working with and across our differences:

> *The sharing and co-learning that was facilitated among this CoP stood out to me as a particularly powerful tool for working to address the problematic nature of fitness. The ideas generated from imparting our diverse experiences were instrumental in creating new knowledge. This has led me to wonder whether consideration of the uniqueness of each person's experiences is what makes a CoP particularly powerful with respect to solving problems and facilitating best practices.*

Rather than thinking about difference as a force that undermines our CoP, we consider it generative and energising, and our work as thriving amid ambiguity and contradiction. In her reflexive writing for this paper, Meredith further elaborates on what the project space felt like for her:

> *When I think of a community of practice or care, I think about people coming together around a common goal or objective, and caring for each other through the process, even when things are sticky or challenging or hard. ReVisioning Fitness has felt like such a community, even from our very first meetings, as a place where we can imagine things together, and where we can come together to resist dominant norms and ideas about fitness, even when we might have different ideas about how exactly to make that happen. It has felt like a place of vulnerability, where I can share about myself and my experiences and feel supported and held by the people in the group.*

When friction arose in our work, permission to refuse and contest created the possibility for deeper, more generative understandings of the concepts we tried to unpack. For example, in one of our team meetings, we discussed the concept of "inclusion" in fitness and created a word-cloud of terms we associated with the phrase. Most of the words proposed were relatively positive, such as "belonging", "expansion", "exciting", "acceptance", "happy", and more. In contrast, Salima contributed words such as "inauthenticity" and "fraught." Later, in a one-on-one interview with Aly, Salima elaborated on her word choices (and what she described as a "grumpy moment" during our meeting), explaining that inclusion is painful and violent for her since fitness spaces often assume what people need without meaningfully engaging with them about their access needs. In her experience, the word inclusion is rarely used in a genuine way but rather is mobilized as a marketing ploy:

> *...with the inclusion part, in terms of it being weaponized, I think that something I'm definitely hyper-aware of is that social responsibility checkmark [version of] inclusion...pretending you care and having the scripts and knowing the right things to say, but it's really just surface level, and for me, I'd rather you not do that at all, then to pretend to seem like a good person or seem like a good company... unless you're willing to do the structural changes to actually [alter] that.*

Salima alludes to neoliberal inclusionism, describing it as a marketing strategy of commercial enterprises that asks/expects bodies of difference to assimilate to the norm through so-called "inclusion" tactics that merely expand tolerance rather than meaningfully building difference-affirming spaces (Bailey et al. 2023; Jones et al. 2022; Mitchell and Snyder 2015). In her interview, she also highlighted the entangled nature of inclusion and racial and disability justice, where hiring "folx that live at various intersections that might have a better way of connecting to people" can contribute to establishing more meaningfully inclusive spaces. Salima goes on to note that as someone with a disability, she needs a fitness trainer who can understand both the physical and the emotional aspects of fitness, as well as her need to rest and not be constantly pushing herself. Salima's disruptive understanding of inclusion became a pivotal moment in the project, propelling us to interrogate our assumptions about inclusion and turn a critical lens on the sudden uptick of "inclusive" physical activity campaigns that surged during the pandemic. We understand contradictions around the meaning of inclusion as generative insofar as they are not easily resolvable, belie any claims of unity, sameness, or homogeneity, and urge us to push into their rubs, tensions, and clashes for clues to what may be required to create inclusive praxis. We follow disability studies' call for alliances that resist normalisation and reorient to difference as political, valuable, and integral—as necessary for imagining alternative fitness worlds where differences are acknowledged as an ever-emerging, foundational part of the flow and movement of life itself (e.g., Kafer 2013; Mingus 2011; Rice 2018; Rice et al. 2021, 2022a).

3. What Unfolded

Our above framework and conditions of possibility—the research team, disability art making, building a community of care, the online nature of our work, and our expansive approach to coalition building—created the container for what unfolded within *ReVisioning Fitness*. We detail the unfolding that occurred within the research space, where we imagined alternative worlds for fitness via relationality, body-becoming pedagogies, access intimacies, and attending to the capacitating effects of our approaches.

3.1. Imagining Alternative Worlds of Fitness

Through our work together, we (re)imagined alternative fitness worlds that centre a politics of difference. Each of us imagined the future of fitness in different ways through our multimedia stories, highlighting the heterogeneity of our work. Skylar shared their relationship with fitness through everyday activities as a non-binary trans masculine person searching for relational meanings of fitness, and Meredith centred the importance of rest and refusal. Salima's story foregrounded the potential of fitness spaces as places where people have agency, while seeley noted the importance of people's dignity within these spaces, especially in changing rooms. Paul's story described his frustrations with a lack of accessibility and accommodations in fitness spaces, while Kayla illustrated how her embodied being works with and through crip time. In her story, Bongi explored her embodied experience of discomfort in a gym as a Black, plus sized woman, while Aly's story focused on implementing everyone's ideas of reimagining fitness through stakeholder involvement, and Tara-Leigh grappled with her complex relationship with fitness, both as something that has brought her joy but that also operates as a site of ongoing and historic harm for others. These accounts highlight what we say "no" to in fitness (e.g., ableism, fatphobia, racism, imperatives of productivity, the gender binary etc.) to make way for alternative possibilities and futures that we can say "yes" to. Stories were also used alongside clips from focus group meetings to create a mini-documentary, a nine minute film showcasing a snapshot of our reimagining of fitness that various team members have already screened in both academic and public presentations.

As a group, we imagined and theorised alternative offerings to the current fitness climate. These offerings encapsulate what has unfolded in our *ReVisioning Fitness* theorizing so far: individualism → relationality, biopedagogies → body-becoming pedagogies, inclusionism → access intimacies, and debilitating → capacitating processes and approaches.

3.1.1. Individualism → Relationality

The current fitness climate is focused on hyper-individualism (e.g., Bailey et al. 2022), but in contrast, community and relationality are central to our revisioning of fitness. Reflecting on our work together, Meredith elaborates on the centrality of relationality in our work—of being in relation with our bodily selves, with each other, and with novel ideas and knowledge, where we collectively think, feel, and move outside of a conventional fitness framework.

> I wonder about how our experience can help to stretch mainstream instrumentalist notions of the purposes of a community of practice or care–not about innovating or always having to move things forward, but as about being present for oneself and each other, even across digital space and incommensurable differences. Our work also necessarily attends to power differentials in fitness spaces and within our group, pushing into challenge and dissent in ways that CoP work has not always done. I recognize, as well, that I hold power in research and fitness spaces, and I wonder about how best to use that power to hold space for difference and challenge norms in the spaces I inhabit.

Disability arts and cultural practices served as a scaffold for our relational exploration of ideas surrounding movement and embodied agency and have given us language to activate alternative concepts of fitness and vitality through a relational lens versus an individualistic one. As a group, we have aimed to become a radical CoP—one where embodied difference and relationality rather than so-called expertise and consensus take the lead, and where normative relations are not reified, allowing knowledge to keep moving. Rather than operating from a place of "aspirational independence", we consider ourselves inherently interdependent, where the making of accessible worlds becomes a "collective human practice" that we all participate in (Valentine 2020, p. 81). Our creation of a relaxed space also likely contributed to this feeling by opening to people missing a meeting, coming late, or leaving early if needed. Members of the collective co-created a culture that welcomed each of us to engage as humans in whatever way made sense in that moment. We have found that reconceptualising CoPs along the lines described by Meredith in her above reflection and in line with the notion of a generative coalition called for within disability studies and activist movements became a necessary step in our shared work to set body-becoming pedagogies in motion.

3.1.2. Biopedagogies → Body-Becoming Pedagogies

CoPs that place significant value on expertise, efficiency, and productivity may become places where practitioners intentionally or unintentionally introduce and reproduce biopedagogies—expert instructions for living informed by moralities (Rice 2014; Rice et al. 2022b). Biopedagogies teach about supposedly morally sound behaviours by coding bodies and minds as good or bad, thereby urging conformity to normative standards through the entanglement of affect with expert knowledge. Our society has become totally pedagogized (Bernstein 2001; Rice et al. 2018), and as such, biopedagogies circulate across all systems, including media, family, education, and healthcare (e.g., Bailey et al. 2022; Bessey and Brady 2021; Friedman et al. 2020). Fitness-related discourses often perpetuate and reinforce biopedagogies, wherein messaging about physical activity reifies moralising ideas about worthy and unworthy bodies (e.g., Bailey et al. 2022).

As part of our relational and difference-affirming approach to CoP, we intentionally work to subvert biopedagogies and take up body-becoming pedagogies instead. Body-becoming involves the artful and improvisational possibilities of affirming embodiment and bodily differences (e.g., Rice 2015). Rather than relying on normative ideas of the human bodymind or on traditional notions of expertise, becoming pedagogies value our embodied differences and knowledge and our own felt understandings of our bodies' capacities as we explore our bodily capacities in spaces designed to proliferate them (Rice et al. 2018, 2021). Taking a disability arts and culture approach to revisioning fitness in a difference-centred and relational CoP has capacitated us by broadening the script for what fitness and movement might mean and how we can communicate alternative understandings to fitness stakeholders.

For Aly, who worked in the fitness industry for over a decade, *ReVisioning Fitness* provided space and opportunity to explore becoming (physically and otherwise) outside the punishing expectations of the fitness world and to resist pressures to practice fitness in the ways that she had undertaken previously. She reflects,

My "fitness" journey has had to transform, from subscribing to normative impulses, to refusing heteronormative, sanist, and ableist rhetoric. As a queer woman who identifies as Mad and has episodic disability, I have had to slowly reclaim fitness for myself. I was able to do this with the coalitional work we have done together across our differences. For me, that is the power of a relational CoP that embraces difference. Prior to ReVisioning Fitness, I never had a safe place to resist the harms of fitness practices and instead had to conform to the norm the best way I could to survive. As a fitness instructor, it was my job to uphold, validate, and confirm the importance of fitness from a biomedical perspective. Not only did this stifle my own growth, but it harmed others too. A radical CoP energises you to resist what feels impossible to resist, and that is body-becoming for me. But CoP is a fluid concept, with ebbs and flows, that needs patience and nurturing and although our team felt connected almost immediately, that may not always happen.

ReVisioning Fitness continues to offer a space where we can "becom[e] together", where we reflect on and tell our stories and have them listened to in new and different ways (Rice et al. 2018, p. 674). We conceptualise this becoming-together as a form of access intimacy, collective care and strength, and as a fruitful alternative to individualism and neoliberal inclusionism.

3.1.3. Inclusionism → Access Intimacies

In our embrace of disability politics, participant co-researcher, Kayla, brought forward the idea that access intimacies can *crip* CoPs, and counter neoliberal inclusionism that pervades fitness spaces (Mingus 2011; Mitchell and Snyder 2015). We embrace access intimacy as "the kind of eerie comfort that your disabled self feels with someone on a purely access level" (Mingus 2011, para. 4), and as an exciting way to re-think fitness practices. Access intimacy emerges from deep relationality that allows a non-normatively embodied person to relax in the presence of those who "get" their access needs (Mingus 2011). Kayla reflects on how access intimacies capacitate her physically, emotionally, and ethically:

I don't use a medical mobility aid. Rather, I see "mobility aid" as something relational rather than a physical object. What I mean is, when I am out with a trusted friend or family member, and we understand one another's needs, they know that I will need a hand or an arm up a flight of stairs, or over an icy sidewalk. When "patterned-access intimacy" (Valentine 2020, p. 83) is present in my interpersonal relationships, I feel, to co-opt a term from the fitness world, that I have better physical and emotional endurance. Patterned access intimacy ensures that the maintenance it takes to inhabit a disabled body is more of a relay race than an individual sprint, and "helps develop an ethical orientation to the world that is relational and interdependent in nature". (Valentine 2020, p. 84)

ReVisioning Fitness took place entirely digitally, so no one in the virtual room could reach out physically using touch to meet another's access needs. However, we note the body-technology interface here—the nature of our online meetings meant that the physical space of the meetings, people's homes, were already accessible to them. People had technologies at home that provided the support and rest that their bodyminds required; for Kayla, this included an electric standing desk, a robot vacuum, soft furniture, and yoga supports. In the absence of touch as a mobilising force, the politic of access intimacy may be enabled via a two-fold approach: remote meetings where we have a commitment to "'staying-with' the constant struggle of inaccessibility" (Valentine 2020, p. 84) and curating our working environments to suit the needs of our bodies and minds.

We propose that fitness stakeholders meet access needs through a process of curation. The mainstream fitness community has much to learn from disability arts. By engaging with the politics of disability arts, fitness practitioners might learn how urging homogeny and "mastery" of a physical or artistic form can become violent. For example, in Kayla's past role as Public Education Coordinator at Tangled Art + Disability, she worked with a team of disability-identified people to co-create greater accessibility in the arts world. Her work with the Tangled CoP illustrates access intimacy in action: the sharing of access knowledge between senior and junior staff members, welcoming the disruptions of disability that lead to creative innovation, and being open to others who move or think in an unexpected way, even or especially when it is unsettling. The creation of disability artworks is necessarily collaborative; to enact access, we must draw on one another's embodied knowledge of how to make art legible to a public with a diverse range of physical, mental, and sensory needs. The work of access is iterative; a checklist model of competence or compliance will always fall short of giving *everyone* what they need (e.g., Chandler et al. 2022). This line of thinking, when applied to mainstream fitness, reminds us that there is no "right way" to move or "right way" to form habits. Instead, habits can be thought of as "physical anchors that can be used as launching points for the imagination" (Hamington 2004, p. 96, quoted in Valentine 2020, p. 91).

Disability aesthetics provides an exciting tie between access to art and fitness, in that access practices innovated in disability cultural spaces can be mobilized for reimagining access and inclusion within fitness. Disability aesthetics rejects an ableist ideal in favour of a processual relationship to "desired outcomes", end goals, and the illusion of perfection. Sean Lee's (n.d.) concept of "the crip horizon" encourages us to move "away from the typically beautiful towards 'the ugly'—towards the magnificence of our imperfections—and towards an aesthetic uniquely situated and held in disability art" (para. 6). Imperfection is antithetical to the aims of mainstream fitness, which seeks to rid us of, or at least obscure, our disabilities and other bodymind differences. The embrace of disability aesthetics played a capacitating role in our work together, as did community, rest, and support, as we explore in the next section.

3.1.4. Debilitating → Capacitating

As noted above, capable bodies comprise bodies coded as productive and capable of life (Puar 2012). Within our neoliberal political economy, disabled and other non-normative bodies become debilitated or under resourced via economic and social processes that simultaneously capacitate or enable only those bodies that reproduce the hegemonic order (white, non-disabled, straight, etc.). Puar (2012) argues that queer bodies and "other bodies heretofore construed as excessive/erroneous" can also be constructed as "on the side of capacity", enabling queerness to operate "as a machine of regenerative productivity" (p. 153) when certain people are absorbed into the body politic, recuperated as good citizens, and can thus generate wealth for the nation. However, we wonder what it might mean to think about capacity differently, outside of the constraints of neoliberal ideas of productivity. The CoP that we created welcomed in difference in a regenerative way in a move towards capacitating bodies in our revisioned approach to body-becoming fitness. Creating these sorts of supportive community spaces may be one way of enacting access intimacy within the context of fitness moving forward. Meredith reflects on what capacitates her,

> *Something that capacitates me in movement practices is community and support, which has felt lacking at many points throughout the pandemic (in part due to the requirement to shift to online fitness classes, and in part due to my former yoga studio closing and feeling severed from many members of that community). ReVisioning Fitness has often helped to fill that gap, even though we were meeting online. I think back to our conversations often as I move through my yoga practice or go for a walk or spin my legs on a bike. I often "allow" myself to move in whatever ways feel intuitive for me in that moment and encourage that for the students in my yoga classes, rather than thinking about what is "right." Being connected to a group of like-minded people who have challenged my notions of fitness continues to capacitate me in my day-to-day movement practices.*

This experience of feeling and being capacitated within *ReVisioning Fitness* was in many ways oppositional to the experience Meredith portrays in her multimedia story about colonized yoga, where she did not feel capacitated to move within her own bodily potential and did not feel empowered to say no or to disengage from movement in order to rest. Respecting no in a fitness space might mean taking a rest pose despite what the teacher is instructing, which can be challenging in a group dynamic and is likely amplified if one already feels othered in that space. Access intimacy in the fitness context might mean creating spaces that welcome deviations from the expectation or norm, including all expressions of movement or rest at any given time. This openness might help to create an affective atmosphere wherein the collective addresses access needs explicitly and processually, taking the burden off non-normatively embodied people to have to advocate for accommodations or inclusion (Mingus 2011). Rather than having someone feel humiliated or like a burden, access intimacy can leave someone feeling free, light, and cared for (Mingus 2011).

A tangible example of enacting the capacitating effects of access intimacy that we imagined as a group was the idea of a fitness doula, or fitness facilitator (a gender-neutral alternative). As another co-investigator, Carla, explained in one of our meetings together, a fitness doula is:

> ...somebody [who could] help me learn how to move, and how to be in my body in the ways... that I want to, I want to expand, that I want to move... and someone who's going to work with me to co-create that, as opposed to always being the expert and telling me what I need to do in order to accomplish something, because I have... experiential knowledge of my body, and I want that to be taken seriously, and not for me to be put in some... sort of box.

We imagine a fitness doula as someone who has a capacitating role in a fitness space and who helps support folx in exploring their own bodily potential outside of what is normatively expected. This concept is drawn from the notion of crip doulaship in disability communities, whereby crip doulas mentor other disabled people and facilitate their access to disability community by supporting their navigation in the ableist world (Valentine 2020). Crip doulaship relies on the wealth of knowledge and skills that disabled people possess as a function of having to navigate a world that lacks supportive structures. "Crip wealth" and crip doulaship are both key to access intimacy, in our view, and capture ways in which our bodily freedom can be enhanced in ableist spaces (Valentine 2020, p. 91). Through the lens of access intimacy and crip doulaship, access becomes something we do or practice together, rather than something that we are striving to achieve or complete.

Furthermore, we envision love, care, connection, support, and a move towards pleasure and desire as being part and parcel of our reconceptualisation of fitness. As one participant co-researcher, Skylar, said during a group meeting, "fitness is feeling good in my body" and "when I feel good in my body, that's when I feel like I am fit." This expands what fitness can look/feel like beyond dominant norms and prompts us to reflect on the conditions or elements that can enable people to think about fitness and movement in relation to their own positive bodily experiences and desires. What if people were supported to move in a way that feels good, whatever that means for them, rather than in trying to subscribe to a narrow idea of "exercise"? How can we best support people to move towards the edges of their embodied needs and desires in ways that are capacitating?

4. Final Remarks

The fitness world is preoccupied with the ableist, capitalist notion of "moving things forward": harder, better, faster, stronger. The *ReVisioning Fitness* CoP rejects this model in favour of moving together at an artful, variable pace across space, time, and difference. This is one way that access intimacy functioned and continues to function for us. The innovation of this CoP, then, lies not in its speed or forward motion but rather in its ability to meet each of its members where they are (even if that is at home on their couch or bed). Our very process of working on this article operated in crip time, in that it required slowness and care to allow our ideas to develop, urging us to reject the need to always be moving ahead quickly to reach academic deadlines.

Within the delimited container of the project, a CoP that enabled dissent, body-becoming pedagogies, and access intimacies unfolded, a space where team members felt capacitated by the community and the support available therein. We recognise that this work is still in a process of unfolding, shifting, and becoming, and just like all participatory community-based work, we may experience collapse at any point in the journey. At this moment, we are left pondering the "big" questions: How might fitness take lessons from disability culture with its enactment and mobilisation of access intimacy to transform approaches to accessibility? And, building on learnings from *ReVisioning Fitness* and the knowledge held by disabled people, what might the fitness world do to create the conditions for difference-affirming and relational fitness experiences?

We also encourage researchers and leaders in fitness spaces to keep in mind that no experiment with access will materialize in exactly the same way given the fluidity of body-worlds and the fact that the specific bodies and forces acting on them will never be precisely the same, making a prediction of outcomes difficult, if not impossible. While it is feasible to anticipate some access needs (e.g., difference-affirming language use, creating a relaxed space), difference is always making a difference, meaning that when one creates the conditions of possibility for difference to emerge, difference will surface in different ways and in ways specific to individualities and group configurations. Thus, one could replicate or inherit many of the conditions we describe here and have an entirely different outcome, leading us to suggest a general philosophical engagement with the concepts we present rather than strict adherence to our approach.

5. Conclusions

Our centring of disability arts and culture helped to create the conditions of possibility for team members to go to the edges of and make meaning from their unique embodied needs, interests, and desires. A difference-affirming context derived from a belief in relationality allowed us to consider the movement practices we wanted to engage in and the conditions under which we might access and experiment with them. Rather than considering fitness as an instrumental praxis for achieving an individualistic or standard ideal of body functionality, our focus on the physical through the lens of disability arts and culture became a creative exploration of perception, movement, and embodiment. This exploration enables us to engage in (re)making the world of fitness through the lens of queering, cripping, and thickening fitness practices. Fitness leaders can learn from disability art making, our relational conceptualisation of CoP, and principles of body-becoming and access intimacy, and we call on them to do so and to open conditions of possibility in fitness through a radical embrace of difference.

Author Contributions: Conceptualization, M.B., K.A.B., K.B., C.R., S.P. and T.-L.F.M.; methodology, M.B., K.A.B., C.R. and T.-L.F.M.; formal analysis, M.B. and K.A.B.; investigation, M.B., K.A.B., C.R. and T.-L.F.M.; resources, K.A.B. and C.R.; writing—original draft preparation, M.B., K.A.B. and K.B.; writing—review and editing, M.B., K.A.B., K.B., C.R., S.P. and T.-L.F.M.; supervision, K.A.B., C.R. and T.-L.F.M.; project administration, K.A.B. and M.B.; funding acquisition, K.A.B., C.R. and T.-L.F.M. All authors have read and agreed to the published version of the manuscript.

Funding: This research was funded by the Social Sciences and Humanities Research Council of Canada grant number 430-2020-00030.

Institutional Review Board Statement: This research was approved by the University of Guelph Research Ethics Board (protocol # 20-10-005, approved 15 December 2020).

Informed Consent Statement: Informed consent was obtained from all participants involved in the study.

Data Availability Statement: Please contact the corresponding author if you are interested in any of the data mentioned in this article.

Acknowledgments: The authors would like to thank the Re•Vision Centre for Art and Social Justice for their support in the multimedia storytelling workshop, specifically the workshop facilitators, Hannah Fowlie and Calla Evans, and the managing director, Ingrid Mündel. The authors would also like to acknowledge the other members of the ReVisioning Fitness team who did not have capacity to contribute to this article but have given in important ways to the project as a whole: these are Bongi Dube, Evadne Kelly, seeley quest, Skylar Sookpaiboon and Paul Tshuma. We are also grateful for the contributions of Ash McAskill in the early stages of this project as she was integral in connecting the members of this group. Lastly, we thank the guest editors of this special issue, Nadine Changfoot, Carla Rice, and Eliza Chandler, for curating this important collection of articles and reviewing our manuscript.

Conflicts of Interest: The authors declare no conflict of interest.

Notes

1. We acknowledge that the term "crip" is a unique political position and that not all disability and access folx adopt this politicised language.
2. Captioning is an accessibility practice and can also be an important storytelling device. Creative captioning adds playfulness and draws attention to specific aspects of a story (e.g., the use of bold or coloured font). See the Re•Vision Centre website for an example.

References

Bailey, K. Aly, Meridith Griffin, Kimberly J. Lopez, Serena Habib, Nosaiba Fayyaz, and Amm Fudge Schormans. 2023. Building Community or Perpetuating Inclusionism? The Representation of "Inclusion" on Fitness Facility Websites. *Leisure/Loisir*, September 5. [CrossRef]

Bailey, K. Alysse, Carla Rice, Melissa Gualtieri, and James Gillett. 2022. Is #YogaForEveryone? The Idealised Flexible Bodymind in Instagram Yoga Posts. *Qualitative Research in Sport, Exercise and Health* 14: 827–42. [CrossRef]

Bernstein, Basil. 2001. From Pedagogies to Knowledges. In *Towards a Sociology of Pedagogy: The Contribution of Basil Bernstein to Research*. Edited by Ana M. Morias, Isabel Neves, Brian Davies and Harry Daniels. New York: Peter Lang, pp. 363–68.

Bessey, Meredith, and Jennifer Brady. 2021. "God Forbid You Bring a Cupcake": Theorizing Biopedagogies as Professional Socialization in Dietetics Education. In *Weight Bias in Health Education: Critical Perspectives for Pedagogy and Practice*. Edited by Heather Brown and Nancy Ellis-Ordway. Oxfordshire: Routledge, pp. 51–62.

Bodies in Translation. n.d. About. Available online: https://bodiesintranslation.ca/bodies-in-translation/ (accessed on 10 August 2022).

Chandler, Eliza, Lisa East, Carla Rice, and Rana El Kadi. 2022. Misfits in the World: Culture Shifting Through Crip Cultural Practices. *Revista Mundau*, Paper under review.

Chandler, Eliza, Megan Johnson, Chelsea Jones, Elisabeth Harrison, and Carla Rice. Forthcoming. Enacting Reciprocity and Solidarity: Critical Access as Methodology. *Australian Feminist Studies Journal*.

Chandler, Eliza, Nadine Changfoot, Carla Rice, Andrea LaMarre, and Roxanne Mykitiuk. 2018. Cultivating Disability Arts in Ontario. *The Review of Education, Pedagogy, and Cultural Studies* 40: 249–64. [CrossRef]

Collins, Kimberlee, Chelsea Jones, and Carla Rice. 2022. Keeping Relaxed Performance Vital: Affective Pedagogy for Accessing the Arts. *Journal of Literary & Cultural Disability Studies* 16: 179–96. [CrossRef]

Contu, Alessia, and Hugh Willmott. 2003. Re-Embedding Situatedness: The Importance of Power Relations in Learning Theory. *Organization Science* 14: 283–96. Available online: https://www.jstor.org/stable/4135137 (accessed on 26 November 2021). [CrossRef]

Cooper, Charlotte. 2021. *Fat Activism: A Radical Social Movement*, 2nd ed. Bristol: Intellect Books.

Cox, Andrew. 2005. What are Communities of Practice? A Comparative Review of Four Seminal Works. *Journal of Information Science* 31: 527–40. [CrossRef]

Curnow, Joe. 2013. Fight the Power: Situated Learning and Conscientisation in a Gendered Community of Practice. *Gender and Education* 25: 834–50. [CrossRef]

Dokumaci, Arseli. 2019. A Theory of Microactivist Affordances: Disability, Disorientations, and Improvisations. *The South Atlantic Quarterly* 118: 491–519. [CrossRef]

Eales, Lindsay, and Danielle Peers. 2016. Moving Adapted Physical Activity: The Possibilities of Arts-Based Research. *Quest* 68: 55–68. [CrossRef]

Evans, Calla, Hannah Fowlie, Chelsea Jones, Lilith Lee, Ingrid Mündel, and Carla Rice. 2022. Re•Vision Online Story-Making. *E-Campus Ontario*. Available online: https://revisionstorymaking.ca (accessed on 15 May 2022).

Friedman, May, Carla Rice, and Jen Rinaldi, eds. 2020. *Thickening Fat: Fat Bodies, Intersectionality and Social Justice*. New York: Routledge.

Garland-Thomson, Rosemarie. 2017. Eugenic World Building and Disability: The Strange World of Kazuo Ishiguro's *Never Let Me Go*. *The Journal of Medical Humanities* 38: 133–45. [CrossRef]

Griffin, Meridith, K. Alysse Bailey, and Kimberly J. Lopez. 2022. #BodyPositive? A Critical Exploration of the Body Positive Movement Within Physical Cultures Taking an Intersectionality Approach. *Frontiers in Sports and Active Living* 4: 908380. [CrossRef] [PubMed]

Hamington, Maurice. 2004. *Embodied Care: Jane Addams, Maurice Merleau-Ponty, and Feminist Ethics*. Urbana: University of Illinois Press.

Jones, Chelsea, Kim Collins, and Carla Rice. 2022. Staging Accessibility: Collective Stories of Relaxed Performance. *Research in Drama Education: The Journal of Applied Theatre and Performance* 27: 490–506. [CrossRef]

Kafer, Alison. 2013. *Feminist, Queer, Crip*. Bloomington: Indiana University Press.

Kelly, Evadne, Seika Boye, and Carla Rice. 2021. Projecting Eugenics and Performing Knowledges. In *Narrative Art and the Politics of Health*. Edited by Neil Brooks and Sarah Blanchette. London: Anthem Press, pp. 37–62.

LaMarre, Andrea, and Carla Rice. 2016. Embodying Critical and Corporeal Methodology: Digital Storytelling with Young Women in Eating Disorder Recovery. *Forum: Qualitative Social Research* 17. [CrossRef]

LaMarre, Andrea, Carla Rice, and Kayla Besse. 2021. Letting Bodies Be Bodies: Exploring Relaxed Performance on the Canadian Performance Landscape. *Studies in Social Justice* 15: 184–208. [CrossRef]

Lave, Jean, and Etienne Wenger. 1991. *Situated Learning: Legitimate Peripheral Participation*. Cambridge: Cambridge University Press. [CrossRef]

Lee, Sean. n.d. Crip Horizons: Disability Art Futurism. *Akimblog*. Available online: https://akimbo.ca/akimblog/crip-horizons-disability-art-futurism-by-sean-lee/ (accessed on 10 June 2022).

Limatius, Hanna. 2019. "I'm a Fat Bird and I Just Don't Care": A Corpus-Based Analysis of Body Descriptors in Plus-Size Fashion Blogs. *Discourse, Context & Media* 31: 100316. [CrossRef]

Lorde, Audre. 1997. *The Cancer Journals: Special Edition*. San Francisco: Aunt Lute.

McRuer, Robert. 2016. Compulsory Able-Bodiedness and Queer/Disabled Existence. In *The Disability Studies Reader*, 5th ed. Edited by Lennard J. Davis. New York: Routledge, pp. 301–8.

Mingus, Mia. 2011. Access Intimacy: The Missing Link. *Leaving Evidence*. May 5. Available online: https://leavingevidence.wordpress.com/2011/05/05/access-intimacy-the-missing-link/ (accessed on 16 August 2022).

Mitchell, David T., and Sharon L. Snyder. 2015. *The Biopolitics of Disability: Neoliberalism, Ablenationalism, and Peripheral Embodiment*. Ann Arbor: University of Michigan Press. [CrossRef]

Piepzna-Samarasinha, Leah Lakshmi. 2021. Cripping Healing. In *The Care We Dream Of: Liberatory and Transformative Approaches to LGBTQ+ Health*. Edited by Zena Sharman. Vancouver: Arsenal Pulp Press, pp. 72–92.

Price, Margaret. 2015. The Bodymind Problem and the Possibilities of Pain. *Hypatia* 30: 268–84. [CrossRef]

Puar, Jasbir K. 2012. Coda: The Cost of Getting Better. Suicide, Sensation, Switchpoints. *GLQ: A Journal of Lesbian and Gay Studies* 18: 149–58. [CrossRef]

Rice, Carla. 2014. *Becoming Women: The Embodied Self in Image Culture*. Toronto: University of Toronto Press.

Rice, Carla. 2015. Rethinking Fat: From Bio- to Body-Becoming Pedagogies. *Cultural Studies « Critical Methodologies* 15: 387–97. [CrossRef]

Rice, Carla. 2018. The Spectacle of the Child Woman: Troubling Girls and the Science of Early Puberty. *Feminist Studies* 44: 535–66. [CrossRef]

Rice, Carla. 2020. Digital/Multi-media Storytelling. In *The Routledge Companion to Health Humanities*. Edited by Paul Crawford, Brian Brown and Andrea Charise. Abingdon: Routledge, pp. 341–46.

Rice, Carla, and Ingrid Mündel. 2018. Story-Making as Methodology: Disrupting Dominant Stories Through Multimedia Storytelling. *Canadian Review of Sociology* 55: 211–31. [CrossRef] [PubMed]

Rice, Carla, and Ingrid Mündel. 2019. Multimedia Storytelling Methodology: Notes on Access and Inclusion in Neoliberal Times. *Canadian Journal of Disability Studies* 8: 118–48. [CrossRef]

Rice, Carla, Eliza Chandler, Elisabeth Harrison, Kirsty Liddiard, and Manuela Ferrari. 2015. Project Re•Vision: Disability at the Edges of Representation. *Disability & Society* 30: 513–27. [CrossRef]

Rice, Carla, Eliza Chandler, Kirsty Liddiard, Jen Rinaldi, and Elisabeth Harrison. 2018. Pedagogical Possibilities for Unruly Bodies. *Gender and Education* 30: 663–82. [CrossRef]

Rice, Carla, K. Alysse Bailey, and Katie Cook. 2022a. Mobilizing Interference as Methodology and Metaphor in Disability Arts Inquiry. *Qualitative Inquiry* 28: 287–99. [CrossRef]

Rice, Carla, Meredith Bessey, Andrea Kirkham, and Kaley Roosen. 2022b. Transgressing Professional Boundaries through Fat and Disabled Embodiments. *Canadian Woman Studies* 35: 51–61.

Rice, Carla, Sarah Riley, Andrea LaMarre, and K. Alysse Bailey. 2021. What a Body Can Do: Rethinking Body Functionality through a Feminist Materialist Disability Lens. *Body Image* 38: 95–105. [CrossRef]

Richardson/Kianewesquao, Catherine, and Vicki Reynolds. 2014. Structuring Safety in Therapeutic Work Alongside Indigenous Survivors of Residential Schools. *Canadian Journal of Native Studies* 34: 147–64.

Rinaldi, Jen, Carla Rice, Emma Lind, and Crystal Kotow. 2020. Mapping the Circulation of Fat Hatred. *Fat Studies: An Interdisciplinary Journal of Body Weight and Society* 9: 37–50. [CrossRef]

Roberts, Joanne. 2006. Limits to Communities of Practice. *Journal of Management Studies* 43: 623–39. [CrossRef]

Samantrai, Ranu. 2002. *AlterNatives: Black Feminism in the Postimperial Nation*. Redwood City: Stanford University Press.

Saxton, Marsha. 2018. Hard Bodies: Exploring Historical and Cultural Factors in Disabled People's Participation in Exercise; Applying Critical Disability Theory. *Sport in Society* 21: 22–39. [CrossRef]

Valentine, Desiree. 2020. Shifting the Weight of Inaccessibility: Access Intimacy as a Critical Phenomenological Ethos. *Journal of Critical Phenomenology* 3: 76–94. [CrossRef]

Viscardis, Katharine, Carla Rice, Victoria Pileggi, Angela Underhill, Eliza Chandler, Nadine Changfoot, Phyllis Montgomery, and Roxanne Mykitiuk. 2019. Difference Within and Without: Health Care Providers' Engagement with Disability Arts. *Qualitative Health Research* 29: 1287–98. [CrossRef]

Wenger, Etienne. 1998. *Communities of Practice: Learning, Meaning, and Identity.* Cambridge: Cambridge University Press. [CrossRef]

Williams, Oli, Sophie Sarre, Stan Constantina Papoulias, Sarah Knowles, Glenn Robert, Peter Beresford, Diana Rose, Sarah Carr, Meerat Kaur, and Victoria J. Palmer. 2020. Lost in the Shadows: Reflections on the Dark Side of Co-Production. *Health Research Policy and Systems* 18: 43. [CrossRef] [PubMed]

Disclaimer/Publisher's Note: The statements, opinions and data contained in all publications are solely those of the individual author(s) and contributor(s) and not of MDPI and/or the editor(s). MDPI and/or the editor(s) disclaim responsibility for any injury to people or property resulting from any ideas, methods, instructions or products referred to in the content.

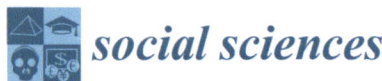

Article

"It Really Put a Change on Me": Visualizing (Dis)connections within a Photovoice Project in Peterborough/ Nogojiwanong, Ontario

Rosa Lea McBee

Department of Sustainability Studies, Trent University, Peterborough, ON K9L 0G2, Canada; rlmcbee@uvic.ca

Abstract: Photovoice is an arts-based participatory action research method that uses photography as a means for individuals, usually those facing marginalization, to document and foster group dialogue around the stories of their valuable lived experiences. This paper details a photovoice project run under the participatory planning project NeighbourPLAN, in Peterborough, Ontario, with the residents of the Downtown Jackson Creek group. The focus of the photovoice project was working with residents facing various forms of marginalization and barriers to reflect on what (dis)connections look like in their community. The findings conclude that photovoice generated new subjectivities, as residents reported feeling more connected to their community after taking photos. The process was generative in that it reminded residents of other creative outlets that they enjoyed doing and inspired them to engage with creative reflection in other ways. The findings also determined that green spaces, non-judgmental institutions, accessible amenities, safe housing, and well-maintained streets were critical for resident researchers' feelings of connectedness. I conclude with recommendations from the residents' feedback on the method and project, along with highlighting the promising potential of arts-based and storytelling methods when conducting research with marginalized groups.

Keywords: photovoice; arts-based methods; social connectedness; participatory planning; community engagement

Citation: McBee, Rosa Lea. 2023. "It Really Put a Change on Me": Visualizing (Dis)connections within a Photovoice Project in Peterborough/ Nogojiwanong, Ontario. *Social Sciences* 12: 488. https://doi.org/ 10.3390/socsci12090488

Academic Editors: Nadine Changfoot, Eliza Chandler and Carla Rice

Received: 28 December 2022
Revised: 14 July 2023
Accepted: 18 August 2023
Published: 31 August 2023

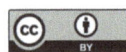

Copyright: © 2023 by the author. Licensee MDPI, Basel, Switzerland. This article is an open access article distributed under the terms and conditions of the Creative Commons Attribution (CC BY) license (https:// creativecommons.org/licenses/by/ 4.0/).

1. Introduction

With growing concern around economic, social, and environmental inequities affecting communities across Canada, participatory engagement methods have become a growing practice in academia, health initiatives, city planning, and beyond. Participatory action research (PAR) principles are commonly drawn upon to examine the link between public health and urban development, especially among vulnerable groups (Arcaya et al. 2018). PAR reframes the traditionally silenced "subjects" of research as key "knowledge producers", aware of their experiences, capable of self-representation, and entitled to mutual benefit that should be generated during and after any research process (Askins and Pain 2011). Concurrently, a growing awareness of the health impacts of loneliness (Griffiths et al. 2007; Hari 2018) and subsequent desire to heal the atrophying social spheres and sense of connectedness in communities, guided this research paper to explore the potential of PAR to address deteriorating social trust and engagement. *Photovoice* is a qualitative, arts-based participatory research method first introduced and implemented by researchers Wang and Burris (1997), who draw inspiration from Paolo Freire's concept of *conscientização* or critical consciousness-raising. Freire's critical pedagogy often started with community members drawing or photographing their community to encourage reflections on the social and political systems that negatively impact them (Freire 1970). Photovoice realizes the spirit of PAR as it invites participants to identify, collect, and analyze their world, realities, and experiences by taking photographs. The photographs encourage creative and visual representations of assets and challenges in a community, which is accompanied by critical dialogue through focus groups, or public exhibitions around selected images (Hergenrather et al. 2009; Joyce 2018; Wang and Burris 1997).

This article details a photovoice project conducted under the umbrella of a multi-year participatory planning project, NeighbourPLAN, while exploring relationship-building within PAR activities, and how building social connectedness can be intentionally fostered within research. Beauregard et al. (2020) define connectedness as the quality and number of ties individuals maintain with others, embracing "areas such as family, peers, school, and community" that "promotes well-being, increases adaptive capacity, and enhances a sense of belonging" (p. 438). Community engagement is becoming central to planning on a local level, and storytelling is more important than ever (Walljasper 2018, p. 29); thus, not-for-profits, researchers, community organizers, and planners are increasingly adopting PAR methodologies when working with local citizens or "lay experts" to create more equitable involvement and reciprocal outcomes (Arcaya et al. 2018). The focus of the photovoice project was to create opportunities for storytelling and reflections on connectedness within a larger participatory project by visually capturing what (dis)connections look like in a low-income neighbourhood facing various forms of marginalization. The findings of this project show that through the process of documentation and photo-storytelling, residents shifted their experience of their community to feel *more* connected than before and clarified the spaces and places that offered safety and those that did not. Photovoice, particularly in participatory planning initiatives, excels at giving narrative support to intangible feelings and experiences for more textured, nuanced, and complex meaning to emerge that is generative of new possible understandings for participants and facilitators. The photovoice project made participants' worlds within Peterborough more visible to themselves, to one another, and to the other stakeholders in the larger NeighbourPLAN project.

2. Background

GreenUP, a Peterborough/Nogojiwanong, Ontario-based non-profit focused on urban environmental sustainability, launched the three-year participatory planning project 'NeighbourPLAN' in 2017, with the vision that there is a mutual benefit when residents are included as planning partners (Nasca 2016). NeighbourPLAN worked with 3 neighbourhoods, 18 organizations, 2 Universities, and numerous city councillors, planners, and architects as they sought to be a third-party broker between city planning and underrepresented, marginalized neighbourhoods. Macedo (2000) warns against using euphemisms like "marginalized" or "disenfranchised" instead of "oppressed" because it risks making the Oppressor invisible. While we can and should expose oppressive institutions and those perpetuating them, I am uncomfortable referring to the people I met through this NeighbourPLAN as "oppressed" as it does not make apparent the agency, skills, power, and creativity of the people I spoke with. For this reason, I will use the term "marginalized" to refer to any group that lives outside the white cisgender, heteronormative, able-bodied, financially secure norm, understanding that this phrase is insufficient and risks obfuscating the severity of many realities.

Within the initial surveys within the Downtown Jackson Creek (DTJC), residents wished for safe, accessible spaces where "residents are able to make new relationships and feel connected to one another through participating in the project (GreenUP Association and The Centre for Active Transportation 2019, p. 6). As a graduate student recruited into NeighbourPLAN to conduct embedded research and an evaluation of the program, this anticipated outcome piqued my curiosity about the social ties and networks formed through participatory processes. Since NeighbourPLAN primarily sought feedback from residents through focus groups, pop-ups, and surveys, I was intrigued by what residents would think about an arts-based methodology. I used photovoice to address how NeighbourPLAN participants would define social connectedness and what connections look like in their communities. I use "connectedness" when referring to relationships, or the social 'glue' in a community, rather than the more prevalent term "social capital", coined by economist Glenn Lour, as the latter is often co-opted by neoliberal discourse (Small 2009). This discourse can assume that if people living in poverty networked better and made "good" 'investments' through relationships, their social circumstances would improve, bypassing speaking to systemic issues such as class relations or the state's role in developing or inhibiting connectedness in communities. (Mohan and Stokke 2000).

2.1. Downtown Jackson Creek (DTJC)

While NeighbourPLAN worked in three neighbourhoods across Peterborough, this paper focuses on the photovoice project I conducted with the DTJC neighbourhood. DTJC, a highly populated region west of downtown Peterborough, is a diverse, low-income neighbourhood with a higher-than-average unemployment rate of 12.7% compared to 8.9% citywide (GreenUP Association and The Centre for Active Transportation 2019). Within the same report, the 2019 average household income was shown to be 34,058 CAD, and 86.6% of residents are tenants, compared to the 37.9% tenancy average in the rest of Peterborough.

NeighbourPLAN planned three phases in each neighbourhood: the portrait phase, engaging residents to determine concerns and assets; the vision phase, to set out goals and priorities (see supplementary materials); and the action phase, to GreenUP's network to advocate for the ideas generated by residents (Active Neighbourhoods Canada 2015). While NeighbourPLAN supported residents with knowledge creation and mobilization, it could not guarantee any of the project's ideas. It is the city that ultimately decides whether design proposals are 'feasible' or not, leaving much uncertainty toward the project's end, reminding us that "sharing through participation does not necessarily entail sharing in power" (White 1996, p. 143).

2.2. Intentional Connection Building in PAR

The interdisciplinary research and evidence of social connectedness as an important factor for health and wellness is extensive, and factors such as individual and community resilience, diagnoses, and recovery all improve with the presence of meaningful connections (Comes 2016; Griffiths et al. 2007; Hari 2018; Taylor and Wei 2020; Umberson and Montez 2010). According to Small (2009), to examine and minimize inequality in well-being due to network inequities, we must first understand how people's social connections are formed. Despite substantial evidence backing its perceived importance, many academic disciplines take social bonds and the mechanisms that establish them for granted (Mayan and Daum 2016; Small 2009). Even the three most notable and prolific writers on Social Capital, Bourdieu, Lin, and Coleman (in Small 2009), sidestepped the subject of how to develop connections. Within this gap, connection-building is glossed over as serendipitous or dependent on the facilitator's leadership and charisma. Of course, practicing reciprocity, promoting listening and learning, and ensuring continual interactions are important steps to creating the foundation for relationships (Hall and Tandon 2017; Hardy et al. 2018; Kesby 2005; Levkoe and Kepkiewicz 2020); however, there is not much documentation of the intentional decisions behind developing connections through the research process.

Participatory techniques already have the potential to be relational, requiring cooperation and diverse stakeholders to work together, who significantly benefit from existing social networks (Janzen et al. 2016; Kemmis and McTaggart 2005). Levkoe and Kepkiewicz (2020) performed a pan-Canadian evaluation of 12 community engagement initiatives and concluded that after participatory research projects, partners perceived other partnering organizations as better colleagues and friends working towards a common goal and agreed that the process broadened networks, leading to future collaborative works.

However, relationships and connections are difficult to anticipate, explain, and evaluate, which can come at direct odds with the bias among funding agencies' criteria to evaluate investments by citing measurable, observable, and quantifiable change, which is equated to impact in final reports. (Hardy et al. 2018; Levkoe and Kepkiewicz 2020). Hardy et al.'s (2018) case study of Hermosas Vidas is unique in that it seeks to quantify the number of 'lasting' relationships built through the participatory health research project. While evaluating the relationship building of the project by taking a cross-section of the stakeholders, from the families to partnering institutions, they found that the institutional partners of the project reported creating up to five times as many new connections as the project's intended beneficiaries and most vulnerable stakeholders, the families dealing with health issues. The authors argue that this asymmetrical benefit, even if unintentional, contradicts PAR values of benefiting the community first. To explain this disparity, they created a Ripple-Effect Theory Model, which sets up PAR researchers with a framework to anticipate a gap in benefits, conduct cross-sectional evaluations, and adjust accordingly, mid-project.

2.3. Prioritizing Connections through Arts-Based Storytelling

Researchers often fear that they may inadvertently choose a method that causes more harm to vulnerable groups they seek to support. In their evaluation of a national participatory initiative in food security conducted in food banks, Bay and Swacha (2020) found that an electronic survey alienated and angered participants who already felt vulnerable and unseen while waiting in line for food services. The authors admitted how the priority of more data too quickly became extractive and dehumanizing and argue that as researchers, we must intentionally map out a process that encourages people's entanglement and connections, with methods that can also allow for the rich experience of daily life to be seen and heard. Cahill (2007) notes that participatory research is emotional listening and reflects on the therapeutic quality of PAR when sharing personal stories in a "collective space for breaking the silence" (p. 281). Expressing emotions through personal stories helps participants work through the confusion of systemic oppression and create solidarity among the group. This is where arts-based storytelling methods, such as photovoice, find their fit.

The literature about participatory research discusses connectivity and quintessential social networks but does not often explain the decisions on how to develop them. Encouragingly, participatory practitioners discuss this gap using narrative and arts-based strategies that disclose their creative processes and observe social relationships as an outcome. Arts-based and storytelling methods do not sidestep PAR's challenges with power dynamics, co-option, and resource constraints, but they offer a way to circumvent social norms as they demand unique dialogue, listening, and cooperation. They are one mechanism we can turn to when strengthening social networks and a sense of belonging in our communities is a priority.

3. My Research Approach

Despite the claim in the participatory literature that building relationships within participatory projects is essential and leads to more action (Janzen et al. 2016), there is a gap in the participatory literature on how connections and relationships are defined and how they are/were formed. NeighbourPLAN's 'Theory of Change[1]' reasoned that more connected residents would have more collective power to influence the services and spaces that mattered to them. Trying to quantify or qualify relationships is difficult due to their "deeply personal and emotional nature" (Levkoe and Kepkiewicz 2020, p. 233). However, I still wanted to ask, what made residents from the DTJC feel more connected to their community, and what disconnected them?

As part of my NeighbourPLAN evaluation role, I acted as an embedded researcher (Lewis and Russell 2011), participant, and member of the Evaluation Committee. I observed, participated in, discussed, collaborated on, and supported different project tasks, including attending resident meetings, for ten months before initiating the photovoice project with the DTJC resident group.

While I used two focus group evaluations with two neighbourhoods in the NeighbourPLAN project as my primary method to evaluate NeighbourPLAN's activities and to determine a context-specific definition of connectedness for residents, in this paper, I focus on the photovoice project I facilitated in the summer of 2019 with the DTJC neighbourhood group. I refer to all the photovoice residents by pseudonyms, which carries some tension around representation and credit. However, I kept them anonymous as many residents were also in my focus groups and giving critical feedback about the program. There were five women and one man, 30–50 years of age, white, low-income, and three were known to be Ontario Disability Support Program recipients and living with chronic health or disabilities that impact how their bodies move through space.

4. Methodology

In traditional academic frameworks, lived experiences and local knowledge are difficult to translate; however, the methods are "key to deconstructing dominant discourses and social hierarchies" and asking a community to articulate its knowledge with conventional methods risks generating conventional answers (Askins and Pain 2011, p. 806; White 1996). In their article, Bay and Swacha (2020) warn participatory practitioners against weighing the institutional demands for quantifiable data over the value and necessity of slower, engaged, and sensitive research methods when interacting with vulnerable populations. After hearing those critiques, I chose a qualitative research design that would prioritize subjective and intersectional knowledge and allow for deeper experiential understandings (Given 2008). As a form of PAR, photovoice would provide a way to engage with the research process that, hopefully, would feel generative and allow residents to reflect differently than they had done previously through regular meetings, focus groups, events, and surveys. As the creators of photovoice, Wang and Burris (1997) outlined three main goals of the research method: (1) to empower research participants to be the ones to document and cogitate on their lives and circumstances, (2) to encourage critical dialogue and knowledge creation through the photographs with the group, and (3) to mobilize the photos and knowledge created to end up with policymakers.

Residents were recruited based on their interest in NeighbourPLAN, and GreenUP staff contacted the participants first. From there, snowball sampling (peer selection) recruited three more from the initial three participants (I had met with the three over the various meetings and events for the previous eight months). This photovoice project had three phases: an introductory workshop, two weeks to take photos, and a final discussion group where residents shared what they felt, learned, and wanted others to see in their photos. During the introductory workshop, I explained the method, gave quick photography tips such as the rule of thirds, lighting, etc., and distributed disposable cameras and printed out photo journals that prompted an examination of feelings, motivations, and desires. Given the two-week timeframe, I simplified Wang's (1999) popular photo-journaling technique, SHOwED[2] in the photo journals. I then asked residents to photograph and reflect on their neighbourhood's connections and disconnections without any other parameters to avoid limiting the possible manifestations, definitions, and perspectives. For example, despite the recommendations from Kindon et al. (2007) to identify a target audience, such as policymakers or service providers, I did not explicitly state a desired audience. Instead, I asked residents to think about whom they wanted to view their photos and to keep them in mind while they took photos and reflected in their journals. This flexibility led to some interesting outcomes but also some limitations, which I discuss further in the limitations section (see Section 4.1). Finally, I led a 90-min focus group where residents shared their photos, gave feedback on the method itself and then went into storytelling around the photos and used coloured stickers to start us thinking about how thematic analysis works. I iteratively returned to those themes, the transcript, photos, and photo journals, until all the data were categorized.

To be clear, while I evaluated a participatory planning project and conducted a literature review on PAR and arts-based participatory methods, I am not suggesting that the research design of this photovoice project strictly adheres to or meets the criteria of what I believe to be PAR. While photovoice allowed the residents to conduct their own data collection and photo journaling encouraged preliminary analysis, a lack of resources coupled with a concern of over-saturation limited us from being able to spend time together in the planning and analysis phases of research. During the photovoice focus group, residents placed coloured dots on photos based on loose themes, contributing to the final analysis. However, I conducted months of analysis work after that, thus privileging my meaning-making over the residents' (Dassah et al. 2017). Regarding the design of the project, I initially suggested to the residents that they take photos within the neighbourhood boundaries set by NeighbourPLAN; however, residents expressed that those boundaries did not align with their concept of their community, which was an issue reiterated later in the focus groups that evaluated NeighbourPLAN as a whole. Expanding those boundaries to where they visit daily would better show their connections, which we agreed on. GreenUP was concerned that I not put too many demands on residents on top of all the events and activities that NeighbourPLAN was requesting of the residents, so it was always a negotiation of what should be prioritized. Indeed, GreenUP's concern was affirmed when I later conducted a focus group evaluating NeighbourPLAN and residents noted the burden of the work.

The final phase of photovoice typically showcases photos to inform policymakers or the community (Wang 1999; Joyce 2018). Time constraints did not allow for a public show, so the photos were used in the final DTJC Vision document, a public document that ended up on the desks of numerous partnering organizations, city planners, city officials, and more. The group also expressed interest in having their photos in local publications, *The River*, a magazine dedicated to showcasing the creativity and ideas of the marginalized and low-income in Peterborough. After submitting one self-selected photo and journal entry on behalf of each resident, the team at *The River* accepted three entries.

4.1. Limitations with Photovoice and the Research Design

High-quality photovoice projects can be costly, but with an internal grant from Symons Trust and some funds made available by GreenUP, I designed this project with honoraria (100 CAD per resident), cameras, developing film, and refreshments totalling approximately 1000 CAD. When asking for feedback and negotiations of the introductory workshop, I decided against a request from one resident to use personal cameras. I felt that using disposable cameras had benefits, such as forcing us to plan out film usage and ensuring that everyone's photos were the same quality since some residents did not have access to cameras. Several residents were inconvenienced by the technical issues of the disposable cameras, especially those with smartphones or better-quality cameras. I am still uncertain whether my attempt at creating equal conditions among participants outweighed the costs to the project. My hope was no one would feel embarrassment or exclusion due to a lack of resources, but by denying some residents their request to use their personal cameras, I potentially communicated to those residents that they were consultants rather than co-creators of the research design (Liebenberg 2022).

As discussed, I did not specify a target audience to participants which resulted in some interesting insights and drawbacks. While many photos were directed to the broader public or to me as the researcher, one resident addressed many of her photos and journal responses towards her fellow neighbours, inviting them to see the community's strengths by becoming more involved in the events and nearby parks and attractions. This resident identified her neighbours as the key to bringing about the change she wanted. I view this variability in the audience as a generative outcome, as residents had different concepts of where power and "agents of social change" were located, i.e., on either the political or community level (Carlson et al. 2006, p. 849). However, it also potentially created some disadvantages by lacking focus and targetedness when considering the explicit appeal that the methodology has to speak to powerful others to effect change (Liebenberg 2018).

While the photovoice project attracted socioeconomically diverse groups with different abilities who were already part of NeighbourPLAN's more consistent partners, neither NeighbourPLAN nor I were able to engage people of colour and Indigenous peoples in a lasting way, despite their presence in the downtown core. Exploring the absences and rejections surrounding every participation project is a chance to learn, but few research papers account for it. White (1996) says that non-participation can be as empowering as involvement for underprivileged groups if they feel the project will not benefit them. This highlights the limitation of what we offer through participation and how people may feel excluded based on ethnicity. Projects can improve this without abandoning participatory models by directly addressing power, class, race, and gender (Cooke and Kothari 2001; Kesby 2005). Cahill (2007) suggests conceptualizing participatory spaces as "contact zones" that do not erase participants' social, economic, and cultural context while focusing on our tensions, exchanges, and reciprocity and by including more diverse representation within the organizing team (Torre 2010; Murdoch et al. 2016). I do not visibly represent that diversity, and while NeighbourPLAN had diverse gender, sexuality, age, and ability in the organizing team and core groups, they also lacked ethnic diversity.

Finally, half of the photovoice participants identified as living with a disability, but I did not use a disability arts framework for this photovoice project. I did not specifically recruit on the topic of disability; however, considering the themes of accessibility, stigma, and healthcare that emerged throughout the photos, and noting that a tremendous body of literature already exists precisely at the nexus of photovoice, disability advocacy, and rewriting harmful narratives around disability (Newman et al. 2009; Oden et al. 2010), I now see the oversight of not utilizing that framework. Especially as I was working with the DTJC neighbourhood group, where disability and low-income status are intertwined and constantly affecting each other.

5. Findings

During the debrief with residents, the discussion ranged from the personal to the systemic. The group seemed to enjoy what Bay and Swacha (2020) call 'affective time', listening and learning about each other and relating to what they heard, from favourite spots in town to negative experiences in institutions. Residents were optimistic about the project when I asked how the photovoice compared to the other participatory methods employed by NeighbourPLAN, responding that photovoice was "more interactive" and "more personal," and Patty added, "it's good to see your connections, see other people's [connections]". Residents evaluated their neighbourhood connections, prompted by the photos, and shared which judgment-free spaces supported their well-being. Furthermore, but not expectedly from a Frerian-based process, residents' collective reflections and conclusions quickly revealed the broader power deficits they feel negatively impact them, such as inaccessible housing and experiencing stigma in healthcare.

During the second half of the focus group, I asked participants to use stickers to organize their photos into themes and describe the stories they wanted to share through them. The preliminary categories set during this time were green spaces, leisure and activities, housing, heritage buildings and art, accessibility, unsafe spaces, health and wellness, and the places and people that made them feel they belonged. I allotted a 90-min session for this activity because some of the residents have chronic health issues and we needed to consider the discomfort sitting for long periods can cause. Additionally, sharing knowledge can be an intimate and emotionally exhausting process, so I consolidated some of the outlier categories into other existing themes. While having participants co-create the categories would have been preferable, I was aware of the time asks of participants within the greater project. Going forward, I would recommend that time and resources for this kind of co-creation be incorporated into future projects. Categorizing the photos into five categories: 'institutions and organizations', 'green spaces and leisure', 'accessibility', 'shifting subjectivities', and 're-igniting creative outlets', the paragraphs below synthesize conversations during the debrief and excerpts from the photo journals, accompanied by select representative photos.

5.1. (Dis)connections: Institutions and Organizations

The first observation in this category was that residents focused on places they felt connected to during the debrief. They were quick to share resources of people and places that made them feel safe and seen. They took many photos of essential local businesses, services, and institutions, listing the new Public Library, GreenUP, Good Neighbours Care Centre, urban gardening groups, and St Vincent de Paul food bank as "mainstays" with friendly, nonjudgmental staff and individuals. Residents felt connected to churches and historic buildings (see Figure 1), which they thought should be more used and respected. Marie, a resident with mobility impairment, took photos of disappearing amenities near her home, making her feel disconnected because she now had to travel outside her neighbourhood to access those same services.

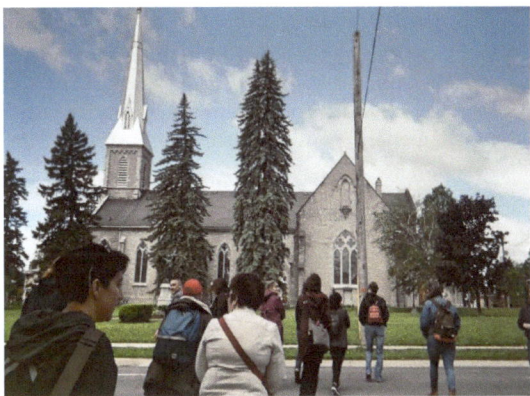

Figure 1. "Trinity Church—Church Row". Marie's entry: This is one of the few churches left still functioning on the row. I am seeing more and more history disappear, and it's disturbing. This church can be used for many other purposes than a place of worship. Let's keep these places of beautiful history running and keep the people going to them. Image Description: Church with tall steeple in background with a group of people crossing the street, walking towards the church.

I noted in the debrief that most participants had photographed the local hospital (see Figure 2). When I asked if this connection was positive or negative, they responded, "negative!" They then shared stories and strategies when being denied care due to stigma and racism. Jessica remarked, "They racially profile", and Patty noted their need to accompany a friend who is Indigenous to the hospital, to which Jessica and Marie agreed. Daniel shared that he had been neglected when visiting the emergency room multiple times in pain for what turned out to be cancer; "that's my problem—they see me and think 'oh, he's a junkie.' They see no teeth, ripped jeans, long hair—but that's just how I look". Through the discussion and journals, it was clear that these residents feel a deep sense of loss in this neighbourhood, taking photos of the hospital and spots where they made memories or visited with friends and family who have since passed.

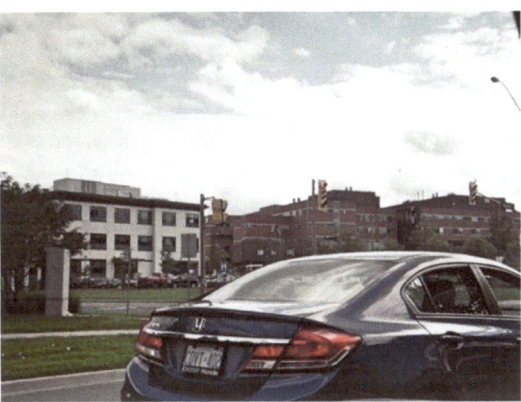

Figure 2. "Peterborough General Hospital". Patty's entry: This is the local hospital. I've taken the pic from a distance because I don't really want to be there. I have been in this hospital for myself and

many friends. Many are not here now. Some are still fighting for life. And I'm in that fight with her/my friend. Don't let anyone die alone. Say what you need to say now. Do what you need to do. There might not be a tomorrow. Image Description: Cluster of large hospital building taken from a car window with a parked car in the lower right corner of the image.

5.2. Green Spaces and Leisure

Green spaces and leisure was a ubiquitous theme within residents' photos for what helped them feel connected. Peterborough's green spaces, trails, urban gardens, rivers, and creeks are plentiful, and residents spoke of their appreciation for beautiful areas to travel to in the city, escape, fish, play, and visit with family (see Figure 3).

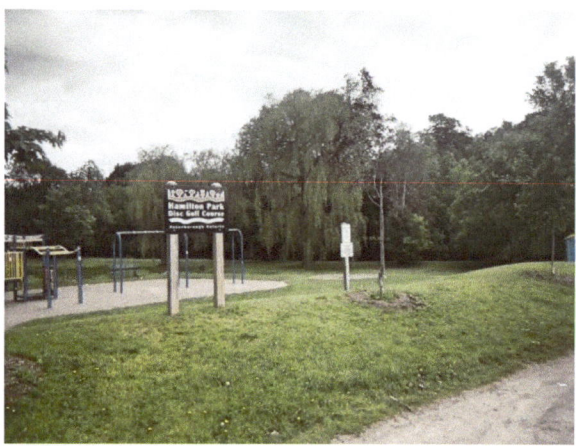

Figure 3. "Hamilton Park". Daniel's entry: Children enjoying themselves when school's out. I love taking my grandchildren. It is a place of happiness, and you leave with a smile. Image Description: A park with a playground in the background. A wooden sign reads "Hamilton Park".

5.3. (Dis)connections: Accessibility

Accessibility and Peterborough's transit system were common themes for residents with disabilities. As demonstrated by Marie's photo (see Figure 4), residents with mobility impairments felt disconnected from neglected areas and streets without sidewalks. Accessible parking spots at the Public Library and drugstores, as well as transit, make the residents with mobility devices and impairments feel more connected as they are able to navigate those spaces they have to frequent regularly. Patty took photos of the bus depot and wrote, "many people use this transit system to stay connected".

Housing accessibility is another critical issue for residents with mobility impairments. Patty took photos of her housing to show all the accessibility ramps into their building, noting it was the only place she could live with her mobility issues, but also the discord she felt, feeling safe having a community but also feeling very restricted and unsafe in the small basement space (see Figure 5). Concern was expressed that residents of diversity groups living in the building were vulnerable to crimes against them.

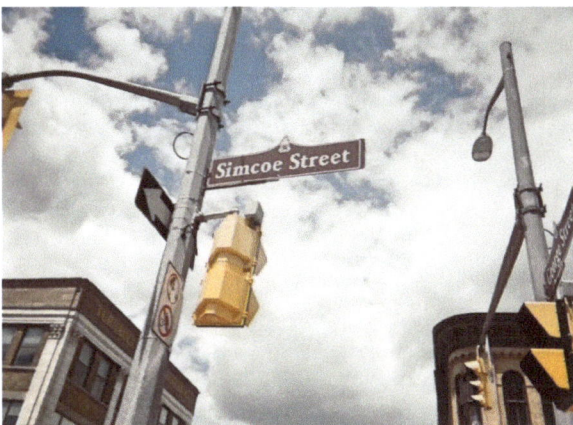

Figure 4. "Sheer Hell". Marie's entry—One of the worst streets in Peterborough for potholes, sinkholes, bad sidewalks. It is horrible for anyone with assisted devices. I use a walker and find it almost impossible to navigate the sidewalks. I want others to become aware of how hard it is to get around on some streets that are not kept up when you have an assisted medical device, not just a vehicle! Image Description: A street sign with a traffic light below it, blue skies, and clouds in the background.

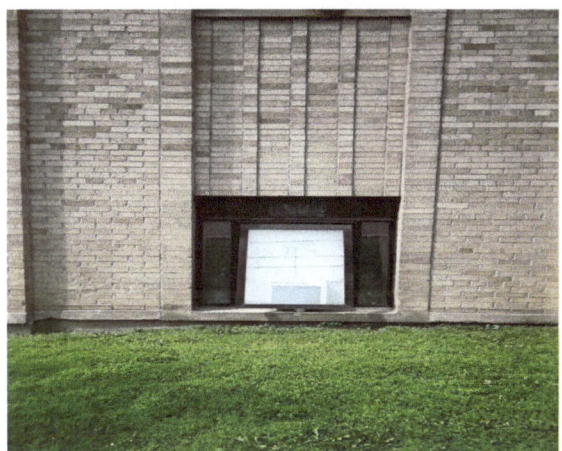

Figure 5. "My only window, ground-floor apartment". Patty's entry—Sometimes, I find this window unsafe. People have knocked and looked in the window, which is frightening. But I need a window so I can see the outside, the weather, the plants, the birds/animals. I need to connect to the outside. Basements are not really healthy apartments to live in! I stay in this apartment and this building because if I didn't and when I become more ill, I will need help from KPP 24-h helpline in the building. Unfortunately, living here is hard. Many of my friends have died. They lived here because they had precarious lives where they needed help. Image Description: Grass leading up to a brick building with one window just inches above the ground, opened from the bottom.

5.4. Shifting Subjectivities

As noted previously, PAR's concept of empowerment is quite vague. Cahill (2007) swaps the word "empowerment" for "shifting subjectivity" to mean redefining marginalized selfhood in a more critical or positive light. Residents in the photovoice project emulated this by describing profound changes in their perceptions of their neighbourhood when they started to think about their connections through a camera lens. Sarah asked herself, "what is my community?" continuing, "I really felt that sense of community. It gave me great pleasure; it really intensified that feeling; it was great!" Marie continued after her, "I always thought where I lived was the building, and I hated it. But no, I live in the community, and I respect it. So, it really put a change on me". Patty said she felt more connected to her community after the activity. Sarah shared a story about an at-risk man in the neighbourhood of whom she took a photo. She shared that she initially was a bit wary of him, but after he shared his story, she saw how "scared and lonely" he was. He has become one of those familiar faces she looks forward to seeing around and fosters a sense of connectedness for her. She observed, "you sometimes connect with those people without even knowing about it. Approaching them with a camera is one way to start talking to someone".

5.5. Reigniting Creative Outlets

Four out of six residents said the process inspired them to reengage with their creative outlets (see Figure 6). Most had not taken photos in a while and enjoyed doing so again. Three residents said the project's photo journal was important; Sarah shared, "I have started journaling again! I used to do it and forgot how much I enjoyed it". Marie said, "I used to make a lot of scrapbooking, and this got me thinking about that again". Patty reflected, "I like to use being creative as therapy—to work out my emotions, my thoughts, and my needs".

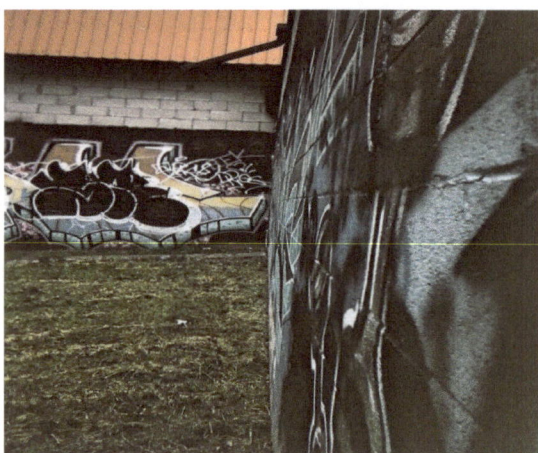

Figure 6. "Graffiti and Vibrant Colors". Sarah's Entry—I walk by so often but never appreciated it up close to really see the writing on the wall. That graffiti is part of a sociological statement. Different painters are combining different thematics, some angry, some playful. I always wanted to be an artist. Image Description: A graffiti wall up close, with another graffiti wall in the background.

5.6. Resident Feedback

Part of the photovoice focus group was dedicated to receiving residents' feedback on the process and gaining future insights for NeighbourPLAN if it wants to use this method in future neighbourhoods. The group shared the following feedback:

- One month, with a two week-window to take photos, worked well timewise.
- Make a list of things to photograph, but also save a few spots for spontaneous photos.
- Visit places you plan to photograph without a camera first. Sarah notes, "not having the camera with me at first was helpful as I backtracked and remembered how I felt about it".
- Taking photos can lead to awkward interactions; plan for what to say if approached.
- Photo journals were an integral part of the process for most participants, but one felt hindered by it; they provide more support or different ways to reflect.

Disposable cameras were a common frustration. They limited photo quality and quantity. "It was nostalgic, but not in a good way", noted Daniel. Others were disappointed by the overexposed or accidentally taken photos. They acknowledged that not providing cameras would be a barrier for those without resources in their neighbourhood. However, they thought people could bring their cameras, and I could coordinate with other organizations to lend out cameras.

6. Discussion

Residents in this photovoice project said seeing the same people, accessibility, green spaces, and cultural events and sites helped them feel connected, while inaccessible design, unaffordable housing, dangerous traffic, and stigmatizing institutions made them feel disconnected. Notably, after photographing their neighbourhood, photovoice participants cited feeling more connected to their neighbourhood. This is a particularly impressive result when comparing it to other NeighbourPLAN engagement activities, about which some of the same residents in the photovoice project later articulated in the evaluation focus groups that those activities did not garner the kind of strong social connectedness they hoped for (McBee 2021). The type of social connectedness residents defined during the evaluation focus groups spoke to more sustained relationships of trust, respect, mutual aid, and support among their neighbours and community. When I asked why connections are so hard to create, some residents from the DTJC felt it was because other residents "don't trust, they're suspicious", or cited a lack of pride in the community and that the participatory engagement strategies that NeighbourPLAN employed felt "too much like work", which led to less long-term participants and less opportunity to develop those relationships (McBee 2021). Rice et al. (2016) write that art "facilitates certain encounters between persons that would not occur otherwise because our communication with one another is so highly regulated" (p. 64), and the literature supports that community artmaking and storytelling can facilitate unique and new connections, especially between stakeholders or individuals whose lives are separated by cultural, social, political, or economic forces (Askins and Pain 2011; Beauregard et al. 2020; Youkhana 2014); however, Lavrinec (2014) highlights how the repetition in playful interactions during large-scale arts-based participatory projects are more helpful in developing emotional connections for a more robust, sustained network.

6.1. "Stuff" and Its Potential for Building Connections

Askins and Pain (2011) write that material-based hands-on methods can be valuable instruments for non-verbal, embodied listening. Material objects can also lower the barriers to interactions with strangers from different socioeconomic groups and thus foster more opportunities to connect than traditional research methods engender. In the participatory planning pilot project 'Stewart Street Active Neighbourhood', Nasca (2016) notes the resident steering committee's unanimous positive evaluation of the 3D asset map as a successful relationship-building tool that allowed neighbours to orbit around a physical, interactive object and engage with others. Social Capital Theorist Small (2009) observes that "relationships often arise around a common object of attention", especially if the item engenders cooperative and non-competitive action (p. 25). This photovoice project supports those findings. Residents seamlessly maneuvered through stories of loss, joys, hobbies, and interests when prompted by photos. Residents then physically interacted with the photos, generating further sharing, and finding commonality in resources, strategies, and ways of seeing their community.

The inquiry into the physical materials in participatory research and their effects on power dynamics are under-theorized in PAR literature (Askins and Pain 2011), despite increasing interest in how spatiality affects outcomes of encounters between diverse groups (Askins 2018; Valentine 2008). Askins and Pain (2011) observe the centrality of materials in physical encounters or 'contact zones' to break down patterns of social interactions. In their case study, interracial youth partook in two phases of an afterschool arts program. The first phase was marked with youth doing the art, requiring the use of materials, which led to positive engagement and a temporary, tenuous collapse of racial divides. In the project's second phase, a local artist designed an art product on behalf of the youth, but in the process, she accidentally made the youth group feel self-conscious by highlighting differences. Without the physical paintbrushes, paints, and paper, fragile bonds fell apart when focusing on otherness. In other words, while it is the act of doing that defines embodied research, the objects we use can serve as helpful catalysts for connection and creating an "axis for emerging citizens' networks" (Lavrinec 2014, p. 59).

Within the photovoice project, the residents moved about and physically interacted with the photos while sharing stories, stimulating further interactions between the group. Through physical images spread across the table, residents could view shared challenges, linking commonalities across photos, thus, situating their personal experiences into broader socio-political realities and biases. This parallels Askins and Pain's (2011) research finding that objects within a contact zone created new knowledge, interactions, and solidarities.

6.2. Strengths, Solidarities, and the Dangers of Photovoice

True et al. (2019) describe that they are continually inspired by how their participants note that photovoice increases awareness of "unmet needs, the strengths, and sources of support that exist in their lives" (p. 24). I also witnessed this sentiment among the DTJC group. Residents expressed an awareness of how connected they were, acknowledged that their connections were assets and articulated when those connections were missing. Residents also reflected on the causes for their missing connections, often scaling it up to larger processes of classism or racial discrimination. Strategies for navigating those realities were also shared with examples including engaging and even starting their own food security initiatives, Peterborough Gleans, to help with chronic illnesses, volunteering, and starting a neighbourhood association to have their voices amplified and accompanying their Indigenous friends and family who needed to go to the hospital as they noted the racism they experienced in health care.

Visiting the spectrum of Freire's foundational model of *conscientização*, which details three levels of consciousness in how people perceive their social and political realities: Magical, when participants have internalized beliefs about their inferiority and remain silent and complicit in their marginalization; Naïve, when participants view others as the problem, placing blame on their peers rather than seeing their role and role of the oppressor; and finally, Critical, when participants become aware of the systems of oppression, and begin to reject harmful representations that are used to justify their disenfranchisement; this photovoice project reached 'critical consciousness' and even inspired some "intentions to act", a fourth phase of consciousness more recently identified by Carlson et al. (2006) when residents stated their intention to continue or start up new creative outlets. However, I would not claim this photovoice project "uncovered" any oppression as residents seemed acutely familiar with the forces that kept them marginalized and struggling in poverty; what it did unveil to residents was how connected they were, and how integral they were in creating connections (i.e., assets) in their communities, while also offering some new insights and unity by sharing their experiences with others.

Participatory storytelling methods like photovoice carry the same potential as any participatory method to unintentionally reproduce dynamics of power, privilege, and harm (Murdoch et al. 2016; Taylor and Wei 2020); in particular, depoliticized art or art that focuses on aesthetics over authenticity can unintentionally objectify, oversimplify, and diminish people's identities (Askins and Pain 2011). By leaning into storytelling, photovoice can be one tool to intentionally build social connections and community. Nevertheless, this research approach does not guarantee participant empowerment, especially if engagement is not meaningful throughout the process (Liebenberg 2018), or attention is not adequately paid to action, power dynamics, and broader political processes. Another risk lies around how much participants are asked to disclose, as this requires caution, education, and training because it can make participants vulnerable and even re-traumatized, especially if antagonistic power relations are present (Beauregard et al. 2020). In Taylor and Wei's

(2020) case study of Story Bridge, participants felt optimistic about building trust, but some left feeling vulnerable and raw, saying they had not shared that deeply in decades. This risk reminds me of Tuck's (2009) call for research to focus on desires, which might include stories of hurt, but also hope and creativity, so as not to fetishize loss and ongoing denigrations. In NeighbourPLAN photovoice project, I saw how readily stories of loss, stigma, and hurt came up, but also stories of connection. Residents were encouraged to decide what they wanted to take photos of and develop self-representational narratives via the photo journals, and they should feel autonomy in what they were choosing to share or not. When undertaken thoughtfully, storytelling methods, such as photovoice, can provide a less extractive exploration of lived experiences, encourage creative thinking, active listening, and connection building (Joyce 2018; Taylor and Wei 2020; Wang 1999), and are possible strategies for mitigating methodological harm.

7. Conclusions

As a highly regarded community organization in Peterborough, NeighbourPLAN leveraged its network to amplify marginalized experiences and perspectives. NeighbourPLAN's commitment to deep engagement allowed ample opportunity to create a feedback-rich environment. NeighbourPLAN included photovoice into their program design upon my suggestion and I recommended that it include more arts-based activities in future projects. Storytelling and arts can be used in participatory planning to capture nuanced human-urban experiences, reveal surprising connections, translate community knowledge into an accessible medium and encourage discussion and visualization of an issue and the next steps for action. Although no quick fix can be guaranteed when trying to foster and sustain relationships, my perspective is hopeful that when undertaken thoughtfully, arts-based research activities can strengthen social networks and senses of belonging while navigating past social norms (Beauregard et al. 2020). Genuinely facilitating storytelling methods creates opportunities for communities to recognize diversity and commonality, building more trusting relationships (Taylor and Wei 2020). These methods can be used to create more meaningful, deeper connections that many participants seek through community engagement. Photovoice participants in this project jointly reflected on their subjectivities and processed systemic injustices by sharing their stories with one another. This project also helped residents animate and express their community's intangible assets, clarify to the residents what spaces felt welcoming or not, and discuss the reasons behind that. In so doing, the worlds of participants within Peterborough became more visible to NeighbourPLAN and to residents/participants themselves. Complex participatory planning projects such as NeighbourPLAN are massive undertakings that require many skills from many passionate people, but ensuring we provide the time and space for marginalized communities to form and share their stories and lived realities beyond a survey has the potential to generate so much more than data.

Supplementary Materials: The final Vision document for the Downtown Jackson Creek Neighbourhood has been published on GreenUP's website. Available online: https://www.greenup.on.ca/wp-content/uploads/2020/04/NP-Vision-DTJC-Web.pdf (accessed on 14 July 2023).

Funding: This photovoice project was funded specifically by the Symons Trust Fund for Canadian Studies (700 CAD), and GreenUP which helped cover 50% of the residents' honorariums (300 CAD of 600 CAD). The overall graduate research and evaluation of NeighbourPLAN and subsequent thesis was funded through Mitacs Accelerate (Application Ref. IT14691) and the Social Science and Humanities Research Council (SSHRC) Joseph-Armand Bombardier CGS Award 766-2019-1463.

Institutional Review Board Statement: The study was conducted in accordance with the Tri-Council Guidelines (article D.1.6) and approved by the Trent University Research Ethics Board (25743, 5 December 2019).

Informed Consent Statement: Informed consent was obtained from all subjects involved in the study.

Data Availability Statement: The data presented in this study are openly available in the Graduate thesis by the author, Rosa McBee, in the Trent University Library and Archives found in http://digitalcollections.trentu.ca/collections/trent-university-graduate-thesis-collection (accessed on 28 December 2022), with the title: Building social connections: Evaluating NeighbourPLAN's participatory planning initiative for increased participant connectedness in Peterborough, Ontario.

Acknowledgments: I want to acknowledge and pay my respects to the traditional territories and the caretakers of the land where I conducted this photovoice project, Curve Lake First Nation's traditional territory and the Mississauga Anishinaabeg people. Thank you to the professors at Trent University. In particular, my supervisor, Nadine Changfoot, who modelled the kind of researcher I wanted to be. I want to thank NeighbourPLAN staff, in particular, who not only helped fund my research in conjunction with Mitacs Accelerate but who always showed openness and support for my thoughts that fostered an environment of mutual feedback and growth. It was an enormous honour to receive the Social Science and Humanities Research Council research award, and I am also indebted to the other external funding that gave me the freedom to do this research. I want to express my gratitude and thanks to the residents who agreed to take part in this photovoice study, Lori, Connie, Jaclyn, Kelly, Kendra and Rick. I found your photos and reflections a source of tremendous motivation throughout grad school, and I hope I represented your perspectives well.

Conflicts of Interest: The author declares no conflict of interest. The funders had no role in the design of the study; in the collection, analyses, or interpretation of data; in the writing of the manuscript; or in the decision to publish the results.

Notes

[1] A theory of change is an evaluation approach that clarifies the underlying hypothesis of social interventions by creating a diagram that visualizes the causal links between activities and short to long-term anticipated or aspirational changes. ToCs have become a predominant approach among evaluations in Canadian non-governmental, governmental, and higher education circles conducting CBR or PAR as a framework to compare the intended versus the actual outcomes (Funnell and Rogers 2011).

[2] SHOwED is an acronym for a series of questions to guide photo journaling for each photograph to identify the strengths and challenges and prompt the photographer to think about how the situation might be improved.

References

Active Neighbourhoods Canada. 2015. *Portrait: Stewart Street Neighbourhood, Peterborough*. Toronto: The Centre for Active Transportation. Available online: https://www.cleanairpartnership.org/wp-content/uploads/2016/08/PBO-portrait-for-web.pdf (accessed on 14 July 2023).

Arcaya, Mariana C., Alina Schnake-Mahl, Andrew Binet, Shannon Simpson, Maggie S. Church, Vedette Gavin, Bill Coleman, Shoshanna Levine, Annika Nielsen, Leigh Carroll, and et al. 2018. Community change and resident needs: Designing a Participatory Action Research study in Metropolitan Boston. *Health & Place* 52: 221–30. [CrossRef]

Askins, Kye. 2018. Feminist geographies and participatory action research: Co-producing narratives with people and place. *Gender, Place & Culture* 25: 1277–94. [CrossRef]

Askins, Kye, and Rachel Pain. 2011. Contact zones: Participation, materiality, and the messiness of interaction. *Environment and Planning D: Society and Space* 29: 803–21. [CrossRef]

Bay, Jennifer L., and Kathryn Y. Swacha. 2020. Community-engaged research as enmeshed practice. *Michigan Journal of Community Service Learning* 26: 121–41. [CrossRef]

Beauregard, Caroline, Joëlle Tremblay, Janie Pomerleau, Maïté Simard, Elise Bourgeois-Guérin, Claire Lyke, and Cécil Rousseau. 2020. Building communities in tense times: Fostering connectedness between cultures and generations through community arts. *American Journal of Community Psychology* 65: 437–54. [CrossRef]

Cahill, Caitlin. 2007. The personal is political: Developing new subjectivities through participatory action research. *Gender, Place and Culture* 14: 267–92. [CrossRef]

Carlson, Elizabeth D., Joan Engebretson, and Robert M. Chamberlain. 2006. Photovoice as a social process of critical consciousness. *Qualitative Health Research* 16: 836–52.

Comes, Tina. 2016. Designing for networked community resilience. *Procedia Engineering* 159: 6–11. [CrossRef]

Cooke, Bill, and Uma Kothari. 2001. The case for participation as tyranny. In *Participation: The New Tyranny?* Edited by Bill Cooke and Uma Kothari. London: Zed Books Ltd., pp. 1–15.

Dassah, Ebenezer, Heather M. Aldersey, and Kathleen E. Norman. 2017. Photovoice and persons with physical disabilities: A scoping review of the literature. *Qualitative Health Research* 279: 1412–22.

Freire, Paolo. 1970. *Pedagogy of the Oppressed*. New York: Seabury Press.

Funnell, Sue C., and Patricia J. Rogers. 2011. *Purposeful Program Theory: Effective Use of Theories of Change and Logic Models*. Indianapolis: Jossey-Bass.

Given, Lisa M., ed. 2008. *The Sage Encyclopedia of Qualitative Research Methods*. Cambridge: The MIT Press. [CrossRef]

GreenUP Association and The Centre for Active Transportation. 2019. A Downtown-Jackson Creek Portrait. Peterborough, Ontario. Available online: https://www.greenup.on.ca/program/neighbourplan/#1630533996171-02d9baa9-2b9c (accessed on 14 July 2023).

Griffiths, Rhonda, Jan Horsfall, Margo Moore, Di Lane, Veronica Kroon, and Rachel Langdon. 2007. Assessment of health, well-being and social connections: A survey of women living in Western Sydney. *International Journal of Nursing Practice* 13: 3–13. [CrossRef]

Hall, Budd L., and Rajesh Tandon. 2017. Participatory research: Where have we been, where are we going?—A dialogue. *Research for All* 1: 365–74. [CrossRef]

Hardy, Lisa J., Elizabeth Hulen, Kevin Shaw, Leah Mundell, and Coral Evans. 2018. Ripple effect: An evaluation tool for increasing connectedness through community health partnerships. *Action Research* 16: 299–318. [CrossRef]

Hari, Johann. 2018. *Lost Connections: Uncovering the Real Causes of Depression- and the Unexpected Solutions*. London: Bloomsbury.

Hergenrather, Kenneth C., Scott D. Rhodes, Chris A. Cowan, Gerta Bardhoshi, and Sarah Pula. 2009. Photovoice as community-based participatory research: A qualitative review. *American Journal of Health Behavior* 33: 686–98. [CrossRef]

Janzen, Rich, Joanna Ochocka, and Alethea Stobbe. 2016. Towards a theory of change for community-based research projects. *Engaged Scholar Journal: Community-Engaged Research, Teaching, and Learning* 2: 44–64. [CrossRef]

Joyce, Hilary D. 2018. Using photovoice to explore school connection and disconnection. *Children & Schools* 40: 211–20. [CrossRef]

Kemmis, Stephen, and Robin McTaggart. 2005. Participatory action research: Communicative action and the public sphere. In *The Sage Handbook of Qualitative Research*. Edited by Norman K. Denzin and Yvonne S. Lincoln. Thousand Oaks: Sage Publications, pp. 559–604.

Kesby, Mike. 2005. Retheorizing empowerment-through-participation as a performance in space: Beyond tyranny to transformation. *Signs: Journal of Women in Culture and Society* 30: 2037–65. Available online: https://www.journals.uchicago.edu/doi/10.1086/428422 (accessed on 14 July 2023). [CrossRef]

Kindon, Sara, Rachel Pain, and Mike Kesby. 2007. *Participatory Action Research Approaches and Methods. Connecting People, Participation and Place*. Abingdon: Routledge.

Lavrinec, Jekaterina. 2014. Community art initiatives as a form of participatory research: The case of street mosaic workshop. *Creativity Studies* 7: 55–68. [CrossRef]

Levkoe, Charles Z., and Lauren Kepkiewicz. 2020. Questioning the impact of impact: Evaluating community-campus engagement as contextual, relational, and process based. *Michigan Journal of Community Service Learning* 26: 219–37. [CrossRef]

Lewis, Susan J., and Andrew J. Russell. 2011. Being embedded: A way forward for ethnographic research. *Ethnography* 12: 398–416. [CrossRef]

Liebenberg, Linda. 2018. Thinking critically about Photovoice: Achieving empowerment and social change. *International Journal of Qualitative Methods* 17: 160940691875763. [CrossRef]

Liebenberg, Linda. 2022. Photovoice and Being Intentional About Empowerment. *Health Promotion Practice* 23: 267–73. [CrossRef] [PubMed]

Macedo, Donaldo. 2000. Introduction. In *Pedagogy of the Oppressed*. New York: Bloomsbury Publishing, pp. 11–27.

Mayan, Maria J., and Christine H. Daum. 2016. Worth the risk? Muddled relationships in community-based participatory research. *Qualitative Health Research* 26: 69–76. [CrossRef]

McBee, Rosa. 2021. Building Social Connections: Evaluating NeighbourPLAN's Participatory Planning Initiative for Increased Participant Connectedness in Peterborough/Nogojiwanong, Ontario. Unpublished Master's thesis, Trent University, Peterborough, ON, Canada.

Mohan, Giles, and Kristian Stokke. 2000. Participatory development and empowerment: The dangers of localism. *Third World Quarterly* 21: 247–68. [CrossRef]

Murdoch, James, Carl Grodach, and Nicole Foster. 2016. The importance of neighborhood context in arts-led development: Community anchor or creative class magnet? *Journal of Planning Education and Research* 36: 32–48. [CrossRef]

Nasca, Francis. 2016. Active Neighbourhoods Canada: Evaluating Approaches to Participatory Planning for Active Transportation in Peterborough, Ontario. Master's thesis, Trent University, Peterborough, ON, Canada.

Newman, Susan, Doug Maurer, Alex Jackson, Maria Saxon, Ruth Jones, and Gene Reese. 2009. Gathering the evidence: Photovoice as a tool for disability advocacy. *Progress in Community Health Partnerships: Research, Education, and Action* 3: 139–44. [CrossRef]

Oden, Kristen, Brigida Hernandez, and Marco Hidalgo. 2010. Payoffs of participatory action research: Racial and ethnic minorities with disabilities reflect on their research experiences. *Community Development* 41: 21–31. [CrossRef]

Rice, Carla, Eliza Chandler, and Nadine Changfoot. 2016. Imagining otherwise: The ephemeral spaces of envisioning new meanings. In *Mobilizing Metaphor: Art, Culture and Disability Activism in Canada*. Vancouver: UBC Press, pp. 54–75.

Small, Mario L. 2009. *Unanticipated Gains: Origins of Network Inequality in Everyday Life*. Oxford: Oxford University Press.

Taylor, Crystal, and Qinghong Wei. 2020. Storytelling and Arts to Facilitate Community Capacity Building for Urban Planning and Social Work. *Societies* 10: 64. [CrossRef]

Torre, Marie E. 2010. Participatory action research in the contact zone. In *Revolutionizing Education*. London: Routledge, pp. 31–52.

True, Gala, Lawrence Davidson, Ray Facundo, David V. Meyer, Sharon Urbina, and Sarah S. Ono. 2019. "Institutions Don't Hug People:" A Roadmap for Building Trust, Connectedness, and Purpose through Photovoice Collaboration. *Journal of Humanistic Psychology* 61: 365–404. [CrossRef]

Tuck, Eve. 2009. Suspending damage: A letter to communities. *Harvard Educational Review* 79: 409–28. [CrossRef]

Umberson, Debra, and Jennifer Karas Montez. 2010. Social relationships and health: A flashpoint for health policy. *Journal of Health and Social Behavior* 51: S54–S66. [CrossRef]

Valentine, Gill. 2008. Living with difference: Reflections on geographies of encounter. *Progress in Human Geography* 32: 323–37. [CrossRef]

Walljasper, Jay. 2018. Planning and the Art of Storytelling. *Planning* 6: 28–31. Available online: https://www.planning.org/planning/2018/jun/artofstorytelling/ (accessed on 1 January 2020).

Wang, Caroline, and Mary Ann Burris. 1997. Photovoice: Concept, methodology, and use for participatory needs assessment. *Health Education & Behavior* 24: 369–87. [CrossRef]

Wang, Caroline C. 1999. Photovoice: A participatory action research strategy applied to women's health. *Journal of Women's Health* 8: 185–92. [CrossRef] [PubMed]

White, Sarah C. 1996. Depoliticising development: The uses and abuses of participation. *Development in Practice* 6: 6–15. Available online: http://www.jstor.org/stable/4029350 (accessed on 15 August 2020). [CrossRef]

Youkhana, Eva. 2014. Creative activism and art against urban renaissance and social exclusion–space sensitive approaches to the study of collective action and belonging. *Sociology Compass* 8: 172–86. [CrossRef]

Disclaimer/Publisher's Note: The statements, opinions and data contained in all publications are solely those of the individual author(s) and contributor(s) and not of MDPI and/or the editor(s). MDPI and/or the editor(s) disclaim responsibility for any injury to people or property resulting from any ideas, methods, instructions or products referred to in the content.

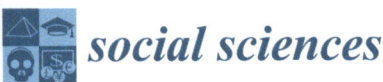

Article

Beyond Utterances: Embodied Creativity and Compliance in Dance and Dementia

An Kosurko [1,*] and Melisa Stevanovic [2]

1 Faculty of Social Sciences, University of Helsinki, 00014 Helsinki, Finland
2 Faculty of Social Sciences, Tampere University, 33100 Tampere, Finland; melisa.stevanovic@tuni.fi
* Correspondence: an.kosurko@helsinki.fi

Abstract: Practices of creativity and compliance intersect in interaction when directing local dances remotely for people living with dementia and their carers in institutional settings. This ethnomethodological study focused on how artistic mechanisms are understood and structured by participants in response to on-screen instruction. Video data were collected from two long-term care facilities in Canada and Finland in a pilot study of a dance program that extended internationally from Canada to Finland at the onset of COVID-19. Fourteen hours of video data were analyzed using multimodal conversation analysis of initiation–response sequences. In this paper, we identify how creative instructed actions are produced in compliance with multimodal directives in interaction when mediated by technology and facilitated by copresent facilitators. We provide examples of how participants' variably compliant responses in relation to dance instruction, from following a lead to coordinating with others, produce different creative actions from embellishing to improvising. Our findings suggest that cocreativity may be realized at intersections of compliance and creativity toward reciprocity. This research contributes to interdisciplinary discussions about the potential of arts-based practices in social inclusion, health, and well-being by studying how dance instruction is understood and realized remotely and in copresence in embodied instructed action and interaction.

Keywords: arts-based research; ethnomethodology and conversation analysis; instructed action; directive–response sequences; dementia; multimodality; intercorporeality; creativity; compliance

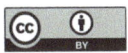

1. Introduction

1.1. Arts-Based Practices and Technology in Ageing and Dementia

Arts-based practices have become an important area of focus due to their potential for social and artistic inclusion, life enrichment, well-being, and quality of life in elderly and dementia care (Chappell et al. 2021; De Medeiros and Basting 2014; Herron et al. 2023; Zeilig et al. 2018). In dementia research, studies of dance and creativity are calling attention to the importance of the embodied expression of agency and self, with implications for new directions in practice (Kontos et al. 2020a, 2020b; Motta-Ochoa et al. 2021). As opportunities to participate in music and dance activities are increasingly mediated by technology, new questions arise as to their access and affordances for diverse abilities. Critical gerontechnology and ageing studies are shifting focus from finding solutions to the health-related problematization of ageing to understanding how complex multimodal relationships of ageing and technology are intertwined. There is keen interest in the community conditions for sharing arts and technologies into existing arrangements of care (Jones et al. 2021; Peine et al. 2021; Skinner et al. 2018). Hills et al. (2022) proposed a methodological expansion to look more closely at the "how" of practice mechanisms, how the various components of an artistic activity are understood, interpreted, and incorporated into activity structures (Hills et al. 2022). Situating our study within these interdisciplinary discussions, our focus is on such mechanisms, in situated interactions of older people, including people living with dementia (PLWD) and their carers, as they participate in dance class through technology. Specifically, we focus on how creative action, which is inherent in artistic practice, emerges in and through participants' variably compliant responses to directive instruction.

1.2. An Interactional Approach to the Study of Remotely Instructed Dances

The arts have evolved through social processes both creative and compliant in forming languages and connecting communities. In ballet, a recognizable form of creative compliance is the plié. A bending and straightening, the plié is an embodied example of how, over time, artforms become collective cultural representations. Through practice in compliance with form, the plié is perfected and prepares the dancer's body to propel itself in performance and expression of technique. Its name derives from the French word *plier*, rooted in both compliance and completion. In etymology, compliance infers a process of joining and bending together in practice—a completion of something—a granted request or wish, a followed direction or instruction. In conversation, compliance is contingent upon the initiation that must precede it. It is a sequential phenomenon which constitutes a central mechanism in interaction that serves the promotion of social solidarity (Clayman 2002). In music, this solidarity is achieved as members keep together, aligning in compliance with rhythm and time (McNeill 1995). A shared beat enables the prediction and coordination of behavior—our synchronous singing and dancing are a feature of our human social adaptation (Merker 2000). Thus, while compliance has come to be associated with obedience to a set of laws, it is not necessarily defined in deference to external regulatory structures that humans obey. Rather, it can be created in interaction socially through coordinated and creative practices.

To look at how the mechanisms of artistic practice are understood and incorporated into structures of interaction in dance activities, we analyze what Garfinkel referred to as the "artful practices" of how people accomplish social action. What characterizes this ethnomethodological approach is how it attends to participants' intelligibility of action (e.g., instructions, directives, and responses) in their displays and interpretations of understanding with each other (Garfinkel 2002). Using conversation analysis grounded in ethnomethodology (thus, EMCA), we seek to reveal the orientations that govern naturally occurring interactions, assuming that this governance is created and complied with in an ongoing manner by the actors themselves. Our objective is to describe the procedures of participants (older people living with dementia, their carers, and their facilitators) as they make sense of their own and others' practices (Heritage 1984; Arminen 2017) in complex relationships of language, embodiment, and the material environment in the creative activity context (Goodwin 2000). Specifically, using multimodal conversation analysis of transcribed video data, we describe sequences of initiating and responsive actions (Schegloff 2007). We focus on responsive, instructed actions (Garfinkel [1967] 1984) in sequential structures of social interaction in an online dance program.

1.3. Multimodality and Embodiment in Instructions and Directives

Instructions initiate responding actions, instructed actions that are interactionally achieved (Garfinkel 2002). In classical conversation analysis (i.e., of talk), responding actions may be considered to complete the second half of an adjacency pair—the key sequential structure that organizes turns of talk (Schegloff 2007). In an adjacency pair, a responsive turn refers to a previous turn and displays understanding of its conditions (Sacks et al. 1974). An instructed action then, as a response to a previous turn, reveals what the social actor finds relevant in the conditions of the instruction.

Closely related to instructions are directives, also a first pair part of an adjacency pair. Directives are used to "get someone to do something" (Goodwin 2006, p. 517). Directives can be verbal or embodied (Goodwin 2000; Goodwin and Cekaite 2013) or combine multimodally to project upcoming action. Using the body in demonstrating an action to be taken contributes multimodally to the evolution of structure (Hofstetter and Keevallik 2020; Keevallik 2010). In turn, responses can be verbal, embodied, and multimodal, implicating the body in action sequences that can be analyzed (Hazel et al. 2014). In the examples of dance interactions that we analyze in this article, instructions and instructed actions are organized in sequences that are initiated by verbal, embodied, and multimodal directives, which, in turn, are responded to and creatively developed, moment-by-moment, by participants in relation to each other.

1.4. On Compliance in Directed Embodiment

Discussions about compliance are relevant to sequence organization, as compliance is considered the interactionally preferred second pair part to a directive (Schegloff 2007). This is the case every time a directive is designed to get someone to do something (see Kent 2012). Craven and Potter (2010) distinguish directives as having tendencies to tell rather than to ask, where noncompliance leads to upgraded directives that highlight the entitlement of the speaker rather than on contingencies of the recipient. Responding actions and response relevance analyses have shown that the design of directives is consequential in how they are met with responses (Stevanovic and Peräkylä 2012; Curl and Drew 2008; Sacks et al. 1974). Stivers and Rossano (2010) analyzed response relevance as a scalar variable and explored the potential of turn design features to increase recipients' accountability in mobilizing response. In response to this, Schegloff (2010) asserted that what is relevant is not necessarily getting somebody to do something or the degree to which turn design features increase compliance but how elements of conduct are shaped in interaction and what their structural organization says about the occasions from which data are taken.

With respect to the structural organization of interactional sequences, Clayman (2002) argued that conversation analysis offers a procedural approach by identifying and analyzing practices to avoid conflict and to promote social solidarity. While some actions constrain responses in how they set them up to agree or disagree, accept or design, answer or follow, etc., response alternatives differ in their cooperativeness, affiliation, and alignment. Sequence organization itself is a form of solidarity in that it provides empirical evidence of how participants promote solidary actions (Clayman 2002). Compliance, in this context then, as a preferred response in sequential organization, is a form of prosocial solidarity. In analysis, the features of a preferred response can be described in terms of their affiliation with what they are responding to (Heritage 1984), as well as their alignment with the structure of the action (Schegloff 2007). Alignment can be considered a structural level of cooperation, and affiliation can be considered an affective level of cooperation (Stivers 2008).

1.5. Previous Research in Multimodal Responses

Our analysis contributes to the growing interests in intercorporeality and creativity in multimodal directive–response sequences. Previous studies on instruction interactions and multimodal response focused on compliance in the sense of accomplishing manual action. Lilja and Piirainen-Marsh (2022) demonstrated how complying bodily actions make relevant the depictive gestures used in multimodal instructions of a second-language cooking class. In the teaching and learning of a skill, Lindwall and Ekström (2012) emphasized that in achieving an instructed action, the skill is learned. Due et al. (2019) showed that, in video-mediated instructional sequences, the embodied demonstration can be designed to be mimicked. In air traffic control, Arminen et al. (2014) deconstructed the multimodal production of second pair parts. In demonstrating bodily quoting in dance correction sequences, Keevallik (2010) showed how the embodiment of a moving form can be understood as a compliant response to a directive in progress. In each of these examples, achievements of the instructed actions involve learning in language or skill. For our analysis, we are interested in how artistic instruction results in creative actions that are constituted socially, in interaction, moment by moment for people living with dementia.

Intercorporeality and creativity have also been investigated in atypical interaction focused on multimodal directive–response sequences. In the context of dementia care, embodied directive–response sequences were analyzed in sequential organization of helping people to sit in a chair (Majlesi et al. 2021); in accomplishing joint activities, such as baking (Majlesi and Ekström 2016); and in achieving wishes within institutional constraints (Kristiansen et al. 2019). In related studies of dance and aquatic activities for adults with intellectual disabilities, Matérne et al. (2022) shared their analysis of the coordinated accomplishments in a range of competencies, using multimodal resources. Hydén et al. (2022) provided evidence that embodiment communicates existing agency of PLWD in their contributions to intercorporeal interaction. Our study builds on this existing knowledge by looking at the embodied directive–response sequences in interactions of PLWD and their carers as initiated remotely in a creative activity. In terms of atypical interaction, our study seeks to understand how PLWD are multimodally afforded interactional resources through a technologically mediated creative activity. By looking at how PLWD embody creativity in variably compliant responses to multimodal directives, we hope to understand how arts practices afford them to do so in mediated settings.

2. Materials and Methods

The video data illustrated in the following analysis were collected at two long-term care facilities in dance classes with people living with dementia and staff and researcher facilitators. We analyzed data from a pilot study of a dance program that was extended internationally from Canada to Finland. The study was approved in Canada by the Research Ethics Boards at Trent University and Brandon University, and in Finland by the University of Helsinki Ethical Review Board of Humanities and Social and Behavioral Sciences, and by participating organizations according to their governance procedures. The study adheres to the ethical considerations when including PLWD (see Skinner et al. 2018; Kosurko et al. 2021). Informed consent for participants was obtained in cooperation with nursing staff and third-party signing authorities (where appropriate) of individual participants. Participants living with dementia were diagnosed at varying stages and types, each with cognitive impairments that affect physical and communicative competencies to degrees unknown to the researcher. Data for this paper include video excerpts from one long-term residential care institution (LTRC) in rural Canada, where eight hours of video were recorded during weekly sessions for eight weeks in 2019; and one excerpt from an LTRC in rural Finland, where five hours of video data were recorded during weekly sessions for five-week periods in 2022. The full corpus of data includes 34 hours of video recordings of online chair dance classes for older people who live with dementia in three (3) institutional settings in Canada and two (2) in Finland. Video excerpts chosen for analysis by the authors were identified as moments in which participants responded to instructions in compliant and creative ways. We considered creativity exhibited as an embodied flourish (also identified as a theme in the Canadian study; see (Kontos et al. 2020a)) or participating in the embodiment of an imaginary narrative scenario. We considered compliance as following instructions closely matched to the OSI or facilitator. The examples chosen do not comprise an exhaustive list of compliant and/or creative responses in the data but are part of an early exploration of the potential of the analytic method. To analyze these excerpts, we used multimodal conversation analysis focused on directive–response sequences (i.e., embodied and multimodal responses of participants to instructions (see Mondada 2011). Actions were transcribed in numbered turns, following multimodal conventions (Mondada 2019), with notations in the talk that follow the system of Jefferson (2004) (see Appendix A).

The Dance Program and Participation Framework

The online program Baycrest NBS Sharing Dance Older Adults (SDOA) was developed by Baycrest and Canada's National Ballet School (NBS) to provide remote access to dance instruction for people with cognitive and physical challenges. The streamed, prerecorded video dance classes vary in length from 20 to 60 min and recur weekly, up to eight weeks. Each class begins with a warm-up, followed by a series of dances to piano accompaniment. In each dance, on-screen instructors (OSIs) first provide a demonstration of a dance movement or sequence, then cue the accompanying musician to start the music, and then cue participants to join with them in the dance. In demonstrating the dances, the OSIs talk through the steps (in English), embodying the movements, with accompanying verbal descriptions of what they are doing. At various points during sessions, in introductions and sometimes during the dance demonstrations, OSIs advise participants that the directives to follow are to be achieved according to the preference of participants by suggesting, "you can follow what I'm doing or feel free to do what you like." As the instructions for the dance are prerecorded and presented to participants on a TV monitor, there is no monitoring, assessment, or evaluation on the part of the dance teacher.

A copresent local facilitator was deployed in each setting to encourage engagement in the online program by modelling the demonstrations in copresence and coparticipating. The goal of the SDOA instruction is not to teach a skill resulting in evidence of learning on the part of the recipient; rather, the purpose of the activity is to bring participants together in a shared dance moment-by-moment within sets of movements and scenarios designed to warm up the body and musicality, to incite creativity and imagination, and to encourage interactions among copresent participants.

3. Analysis and Results

Below, we present five multimodal transcripts that illustrate how participants, including resident older adults, PLWD, and carers (staff/facilitators), respond to the on-screen instruction (OSI) of the seated Sharing Dance program. In each of the settings shown, participants are seated in chairs facing a TV monitor, where the program plays. The OSI is prerecorded and streamed from a remote location, with her chair facing the camera and her gaze to the lens so that her instructions seem directed to the viewer. The facilitator (either the author/researcher or a staff member) is seated close to the screen. As the dance program plays on the screen for participants, the OSI first demonstrates the upcoming movements with verbal descriptions and then cues the music and participants to join with her as she repeats the dances, providing verbal directives with accompanying embodied demonstrations. Each of the dances below (other than the warm-up in the first example) is designed to depict scenarios (i.e., a Broadway chorus line; under the sea; a coffee break; and a trip to the art gallery). The first two examples show how participants' responses to creative direction embody mimicable shapes as directed. In the first, an individual complies with the OSI in a classical (albeit embodied) adjacency pair completion. In the second, a series of adjacency pairs are coordinated in sequential order by a copresent facilitator. The third and fourth examples highlight how participants respond creatively in their instructed actions: one with embellishing flourishes in response to the OSI, and the other improvising according to ability in response to the copresent facilitator. In the fifth example, reciprocal cocreativity is highlighted in a sequence of contingent responses between a participant and a copresent facilitator, as initiated by the OSI. In all cases, instructed action comprises multimodal directives (verbal and embodied) in demonstrations for participants to follow.

In the transcript extracts that follow, multimodal transcription conventions are followed (see Appendix A). Symbols are used to delimit the embodied movements of each participant:

- On-screen instructor (Osi): ¶.
- Facilitator (Fac): +.
- Participant dancers: Δ, ©, ø.
- Gaze for all participants: gz.
- Musical beats (mus) are marked up to eight counts: ♪1, ♪2, ♪3, etc.
- Figures: #.
- Video screen capture images have been anonymized as sketches.
- Green arrows indicate gaze direction (in Figures 2, 3, 5–7 and 9).

3.1. Getting Warmed Up: Following the Leader with Matching Movements

In the first excerpt (1), we analyze how a participant follows the OSI on cue, with matching movements, bodily quoting the OSI (Keevallik 2010) in response to multimodal directives, in coordination with temporal rhythm of the music. As this excerpt begins, a previous sequence of dance movements has finished and is to be repeated. The participant, Anita, is seated among other participants in a side-by-side formation, with her chair facing the screen (shown in rectangular boundary box in Figure 1). Anita follows the directions and matches the knee-tapping movements of the OSI in time, joining together with the OSI as she continuously maintains the rhythm of the music.

(1) OSI: On-screen instructor (¶), Anita(ani): dancer PLWD (Δ), Music (mus) ♪

```
1 OSI          one more time here we go ¶♪1Δtapping, (0.1)#
a  mus         >>piano plays                    ♪1->>
b  osi         >>gz camera                      ¶taps hands on knees ((with music))->>
c  ani         >>gz screen                      Δtaps knees ((in same time)->>
d  fig                                          #Figure 1
```

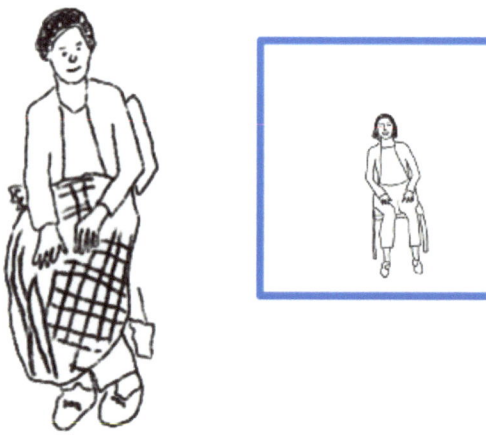

Figure 1. Anita (**left**) matches her movements to the on-screen instructor's (**right**).

Prior to the start of the transcript (1a), the music set the temporal, rhythmic structure for the activity in a predictable, recognizable pattern, made relevant by the OSI, who was oriented to the beat in how she timed her multimodal instruction. The OSI began with a verbal directive that indicated an upcoming action, "one more time," involving "we," with a cue of when to start ("go") and what to do: "one more time, here we go tapping" (1a). The OSI's embodied demonstration of knee-tapping began on the first beat immediately following the verbal directive "go" (1b) that projected the embodied response of the ongoing repeated action "one more time" (see Figure 1). Anita responded in turn, on the beat in the relevant place in the sequence (1c), tapping her knees at the same time as the OSI, with both continuing the tapping in keeping with the music to the end of the sequence.

Within the embodied conversation of the dance class, a bodily move can be equated to a verbal utterance (see Keevallik 2010). As the OSI directed an embodied response from the dancer, this can be seen as the first part of the classic adjacency pair in conversation analysis (Sacks et al. 1974). When Anita responded by following along with the instruction, in time, with matching movements bodily quoting the OSI (Keevallik 2010), the second part of the pair was in compliance with the initiated first part, and completion of the pair. The achievement of the instructed action was directed by the prerecorded OSI using verbal and embodied resources in coordination with the predictable external musical rhythm (see Albert 2015). Anita's subsequent embodied response displayed her understanding of not only what was expected but also how to complete the action in time as the moment progressed, by tapping her knees as demonstrated, immediately upon the beat following the directive "go."

3.2. A Sequence of Depictive Gestures in Turn: Coordinating a Pretend Coffee Break

In the next excerpt (2), we illustrate how coparticipants orient to each other sequentially within a timed musical structure in response to on-screen instructions (OSIs) and as they are repeated by a copresent facilitator. Three participants, Dancer 1, Dancer 2, and Dancer 3, are seated with their chairs facing the screen, and a facilitator sits beneath the screen, facing the participants (see Figure 2). The OSI provides an embodied demonstration of a coffee-pouring and -sharing scenario within a musical structure of eight beats. The coffee pouring takes four beats, and the sharing takes four beats (two beats to reach toward a participant (to hand them a cup) and two beats to return to home position). The eight beats are shown in the transcript as numbered musical notes (♪1, ♪2, etc.). Example (2), below, begins as music playing leads up to the first measure (counted and shown as ♪5, ♪6, ♪7, and ♪8). During the musical lead in, the OSI cues the timing of the projected instructed action, "pour yourself some coffee." The facilitator then "takes the lead" and pours coffee for the three dancers, who each respond in turn.

(2) OSI: On-screen instructor ¶, Fac: Facilitator (staff) +, Dancers 1–3, Da1 ∆ (PLWD), Da2© , Da3 (PLWD) ø

```
1 OSI        ¶   ♪5 Pour yourself♪6 some coffee,♪7
a Osi        ¶ ((mimes pouring))->
P Mus        >>♪piano plays 4/4time ((5,6,7,))♪->>

2 Fac        ♪8¶(0.2) ♪1+Coffee,# (0.3)                    ♪2
p Mus              ♪piano plays 2 beats ((1,2))♪
a Osi        ->¶
a Fac              +((mimes pouring acc to demo))->
b Fac              ->gz own hands
c Da1              ->gz Fac hands
d Da2              ->gz Fac hands
e Da3              ->gz Fac hands
f fig                    #Figure 2
```

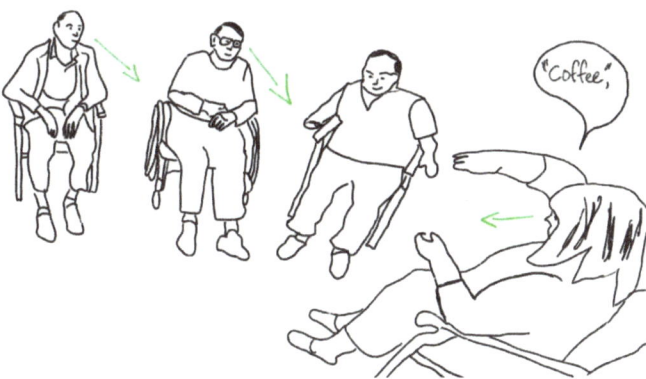

Figure 2. From L to R, Dancers 3, 2, and 1 watch facilitator (R) mime pouring "coffee".

In compliance with the OSI's directive (1), the facilitator depicts with her hands the matching shape of pouring a coffee (2a) and verbalizes "coffee" (2) within the timed structure of four beats (2P—3b). Her gaze is on the shape as she creates it with her own hands (2b) (see Figure 2). The dancers each orient to her movements with his or her gaze, focused on her hands (2d–f).

```
3 OSI     Give¶♪3 it to a friend,                          +¶♪4
P mus            ♪piano plays 2 beats ((3,4)) -------♪
a Osi            ¶♪reaches to camera, flicks wrist    ¶♪((to place coffee))
b Fac     -------------------------->+

4 FAC     (0.2)+for you,♪5 (0.1)+(0.6)♪6Δ      + #♪7 (0.6)+(0.6)         +♪8
P Mus                    ♪piano plays 4 beats ((5,6,7,8))--------♪
a Fac            +reaches ♪to Da1 +puts ♪cup btwn+ #♪""",+reachback+♪
b Da1                                         Δ turns head, opens hands
                                                         gz cup spot->
c fig                                         #Figure 3
```

Continuing with the sequence in time to the music, the OSI initiates the next directive, "give it to a friend," just in time to finish on the fourth beat (3), when the F completes the pouring gesture (3b). Next, on beat five (4), the facilitator reaches toward and "hands" the imaginary coffee to Dancer 1 with a verbal offer, "for you" (4). With a wrist motion, she "places the coffee" (4a) in the space between them on beat seven, reaching back by beat eight. Dancer 1's gaze follows the facilitator's hand and remains focused on the spot where the cup was placed (4b) (see Figure 3).

```
5         (0.1)+♪1Δ      ♪2       ♪3     (1.6)        ♪4+
P Mus              ♪piano plays 4beats ((1,2,3,4))♪
a Fac              +mimes pouring------------+
b Da1              Δgz Fac hands->

6 FAC     For +♪5you, hehehe©#+   (0.6) ©       +♪6 +(0.6)Δ (0.1)
P mus             ♪piano plays 2 beats((1,2))---♪
a Fac             + reaches to Da2+puts cup btwn  +",+reaches back->
b Da2                     ©#nods head©
c Da1                                             Δgz coffee
d fig             #Figure 4
```

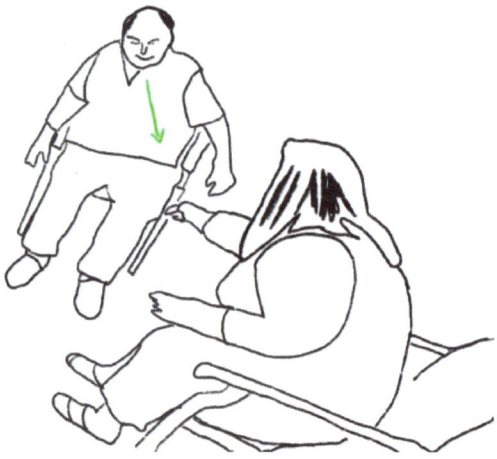

Figure 3. Dancer 2 looks at space where facilitator puts imaginary coffee.

Starting again on beat one of the next musical measure and over the course of four beats, (5) the facilitator repeats the coffee-pouring motion (5a) and verbalization "for you" (6) that she did in her first turn (2,2a); again, similarly to her previous turn (4a), the OSI reaches with the coffee on beat five, but this time to Dancer 2, (6a) who sits next to Dancer 1. Dancer 1 shifts his gaze to the spot where the coffee was placed for Dancer 2. Dancer 2 acknowledges receipt of the coffee with a head nod (6b) toward where the coffee was placed (see Figure 4).

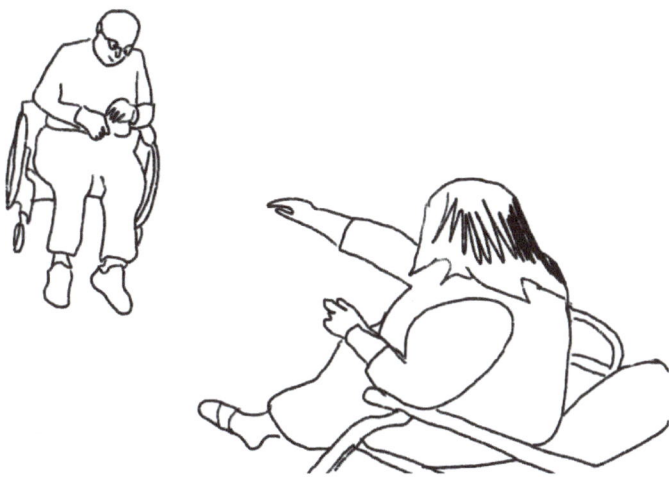

Figure 4. Dancer 2 nods head as facilitator hands him imaginary coffee.

On beat seven, Dancer 2 looks down at his hands (7a) and shapes them as if around an imaginary cup (7b) (see Figure 5). Then, within the next and eighth beat, Dancer 2 breaks his hands apart (making the cup disappear) and looks up (8a) with an eye roll, smiling (8b) (see Figure 5), making visible to coparticipants his stance on the creative practice, within the structure of the musical measure.

```
9  FAC      ♪1+hehehe☺(0.6)∆ (0.6)                    ♪4
P  Mus      ♪piano plays 4beats ((1,2,3,4) ♪
a  Fac            +mimes pouring coffee->
b  Da2                       ☺gz Fac, smiles->
c  Da1                             ∆gz dancer3->

10         ♪5+(0.6)☺∆#            +ø (0.3)     ♪6+ (0.3)ø+ (0.3)        ø+♪7
P  mus      ♪piano plays 3 beats ((1,2,3)) ---------------♪->>
a  Fac            +reaches#to Da3+ places cup    +„„„,+reaches back +
b  Da3                                            øreaches coffee„„„øcloses thumb ø
c  Da2            ->☺gz Da3 hand->
d  Da1            ->∆gz Da3 hand->
e  fig                  #Figure 5
```

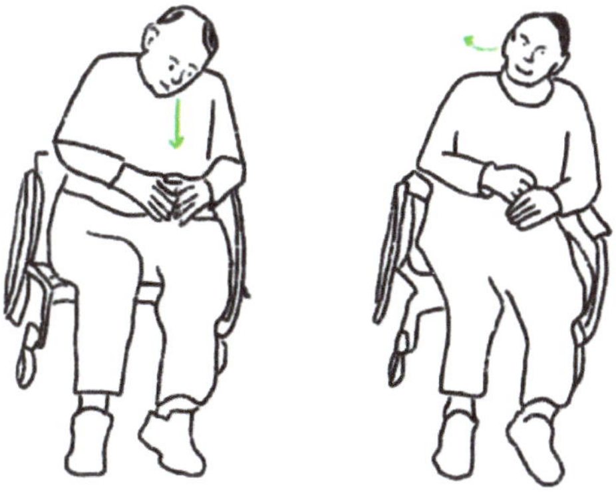

Figure 5. Dancer 2 looks at hands shaping, then looks up with a smile.

On the first beat of the next musical measure, the facilitator laughed (9) in response to Dancer 2's stance display. Dancer 2 shifted his gaze to the facilitator (9b) and smiled. At the same time, within the four-count measure, the facilitator repeated the mimed pouring of coffee (9a). Halfway through this measure, before the facilitator was finished pouring, Dancer 1 oriented his gaze to Dancer 3, displaying understanding of whose turn was projected to receive the next cup. In the same pattern as the previous two turns, on the fifth beat (10), the facilitator reached toward the next seated participant, Dancer 3 (10a). Dancer 3 reached toward the placement of the imaginary coffee and then closed his thumb as if around an invisible handle on the seventh beat (10b). Dancers 2 and 1 were both focused with their gaze at the space where the cup was being shaped (10c,d). At this point, all four of the coparticipants were oriented toward the imaginary cup (see Figure 6).

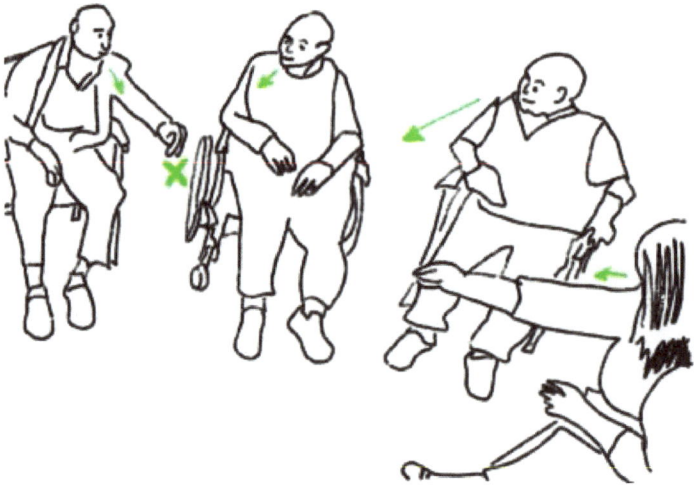

Figure 6. Group focuses on Dancer 3's hand as he reaches for "imaginary coffee cup".

Over the course of the coffee-time scenario, the coparticipants shared a joint focus of attention on the facilitator, and each displayed an understanding of being handed something in their turn, as well as an understanding of the next participant's upcoming turn. The facilitator repeated the pattern of the movement sequences in time with the rhythm established by the OSI for a total of three times. In each iteration, the OSI poured the coffee from beats one to four, and then on beats five to six, she handed it to each participant in turn. On beat seven, in all three instances, the dancers embodied receipt of the facilitator's offered object within the timed structure of the musical rhythm. Each dancer's embodied response was individually enacted. Dancer 1 opened his hands (4b), Dancer 2 brought his hands together in a shape around the invisible object, and Dancer 3 reached and closed his thumb. Each performed their receipt on the same seventh beat in the musical structure in a coordinated, taking turns. While the OSI initiated the embodied directive to "pour yourself some coffee" (1) and "give it to a friend" (3), each participant, in coordination with the facilitator, was given his moment in a measured musical beat to create a signature move in response. By the eighth count of each iteration of the coffee-pouring and -sharing sequence, the group focus of the movement shifted in orientation to the next dancer in turn. While initiated by the OSI, then led by the facilitator, the rhythm of the music provided an external interactional resource in a predictable structure (Albert 2015) with which each individual aligned in sequence. By the end of the sequence, each dancer had contributed a unique movement to the creation of a shared dance, which was led by the facilitator, in alignment with the ongoing instructed action (Stivers 2008). Coparticipants, in turn, each displayed alignment with the musical beat as the facilitator-initiated responses in a chain of sequentially contingent actions (Schegloff 2007). The creativity afforded to each individual was structured yet improvised according to individual interpretation and ability. Their responses were compliant in aligning with the predictable structure of the turns in sequence and creative in their individual expressions of receiving their "coffees" in turn.

In the two examples above, participants used bodily quoting in alignment with sequential and musical structures to achieve instructed actions. Participants' responses to creative direction were achieved in interactional compliance with matching movements. In the first, Anita complied with the OSI in a classical (albeit embodied) adjacency pair completion. In the second, a series of embodied adjacency pairs were coordinated in sequential order by a copresent facilitator. In both examples, the temporal structure of the music provided a resource to cue participants as to when to move. In the second example, the facilitator responded to the OSI's multimodal directive on cue to the beat, and repetitively, in quoting the OSI's bodily movements (Keevallik 2010). In sustaining the rhythm of the OSI choreography, the facilitator used the music as a resource to organize the turn-taking sequence that projected a visible predictability of upcoming action for her coparticipants. The inherent artistic creativity of the dance was realized in both cases through participants' compliant turn-taking responses to the instructions.

3.3. Being Dramatic on Broadway: Embellishing Flourishes

In the next example, we analyze how a participant creatively embellished the instructed movements in response to directives. In the transcript (3) below, Dan is seated facing the screen. The OSI demonstrates the Broadway chorus line choreography in which she depicts that she is clasping a top hat in her hands, held at the torso. The OSI directs participants to depict and present their own imaginary hats by pushing them out (reaching) and bringing them back in. Dan complies by following the instructions and adding his own embellishments.

```
(3) OSI: On-screen instructor (¶), Dan:   dancer PLWD (Δ)

1 OSI        and ¶re:ach, (0.3)Δ and (0.2)     ¶in, (0.3)Δ           ¶           Δ
a Osi                ¶pushes hands out                  ¶pulls hands in ¶
b Dan        >>gz screen             Δpushes hands right---Δpulls hands inΔ

2 OSI        and then can you (0.3) ¶↑throw it away ¶
a Osi                                        ¶flicks wrist up¶

3              (0.3)Δ(0.3)                        # Δ
a Dan                 Δflicks hand to side     Δ
b Dan                   ->gz imaginary hat#
c fig                                                 #Figure 7

4 OSI        ↑nice and dramatic Δ like on Broadway#
a Dan                             Δ suspends raised arm, turns torso->
b Dan                             ->gz follows hat above arm and R->
c fig                                                       #Figure 7
```

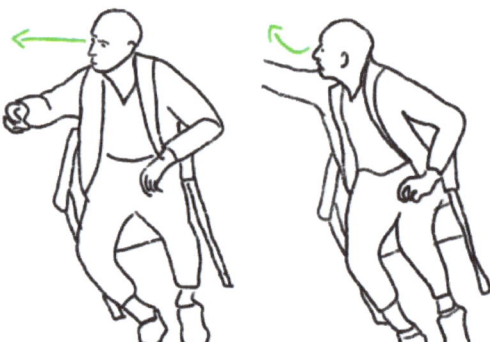

Figure 7. Dancer reaches for imaginary hat.

From the beginning of the sequence, a compliant embodied response was projected by multimodal instructions composed of verbal directives—"and reach" (1), followed by "and then can you throw it away" (2)—accompanied by an embodied demonstration of reaching (1a) and then flicking wrists (2a) movements by the OSI. Dan showed his understanding of what was expected by matching his arm movements to those of the OSI (1b). When Dan responded with the compliant embodied flick, he additionally moved his gaze to where the hat would be thrown away (3a). This extension of his gaze was not an instructed action but an embellishment of his own. Next, the OSI verbally directed the movement to be "nice and dramatic" (4). In response, Dan extended his arm and gaze, twisting his body to watch the hat fly away. Within the sequence, Dan complied with the directed action, created his own flourish, and embellished it on cue according to what was directed, "to be dramatic." Within the sequence, Dan displayed his unique expression of individual creativity. His emphasized embodiment made relevant the OSI's directive to be dramatic and displayed his understanding of what was expected of him in his individual performance of throwing the hat (4b) (see Figure 7). He was compliant in his response to the instruction and creative in his individual interpretation. As Kontos et al. (2020a) pointed out, the creative flourish is often associated with the accomplished artist; this example showcases a person living with dementia performing an artistic embellishment with his own signature. Our analysis illustrated how this was achieved in response to multimodal directives in the creative instruction.

3.4. Individual Expression: Improvising Seaweed Movements

In the next example (4), we focus our analysis on how one participant improvises an unplanned movement of his own, within the structure of the activity, in response to the copresent facilitator's encouragement. The participant, George, is part of a group of seated dancers facing the screen. A facilitator (staff) sits below the screen facing the dancers and demonstrates the movements in copresence. The sequence begins as a dance session is in progress and the on-screen instructor (OSI) has directed participants to move their arms and upper body like seaweed. The facilitator encourages George to comply with the instructed movements and provides an embodied demonstration similar to the OSI. George complies with the instructed movement by copying the facilitator's movements at first. Then, he deviates from the demonstration and moves his hands his own way.

(4) OSI: On-screen instructor ¶, FAC: facilitator +, Dancer George (Geo) ø (PLWD)

```
1 OSI          Now ¶we have our seaweed,
a Osi              ¶sways torso, twists arms upward->>

2 FAC          (0.2) O:ohh+seaweed (1.0) C'mon George be some seaweed
a              >>gz screen+gz George
b                           +sways torso, twists arms upward->

3 FAC          (1.0)øSome seawee=ø =thats# it(.)good one George(.)good one(.)
a Geo              øgz Fac      ø sways#torso, swings arms to sides->
b fig                                              #Figure 8

4 GEO          (1.0) ø(0.3)+(I can say I'm just doing this)# ( )follow yours
a Geo             ->øwrings hands together->>              #
a Geo              gz hands
b fig                                                      #Figure 8
c Fac                      +stands, leans into George->

5 FAC          You just can't do it +well you do what +your body can do, right,
a                                 ->+sits back in seat+
```

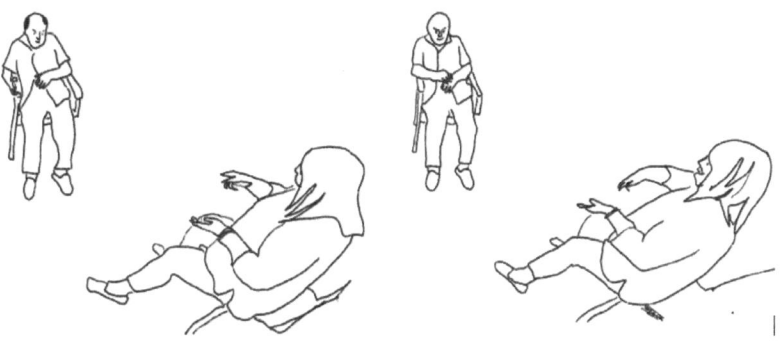

Figure 8. Dancer complies with directive and improvises his hand moves.

Continuing an ongoing instruction sequence, the OSI gave the verbal directive, "now we have our seaweed" (1), with an embodied demonstration, twisting her arms in upward motions (1a), comprising the multimodal instruction. This projected a relevant next in the dance sequence. "Now" provided the cue in the timing, along with the embodied demonstration of what "we" the participants following were to be doing in this moment, "our seaweed." Neither did the depictive gesture nor the verbal directive alone represent a recognizable instruction; together, they constituted the formation of the action (Lilja and Piirainen-Marsh 2022). The response of the facilitator produced the instructed action (Garfinkel 2002) in her compliant embodied replication of moving and swaying her arms similarly to the OSI (2a). Her verbal "o:ooh" (2) produced an affiliative stance display that positively endorsed the movement, while her embodiment of seaweed aligned with the structure of the ongoing activity (Stivers 2008). The facilitator reformulated the OSI directive as an invitation with a summons, "C'mon George, be some seaweed," as she quoted the OSI depictive gesture of seaweed (2). When George responded to the summons with shifting gaze, matching the facilitator's movements (3a), he made the facilitator's reformulated instruction understandable and aligned with her directive in compliance (see Figure 8). After a beat, George changed his hand movements to his own unique wringing movements, not demonstrated by the OSI or the facilitator (4a) (see Figure 8). He accounted for this verbally, with a deictic reference, "I'm just going like this," and his gaze pointed toward his hands (4a). The facilitator responded to George with an affirmation of his approach, "well you do what you can, right," (5) showing agreement with George's change of movement and affiliation that his action was right based on his physical ability.

In breaking away from following the lead of the facilitator and improvising his own movement, George initiated a response from the facilitator (5), who complied with affiliating agreement to his approach. As Kontos et al. (2020b) highlighted, creative action can emerge from practical involvement in a task, not only as an individual cognitive trait. This example illustrated George's improvisation in response to the facilitator's creative direction to "be some seaweed" in relation to what he had to work with using his own hands. George's verbal turn reformulated his ongoing action as self-motivated rather than according to the facilitator's multimodal directive. In this way, his accounting for his incipient compliance (see Kent 2012 allowed him to maintain autonomy of his own conduct according to his ability. George's account of his interpretation can be analyzed as a prosocial action in explaining his potentially misaligning move (Schegloff 2007), afforded in interaction by the copresence of the facilitator. In this example, the copresent facilitator's affiliating stance afforded the opportunity for George's improvised movement to be sanctioned as allowable within the parameters of the activity.

3.5. When Pointillism Becomes Pointing at Each Other: Cocreating Embodied Reciprocity

Our final example showcases how a facilitator and participant reciprocate and build upon each other's movements and affective stances in the cocreation of their own dance in response to instructions. In the excerpt (5) below, the copresent facilitator is seated in a circle, along with residents and staff, oriented toward the screen, where the prerecorded dance is in progress. The scenario is a trip to the art gallery, and the movements represent different techniques of painting. Where the transcript begins below (5), the OSI directs dancers through the pointillism technique, depicting repetitive pointing gestures into the air. The facilitator is pointing into the air, as instructed by the OSI, while monitoring participants. One of the dancers, Joe, watches the facilitator before joining in with matching his movements to the facilitator's. The facilitator sees Joe watching her and points toward him. What follows is a reciprocal exchange of movements that lead to the dyadic dance cocreated by Joe and the facilitator.

(5) OSI: On-screen instructor ¶, Fac: Facilitator (researcher) +, Joe: Dancer (PLWD) Δ

```
1 OSI         and now we ¶make our fine details+
a Osi                    ¶points fingers repeatedly->>
b Fac                                    +points fingers repeatedly->>

2             (1.0)+ (0.3) +          Δ    (1.3) +
a Fac              +gz Joe +raises eyebrows +gz own fingers->
b Joe         gz Fac->>                Δlifts hands->

3             (1.0)Δ(0.6)+*(1.0)                                    +
a Joe           ->Δ pokes fingers into air repeatedly toward Fac->>
b Fac             ->+gz Joe's fingers, raises eyebrows+
c Fac                 *nods, turns torso and pointing toward Joe->>

4 Fac         + (1.8) Δ(1.0) hehehe#                    +
a Fac         +gz Joe, shrugs shoulders toward Joe+
b Joe              Δsmiles at Fac, shakes shoulder in silent laugh->>
c fig                       #Figure 9
```

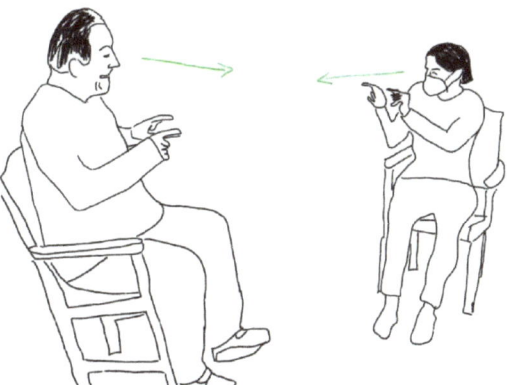

Figure 9. Dancer and facilitator reciprocate pointing movements and smiles.

From the beginning of the sequence, an instructed action was projected in response to the OSI. Following the OSI's verbal directive, "now we make our fine details," accompanied by embodied demonstration of pointing fingers (1,1a), the facilitator made repeated pointing gestures (1b), demonstrating the OSI's embodied directive (1,1a) as Joe watched (1b). The facilitator raised her eyebrows at Joe and, using her gaze, shifted her focus to her pointing fingers (2a). When Joe started to join the action with his own pointing fingers, (3a) the facilitator returned her gaze to Joe and raised her eyebrows in his direction (3b), turning her movements toward him in alignment with his joining the activity. The facilitator's shrug and laughter directed toward Joe (4) displayed an affective stance to which Joe's contingent response was an affiliative smile. The result was a collaborative achievement of joining together in a cocreated response to instructions in a shared moment of laughter. Their shared moment of pointing at each other was collaboratively achieved in a sequencing chain, in reciprocity. The resulting escalation unfolded as the two oriented to each other's movements and responded in turn to their affiliative stance displays, in the service of experience sharing (Stevanovic and Peräkylä 2015). In their compliance within a chain of sequentially and reciprocally contingent actions, as initially directed by the OSI, they cocreated their own shared work of art—in an intercorporeality that neither could have accomplished without the other.

In summarizing the five excerpts we presented above, each of the examples illustrated sequences initiated by an onscreen instructor, followed by variably compliant responses and different types of creativity. We organize these below on axes of compliance and creativity to demonstrate how they are related to the dance instruction.

Anita's warm-up was a precise following in the matching movements of instructed action, demonstrating a prosocial second pair part embodied by the participant in response to the OSI. The coffee break was similarly prosocial, with the facilitator taking the lead and participants coordinating their matching, yet individual movements in a turn-taking structure (Schegloff 2007). Both of these examples were in alignment with the activity structure as instructed by the OSI and facilitated by copresent staff. The first was compliant with the OSI, and the second was compliant with the copresent facilitator, increasing the complexity and cooperative nature of the social interaction.

The next two examples highlight the nature of the creativity in relation to the dance activity. Dan complied with OSI directions, embellishing flourishes—as instructed and of his own accord, given space in the sequence to do so. Dan was compliant similarly to Anita in response to the OSI and added a level of creativity in his embodied self-embellishments, exaggerating dramatically "in the Broadway chorus line." George went even further in his artistic expression in improvising his seaweed movements, adding a creative touch and an interactional turn to the sequence in response to the facilitator.

In the final example of the pointillism dance, a facilitator and participant each responded to each other in reciprocated instructed movements in what became a pointing at each other in their own shared creation of a pointing dance. Both creative and compliant, this example illustrated how the dance instructions were achieved in a sequential chain and built reciprocally, as each contingently responded to each other in alignment with the structure of the activity and in affiliation with each others' stance displays (Stivers 2008).

We organized each of the examples in a figure (Figure 10) below that illustrates the different types of creativity (in the activity of the dance) and compliance (in the instructed actions). Along the axis of creativity are the actions of embellishments that built upon the dance instruction, first in embellishing and then in improvising. Along the axis of compliance are the actions that increase in complexity of coordination with coparticipants, from following OSI movements as an individual to following in sequential turn-taking. Somewhere in between the intersections of artistic creativity and interactional compliance, cocreativity is realized, as indicated in our final example (see Figure 10).

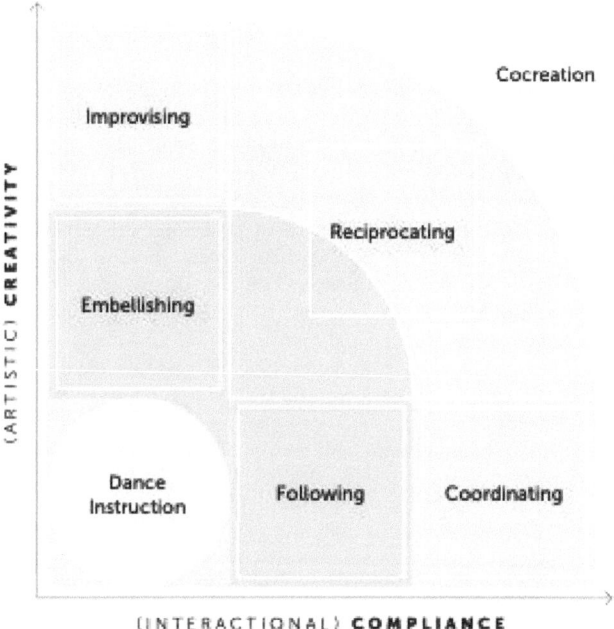

Figure 10. Participant's creative and compliant actions in response to dance instruction.

4. Discussion

In each of the examples above, the instruction was designed to be mimicable remotely with verbal and embodied directives (Due et al. 2019). These, together within the temporal structure of the music, allowed the inherent artistic creativity of the dance to be realized through participants' compliant responses to the instructions both in copresent and mediated interactions. Participants' compliance in response to the multimodal directives of the OSI and then the facilitator displayed alignment with the ongoing structure of the activity (Schegloff 2007; Stivers 2008) regarding when and how they were accomplished, resulting in their compliant and creative contributions to the progressivity of the instructed activity. Actions were not separable from instructions and, as such, were examples of instructed action (Garfinkel 2002).

As pointed out by Lilja and Piirainen-Marsh (2022), a multimodal instruction comprises a directive and depicted gesture to demonstrate how something should be performed to achieve a desired result in a second-language cooking class. In the cases of our data, verbal directives contributed to a multimodal instruction of a creative goal in how an embodied depictive gesture can be embellished. In a second-language (L2) context, this raises questions about the understandability of verbal directives, drawing attention to the order of priority of various modes in multimodal instructions toward different types of goals (i.e., cooking vs. aesthetic objectives). The dance program, in this case, was not intended for an L2 audience or purpose. In terms of second language, the verbal directives as "creative cues" to induce the narrative scenario or imagery of the art gallery or being under the sea are necessarily understood through the talk. In our one example of a foreign-language setting, the focus was on the embodied exchange in turn-taking between the facilitator and the participant. While the OSI may have led the movements of the group in an imaginary narrative of a trip to the art gallery, the pointillism technique shared between the two participants became pointing at each other in a dance of their own making.

Not surprisingly, our results illustrate how the complexity of the interactions increased with the copresence of the facilitator who initiated and encouraged responses of PLWD. The role of the facilitator was implicated in both creative and interactional compliance in the progressing activity. Notably, the opportunities for affiliation with affective stance displays (Lee and Tanaka 2016). (Stivers 2008) were afforded by the copresence of the facilitator, but not the OSI in our examples. Further exploration is warranted into the participation framework and the role of the copresent facilitator (as staff, family, or volunteer), as well as the interactional space in the material environment. As our results show how facilitators were instrumental in initiating copresent interactions, it would be interesting to study further in what circumstances PLWD initiate the same and with each other.

There are many contributions that dance makes to health and well-being, including embodiment, affective responses, and creativity, among others (Chappell et al. 2021). The authentic presence of being with a person, the moment of connection and holding on to it, acceptance of fictional truths, and spontaneous interactions have each been identified as qualities of social communion through art (Balfour 2019). By looking closely at the interactional mechanisms of how these social actions are accomplished, we can identify practices and methods to incorporate these artful processes increasingly into everyday lives in the context of long-term residential care for PLWD. With the overarching directive to "be creative" or to "do what you can," individuals are allowed to bring their own ideas to play in alignment with the structured activity in which they agree to participate.

Importantly, while this research involves a sample demographic of PLWD in institutional settings, our findings are not only relevant for applied conversation analysis (see Antaki 2011), atypical interaction, or ageing studies. These findings contribute to ongoing discussions in the literature regarding compliance and creativity in interaction, multimodal instructed actions, and directive–response sequences in multimodality, embodiment, and intercorporeality in conversation analysis. Contributing to discussions concerning response relevance and recipiency relevance (Schegloff 2010; Stivers and Rossano 2010), we do not assert creativity or compliance in scalar terms but that complexity and diverse combinations of multimodal resources may be drawn upon in instructed actions in consideration of diverse participant abilities and contingencies. The recognition of embodied pair parts as drivers of action as much as utterances (Keevallik 2010) is an important contribution that our work builds upon. Arts-based practices offer environmental contexts within which variably compliant responses are afforded—beyond utterances. How these elements of conduct are shaped in interaction speaks to the artistic and social inclusion practices developing in institutions of health, care, and arts-based research. Including older adults and PLWD in ongoing research in everyday practices for everyone will also be an important consideration for future research on health, well-being, and social inclusion.

5. Conclusions

This article explored the artistic mechanisms at play in an online dance program and how compliance was implicated at a social interactional level. The institutional context of long-term residential care for PLWD was an important setting in which to analyze how arts-based practices contribute to social inclusion, health, and well-being when delivered remotely via technology. Our findings revealed how creativity was achieved in instructed actions that were variably compliant with multimodal directives, from individual following to coparticipants' coordinating. Creativity resulted as participants embellished and improvised in response to directives, building upon dance instruction. At intersections of artistic creativity and interactional compliance, participants' reciprocating actions became cocreative. By demonstrating the sequences of interactions and how they unfolded temporally in the context of the dance, we were able to show how copresent facilitators played an important role in the coordination of compliant and creative instructed actions. Understanding how to support facilitators in institutional contexts will be an important next step in the continued development of remote arts-based programs and practices. Our contribution is about revealing the "how" of the practice mechanisms in bringing arts-based research to dementia care remotely, with a focus on creativity in artistic dance and compliance in interaction.

Author Contributions: Conceptualization, A.K. and M.S.; methodology, A.K.; formal analysis, A.K. and M.S.; investigation, A.K.; resources; A.K. and M.S. data curation, A.K. and M.S.; writing—original draft preparation, A.K.; writing—review and editing, A.K.; visualization, A.K.; supervision, M.S.; project administration, A.K.; funding acquisition, A.K. All authors have read and agreed to the published version of the manuscript.

Funding: As part of "Improving Social Inclusion for Canadians with Dementia and Carers through Sharing Dance" this study was funded by a Canadian Institutes of Health Research/Alzheimer Society of Canada Operating Grant: Social Inclusion for Individuals with Dementia and Carers (CIHR/ASC grant no. 150702). The study also funded, in part, by the Canada Research Chairs program (M. W. Skinner, Trent University; R. V. Herron, Brandon University).

Data Availability Statement: Data is unavailable due to privacy and ethical restrictions.

Acknowledgments: The authors would like to thank the special edition editors as well as reviewers for their comments as well as colleagues who contributed to analysis in data sessions. We would like to give special thanks to Saul Albert for his helpful insights and advice. We also gratefully acknowledge the research sites in Canada and Finland, participants, volunteers, and facilitators, and Canada's National Ballet School for use of the Sharing Dance Older Adults program and research support.

Conflicts of Interest: The authors declare no conflict of interest.

Appendix A

Transcript Conventions

Talk was transcribed according to conventions developed by Gail Jefferson (2004) (see, e.g., Schegloff 2007 for a full description).

gz	gaze
( )	unheard or unclear utterance
[ ]	overlapping speech
↑/↓	sharp rising/falling intonation
(.)	just noticeable pause
(1.0)	timed pauses
,	slight rise of intonation in the last syllable
(( ))	transcriber's comments or descriptions.
wor—	a dash shows a sharp cutoff
wo:rd	colons show that the speaker has stretched the preceding sound
word	underlined sounds are louder, capitals louder still
=	no discernible pause between two speakers' turns

Embodied and multimodal actions were transcribed according to the following conventions developed by Lorenza Mondada: https://www.lorenzamondada.net/multimodal-transcription accessed on 1 January 2021.

Symbol	Description
* *	Descriptions of embodied actions are delimited between
+ +	two identical symbols (one symbol per participant and per type of action)
Δ Δ	that are synchronized with correspondent stretches of talk or time.
*--->	The action described continues across subsequent lines
---->*	until the same symbol is reached.
>>	The action described begins before the excerpts beginning.
--->>	The action described continues after the excerpts end.
.....	action's preparation
----	action's apex is reached and maintained
,,,,	actions retraction
ric	participant doing the embodied action is identified in small caps in the margin.
fig	The exact moment at which a screen shot has been taken
#	is indicated with a sign (#) showing its position within the turn/a time measure.
¶ ¶	On-screen instructor's actions
+ +	Facilitator actions
Δ Δ	Dancer actions (Anita, George, Dancer 1, Joe)
© ©	Dancer 2's actions
ø ø	Dancer 3's actions
♪♪	Within this framework, we added musical beats that count to eight ♪1, ♪2, ♪3, etc.

References

Albert, Saul. 2015. Rhythmical coordination of performers and audience in partner dance. Delineating improvised and choreographed interaction. *Etnografia e Ricerca Qualitativa* 8: 399–428.

Antaki, Charles. 2011. *Applied Conversation Analysis: Intervention and Change in Institutional Talk*. Berlin/Heidelberg: Springer.

Arminen, Ilkka. 2017. *Institutional Interaction: Studies of Talk at Work*. London: Routledge. [CrossRef]

Arminen, Ilkka, Inka Koskela, and Hannele Palukka. 2014. Multimodal production of second pair parts in air traffic control training. *Journal of Pragmatics* 65: 46–62. [CrossRef]

Balfour, Michael. 2019. The politics of care: Play, stillness, and social presence. In *The Routledge Companion to Theatre and Politics*. Edited by P. Eckersall and H. Grehan. London and New York: Routledge, pp. 93–97.

Chappell, Kerry, Emma Redding, Ursula Crickmay, Rebecca Stancliffe, Veronica Jobbins, and Sue Smith. 2021. The aesthetic, artistic and creative contributions of dance for health and wellbeing across the lifecourse: A systematic review. *International Journal of Qualitative Studies on Health and Well-Being* 16: 1950891. [CrossRef]

Clayman, Steven E. 2002. Sequence and solidarity. In *Advances in Group Processes: Group Cohesion, Trust, and Solidarity*. Edited by E. J. Lawler and S. R. Thye. Amsterdam: Elsevier Science, vol. 19, pp. 229–53. [CrossRef]

Craven, Alexandra, and Jonathan Potter. 2010. Directives: Entitlement and contingency in action. *Discourse Studies* 12: 419–42. [CrossRef]

Curl, Traci S., and Paul Drew. 2008. Contingency and action: A comparison of two forms of requesting. *Research on Language and Social Interaction* 41: 129–53. [CrossRef]

De Medeiros, Kate, and Anne Basting. 2014. "Shall I compare thee to a dose of donepezil?": Cultural arts interventions in dementia care research. *The Gerontologist* 54: 344–53. [CrossRef]

Due, Brian L., Simon B. Lange, Mie F. Nielsen, and Celine Jarlskov. 2019. Mimicable embodied demonstration in a decomposed sequence: Two aspects of recipient design in professionals' video-mediated encounters. *Journal of Pragmatics* 152: 13–27. [CrossRef]

Garfinkel, Harold. 1984. *Studies in Ethnomethodology*. Malden: Polity Press Malden. First published 1967.

Garfinkel, Harold. 2002. *Ethnomethodology's Program: Working Out Durkheim's Aphorism*. Lanham: Rowman & Littlefield Publishers.

Goodwin, Charles. 2000. Action and embodiment within situated human interaction. *Journal of Pragmatics* 32: 1489–522. [CrossRef]

Goodwin, Marjorie H. 2006. Participation, affect, and trajectory in family directive/response sequences. *Text and Talk* 26: 4–5. [CrossRef]

Goodwin, Marjorie Harness, and Asta Cekaite. 2013. Calibration in directive/response sequences in family interaction. *Journal of Pragmatics* 46: 122–38. [CrossRef]

Hazel, Spencer, Kristian Mortensen, and Gitte Rasmussen. 2014. Introduction: A body of resources–CA studies of social conduct. *Journal of Pragmatics* 65: 1–9. [CrossRef]

Heritage, J. 1984. Conversation analysis. *Garfinkel and Ethnomethodology* 233: 292.

Herron, Rachel V., Rachel J. Bar, and Mark W. Skinner. 2023. *Dance, Ageing and Collaborative Arts-Based Research*. New York: Routledge. [CrossRef]

Hills, Francince, Ralph Buck, and Rebecca Weber. 2022. Re-imagining 'how' community dance affects the health and wellbeing of older adults. *Dance Articulated* 8: 27–43. [CrossRef]

Hofstetter, Emily, and Leelo Keevallik. 2020. Embodied interaction. In *Handbook Pragmatics: 23rd Annual Installment*. Amsterdam: John Benjamins Publishing Company, vol. 23, pp. 111–38.

Hydén, Lars-Christer, Ali Reza Majlesi, and Anna Ekström. 2022. Assisted eating in late-stage dementia: Intercorporeal interaction. *Journal of Aging Studies* 61: 101000.

Jefferson, Gail. 2004. Glossary of transcript symbols with an introduction. In *Conversation Analysis: Studies from the First Generation*. Edited by G. H. Lerner. Amsterdam: John Benjamins Publishing Company, pp. 13–31. [CrossRef]

Jones, Chelsea Temple, Carla Rice, Margaret Lam, Eliza Chandler, and Karen Kiwon Lee. 2021. Toward technoaccess: A narrative review of disabled and aging experiences of using technology to access the arts. *Technology in Society* 65: 101–537. [CrossRef]

Keevallik, Leelo. 2010. Bodily Quoting in Dance Correction. *Research on Language and Social Interaction* 43: 401–26. [CrossRef]

Kent, Alexandra. 2012. Compliance, resistance, and incipient compliance when responding to directives. *Discourse Studies* 14: 711–30. [CrossRef]

Kontos, Pia, Alisa Grigorovich, An Kosurko, Rachel J. Bar, Rachel V. Herron, Verena H. Menec, and Mark W. Skinner. 2020a. Dancing with dementia: Exploring the embodied dimensions of creativity and social engagement. *The Gerontologist* 61: 714–23. [CrossRef]

Kontos, Pia, Alisa Grigorovich, and Romeo Colobong. 2020b. Towards a critical understanding of creativity and dementia: New directions for practice change. *International Practice Development Journal* 10: 1–13. [CrossRef]

Kosurko, An, Ilkka Arminen, Rachel Herron, Mark Skinner, and Melisa Stevanovic. 2021. Observing Social connectedness in a Digital Dance Program for Older Adults: An EMCA Approach. Paper presented at the Human Computer Interaction International Conference, Washington, DC, USA, July 24–29; Cham: Springer.

Kristiansen, Elisabeth D., Gitte Rasmussen, and Elisabeth M. Andersen. 2019. Practices for making residents' wishes fit institutional constraints: A case of manipulation in dementia care. *Logopedics Phoniatrics Vocology* 44: 7–13. [CrossRef]

Lee, Seung-Hee, and Hiroko Tanaka. 2016. Affiliation and alignment in responding actions. *Journal of Pragmatics* 100: 1–7. [CrossRef]

Lilja, Niina, and Arja Piirainen-Marsh. 2022. Recipient Design by Gestures: How Depictive Gestures Embody Actions in Cooking Instructions. *Social Interaction* 5: 1–30. [CrossRef]

Lindwall, Oskar, and Anna Ekström. 2012. Instruction-in-interaction: The teaching and learning of a manual skill. *Human Studies* 35: 27–49. [CrossRef]

Majlesi, Ali Reza, and Anna Ekström. 2016. Baking together—the coordination of actions in activities involving people with dementia. *Journal of Aging Studies* 38: 37–46. [CrossRef] [PubMed]

Majlesi, Ali Reza, Anna Ekström, and Lars-Christer Hydén. 2021. Sitting down on a chair: Directives and embodied organization of joint activities involving persons with dementia. *Gesprächsforschung* 22: 569–90.

Matérne, Marie, Charlotta Plejert, André Frank, Jessica Bui, Karin Ridder, and Camilla Warnicke. 2022. Interaction and multimodal expressions in a water-dance intervention for adults with intellectual and multiple disabilities. *Journal of Interactional Research in Communication Disorders* 14: 122–53. [CrossRef]

McNeill, W. 1995. *Keeping Together in Time*. Cambridge, MA: Harvard University Press.

Merker, Björn. 2000. Synchronous chorusing and human origins. In *The Origins of Music*. Edited by B. B. Merke and N. L. Wallin. Cambridge: MIT Press, pp. 315–27.

Mondada, Lorenza. 2011. Understanding as an embodied, situated, and sequential achievement in interaction. *Journal of Pragmatics* 43: 542–52. [CrossRef]

Mondada, Lorenza. 2019. Contemporary issues in conversation analysis: Embodiment and materiality, multimodality and multisensoriality in social interaction. *Journal of Pragmatics* 145: 47–62. [CrossRef]

Motta-Ochoa, Rossio, Natalia Incio Serra, Allison Frantz, and Stefanie Blain-Moraes. 2021. Enacting agency: Movement, dementia, and interaction. *Arts & Health* 14: 133–48. [CrossRef]

Peine, Alexander, Barbara L. Marshall, Wendy Martin, and Louis Neven. 2021. Socio-gerontechnology: Key themes, future agendas. In *Socio-Gerontechnology: Interdisciplinary Critical Studies of Ageing and Technology*. London: Routledge, pp. 1–23. [CrossRef]

Sacks, Harvey, Emanuel A. Schegloff, and Gail van Jefferson. 1974. A simplest systematics for the organisation of turn-taking in conversation. *Language* 50: 696–735. [CrossRef]

Schegloff, Emanuel A. 2007. *Sequence Organization in Interaction: A Primer in Conversation Analysis*. Cambridge: Cambridge University Press. [CrossRef]

Schegloff, Emanuel A. 2010. Commentary on Stivers and Rossano: "Mobilizing Response". *Research on Language and Social Interaction* 43: 38–48. [CrossRef]

Skinner, Mark W., Rachel V. Herron, Rachel J. Bar, Pia Kontos, and Verena Menec. 2018. Improving social inclusion for people with dementia and carers through sharing dance: A qualitative sequential continuum of care pilot study protocol. *BMJ Open* 8: E026912. [CrossRef] [PubMed]

Stevanovic, Melisa, and Anssi Peräkylä. 2012. Deontic authority in interaction: The right to announce, propose, and decide. *Research on Language & Social Interaction* 45: 297–321. [CrossRef]

Stevanovic, Melisa, and Anssi Peräkylä. 2015. Experience sharing, emotional reciprocity, and turn-taking. *Frontiers in Psychology* 6: 450. [CrossRef] [PubMed]

Stivers, Tanya. 2008. Stance, alignment, and affiliation during storytelling: When nodding is a token of affiliation. *Research on Language and Social Interaction* 41: 31–57. [CrossRef]

Stivers, T., and Frederico Rossano. 2010. Mobilizing response. *Research on Language and Social Interaction* 43: 3–31. [CrossRef]
Zeilig, Hanna, Julian West, and Millie van der Byl Williams. 2018. Co-creativity: Possibilities for using the arts with people with a dementia. *Quality in Ageing and Older Adults* 19: 135–45. [CrossRef]

Disclaimer/Publisher's Note: The statements, opinions and data contained in all publications are solely those of the individual author(s) and contributor(s) and not of MDPI and/or the editor(s). MDPI and/or the editor(s) disclaim responsibility for any injury to people or property resulting from any ideas, methods, instructions or products referred to in the content.

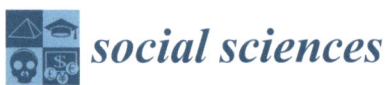

Article

Honouring Differences in Recovery: Methodological Explorations in Creative Eating Disorder Recovery Research

Andrea LaMarre [1,*], Siobhán Healy-Cullen [2], Jessica Tappin [3] and Maree Burns [4]

1 School of Psychology, Massey University, Auckland 0632, New Zealand
2 School of Psychology, Massey University, Palmerston North 4474, New Zealand
3 School of Psychology, Massey University, Wellington 6021, New Zealand
4 Independent Researcher, Auckland 0610, New Zealand
* Correspondence: andrea.m.lamarre@gmail.com or a.lamarre@massey.ac.nz

Abstract: What would it look like to honour differences in eating disorder recovery? Recoveries from eating disorders and eating distress are enacted in relation to discursive, material, and affective flows that open and constrain different possibilities for differently embodied people. Yet, the pull toward establishing consensus on "what recovery is" continues to dominate the landscape of both qualitative and quantitative eating disorder recovery work. While researchers from a variety of perspectives, disciplines, and methodological traditions have sought to establish consensus on what recovery "is", a singular definition remains elusive. Indeed, when researchers continue to adopt the same methodologies—which largely emphasize establishing patterns of sameness—the opportunity to dig into contradictions and tensions that enliven recoveries is missed. In this paper, we reflect on our experiences conducting creative, collaborative, generative research to re-write, re-design, re-draw, and otherwise re-imagine recoveries. The knowledge generated in our research is co-constructed with people with living experience of disordered/distressed eating/eating disorders who spoke back to mainstream recovery discourses (e.g., the idea that recovery is about perfection, that recovery is linear, that one is either recovered or not, that the word "recovered" encapsulates the experience, etc.). We engaged with 12 participants: four in an online group workshop and eight in individual online sessions. Participants held a variety of experiences and backgrounds from Canada, the United States, and Aotearoa New Zealand. We explored their journeys into this conversation with us, the meaning of recovery, and their thoughts on what makes recovery im/possible. Participants were offered several options for creative engagement and took up the idea of "creativity" in ways as different as the stories they shared. Participants created collages, short stories, poems, drawings, and told stories about their experiences. Here, we discuss methodological insights gained from asking participants to lead the creative process. We also explore how this project potentially enables different ways of thinking about and doing eating disorder recovery. Delving into the differences in both *method* and *content* opens up opportunities to take seriously the different relational, material, and affective constellations of participants' living experiences of eating distress/disorder "recovery".

Keywords: eating disorders; recovery; qualitative research; creative methods

Citation: LaMarre, Andrea, Siobhán Healy-Cullen, Jessica Tappin, and Maree Burns. 2023. Honouring Differences in Recovery: Methodological Explorations in Creative Eating Disorder Recovery Research. *Social Sciences* 12: 251. https://doi.org/10.3390/socsci12040251

Academic Editor: Nigel Parton

Received: 4 December 2022
Revised: 17 March 2023
Accepted: 13 April 2023
Published: 20 April 2023

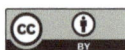

Copyright: © 2023 by the authors. Licensee MDPI, Basel, Switzerland. This article is an open access article distributed under the terms and conditions of the Creative Commons Attribution (CC BY) license (https://creativecommons.org/licenses/by/4.0/).

1. Introduction

Eating disorder recovery is a fraught and contested space/process, without a clear definition but with considerable social currency. People seeking to establish a sense of greater ease in their bodies after struggling with eating and body distress do so in relation to various discourses on what "recovery" is and should look like (Churruca et al. 2019; Holmes 2018; Malson 1998; Saukko 2008; Shohet 2007, 2018). Recovery might be enabled by or performed within particularized, often white, cisgender, heterosexual, female, socioeconomically advantaged matrices (LaMarre and Rice 2017; Rinaldi et al. 2016). These matrices present narrow confines for what "health" might look like and in so doing only provide the conditions of possibility for some recoveries from eating distress—those that toe a fine line between so-called restriction and excess, fat and thin, disordered and healthy (Hardin 2003; LaMarre and Rice 2016; Malson et al. 2011; Musolino et al. 2016). Arguably, the selves recovered in dominant eating disorder recovery discourses align with healthy neoliberal subjects, leaving little room for the articulation of other ways of being. In a society where health has become shorthand for morality (Crawford 1980, 2006) and self- and other-body surveillance is everywhere (Jette et al. 2014; Harwood 2009; Mulderrig 2019; Riley et al. 2016), we must consider how recoveries from eating distress converge with, break off from, reproduce, negotiate, and challenge dominant health norms.

Before we begin our exploration, we offer here a few comments on our terminology and approach. Throughout this piece, we pluralize "recoveries" intentionally to connote the changing, shifting, dynamic, and different experiences of "recovery" people may have. We use recovery in the singular when writing specifically about a piece or body of literature that uses the term in the singular. In this article, we delve into the tensions that arise as we surface differences—differences both in terms of processes we followed in our research and in terms of the stories and artistic renderings participants shared. We explicitly frame difference as affirmative, here, rather than "other" or negative—as something that opens new possibilities and ways of thinking and doing (Braidotti 2013). This orientation aligns with that of others who consider the potential of creative methods "for making dialogue across social problems and uneven power relations possible, but do this in ways that do not erase power, collapse difference or ignore the psychic and material effects of systemic harms" (Rice et al. 2021, p. 346).

2. Methodological Efforts toward Defining and Delineating Recovery

Alongside quantitative approaches aiming to delineate the process and boundaries of recovery (e.g., Bachner-Melman et al. 2006; Couturier and Lock 2006), there is a significant body of qualitative research on recovery that works to provide a contextually situated, detailed account of recovery experiences. This literature employs a wide range of qualitative methods, including discourse analysis (e.g., Hardin 2003; Malson et al. 2011), narrative analysis (e.g., Conti 2018; Dawson et al. 2014; Matusek and Knudson 2009; LaMarre and Rice 2016; Shohet 2007), and thematic analysis (e.g., Hay and Cho 2013; LaMarre and Rice 2017; Lord et al. 2018; Richmond et al. 2020).

There is also qualitative recovery research using life-history approaches (e.g., Patching and Lawler 2009; Redenbach and Lawler 2003) and case study analyses (e.g., Hsu et al. 1992; Lea et al. 2015; Matoff and Matoff 2001; Shohet 2018), as well as grounded theory (e.g., D'Abundo and Chally 2004; Krentz et al. 2005; Lamoureux and Bottorff 2005; Musolino et al. 2016; Woods 2004) and phenomenological or phenomenographic (e.g., Björk et al. 2012; Björk and Ahlström 2008; Jenkins and Ogden 2012) approaches. These studies tell us about some pathways and experiences of people working through change/recovery, often from what has been diagnosed as anorexia nervosa, which is often the experience denoted by the term "eating disorder" despite the variability of distressed eating/embodiment. While the majority of studies noted here were conducted with people who had been diagnosed and/or received clinical treatment, there are also some examples of studies incorporating the recovery stories of those who have not been diagnosed or sought treatment (e.g., Musolino et al. 2016; Shohet 2018; Woods 2004). Nonetheless, efforts toward defining and delineating recovery are most often rooted in clinical practice, with the argument for a consensus definition tied to (in a somewhat circular fashion) the potential for such a definition to provide the foundation for clinical decision-making and research integrity (e.g., Bardone-Cone et al. 2010, 2018).

However, the proliferation of qualitative studies over the course of the past 30 years indicates movement toward incorporating the perspectives of people in recovery into research-based articulations about recovery. Some of this work explicitly integrates attention to how and why discourses around eating disorders and recovery might be resisted by people who would otherwise be labelled with an eating disorder diagnosis (e.g., Musolino et al. 2016; Shohet 2018). The majority of messages proliferated in clinical and general society venues alike about recoveries still hinge on airing particular experiences—those of a largely white, female, thin, cisgender, diagnosed, and treated population. This reflects the significant barriers that continue to exist in diagnostic processes and accessibility to treatment for eating disorders (Cachelin et al. 2001; Gordon et al. 2006; Sinha and Warfa 2013; Thompson 1994), suggesting that large swaths of those experiencing distress may be excluded from such studies.

Further, very little co-designed, creative, and collaborative work provides space for recoveries beyond the confines of "typical" research practice. Those with eating disorders are not typically trusted to tell full or "true" accounts of their experiences (Holmes 2016; Malson et al. 2004; Saukko 2008). Accordingly, what we know about recoveries remains tethered to the dominant discourses researchers, clinicians, and people with eating disorders themselves commonly use to delineate the boundaries between illness and wellness on either "side" of eating disorder and recovery. Further, researchers, and clinicians continue to struggle to find different ways of talking about and doing recovery work, despite years of knowing that (a) existing (particularly residential, hospital, and partial hospitalization) treatment for eating disorders is often ineffective at maintaining wellness in the longer term (Steinhausen 2009; Friedman et al. 2016; Lock et al. 2013) and (b) existing understandings of recovery usually do not present a holistic picture of what recovery is and how to get there, nor an inclusive picture of lived recoveries.

3. Approaching Recoveries Differently

In order to understand, explore, depict, and live recoveries differently, there is a need to approach recoveries in novel ways—methodologically, theoretically, and substantively. Recently, some researchers have begun to employ creative methods to explore recoveries with people experiencing eating disorders, including digital storytelling (LaMarre and Rice 2016) and Photovoice (Saunders and Eaton 2018). However, it is still uncommon for arts-based research to be used to explore—and indeed create—new understandings of recoveries from eating distress. In order to step out of our taken-for-granted ways of knowing, we must look differently at research processes themselves (Levy et al. 2016). Burns (2006) suggests that "attending to embodied subjectivity is both an important ethical consideration for our research activities and offers an exciting resource for enriching our analyses" (p. 4), advocating for an approach to research that conceptualizes "the body as simultaneously material and discursive". As we will demonstrate in this article, creative methods offer an exciting way into engagement with, and analyses of, the constitution of bodies, matter, and discourse, allowing researchers and participants to engage with bodies and the worlds in which they are embedded and impactful. This work aligns with this Special Issue, which is oriented toward "(re)worlding in affective, cultural, imaginative, and justice-attuned (re)ordering ways" (Special Issue CFP) in the way that it pushes forward theorizing around eating disorders and embodied recoveries in entanglement with worlds. As researchers, we were drawn to engage in a deep exploration of how doing research differently and (re)conceptualizing recoveries differently might allow not only for different *theoretical* attunement, but how theory can come to life and enable different ways of *doing and living* recoveries.

Beyond the eating disorders field, creative and arts-based approaches have generated new meanings of disability and difference (e.g., Rice et al. 2017; Rice et al. 2016), cancer (e.g., Frith and Harcourt 2007; Gray et al. 2000, 2003), sexual health (e.g., Crath et al. 2019), HIV/AIDS (e.g., Pietrzyk 2009), and other health-related conditions. Arts-based approaches are particularly well-suited for thinking otherwise about health; as Viscardis et al. (2019) argue, artistic practices can "unsettle the mythical norm of liberal human embodiment—the rational, autonomous, invulnerable subject—that is foundational to health care and informs health care practice" (p. 1287). Arts-based research occurs across paradigms; feminist new materialist and posthuman-oriented arts-based methodologies in particular may offer up the opportunity to engage deeply and differently with embodied issues (Crath et al. 2019;

Renold 2018). Such approaches enable researchers to establish "a more direct connection with, and responsibility for, how research practices come to matter (Barad 2007, p. 89)" (Renold 2018, p. 37). This is of particular interest in the eating disorders field where what we know and how we construct knowledge is so powerfully inflected with tenacious discourses that limit our ability to imagine otherwise. As Levy et al. (2016) note, if we wish to "find new insights" about eating distress, we must "disrupt habitual modes of hearing and seeing research data, with the accompanying biases and blinkers that these habits often entail" (p. 194). One way of engaging differently, Renold (2018) suggests, is to bring together "research creation assemblages" (Manning and Massumi 2014) such that "arts-based research practice can summon new forms of voicing, thinking, feeling and being to emerge" (Renold 2018, p. 40).

4. Our Research

In this paper, we reflect on our experiences of conducting creative, collaborative research with people with living experience of eating distress and eating disorders who spoke back to existing recovery discourses. Collectively, we re-wrote, re-designed, re-drew, and otherwise re-imagined recoveries. Through online sessions, participants engaged with creative modalities to explore "recovery", the meaning(s) of recovery to them, and conditions, feelings, relationships, and experiences that make recovery im/possible. As we will discuss, engaging openly with participants about the idea of "creativity" pushed us to reconsider different ways of doing research. We offer our thoughts on the methodological possibilities of conducting creative eating disorders recovery research and reflect on the different aspects of recoveries made visible or possible through engagement with these methods.

5. Methodological Processes

Our work was designed to foreground new knowledges around recoveries and explore the conditions necessary for these recoveries to coalesce. We align with prior feminist new materialist and posthuman approaches to participatory art-making methodologies in and beyond research contexts, which emphasize the emergent and improvisational nature of all research processes, as well as the need to attend to *non-human* agency and action in this coming-together (e.g., Fullagar and Small 2019; Renold 2018). Accordingly, our focus was on moving toward the creation of "change-making assemblages" (Renold 2018, p. 47). The work took place during a global pandemic; thus, we held all meetings with participants virtually. While this arguably meant a kind of *distance* from participants and their embodied responses, we encouraged participants to turn their cameras off and work on poems or collages or drawings in a way that suited them before returning to the screen to discuss and explore recoveries. In some ways, this may have *facilitated* accessibility in the context of the research, allowing us to do this work across time zones and cities, within spaces where participants could feel more at home (quite literally).

6. Research Team

Andrea LaMarre has been working on eating disorder recovery research for the past ten years, spurred into this work by her own experiences of having and moving through an eating disorder. She is a white, cisgender, heterosexual woman who has benefitted from able-bodied privilege. After receiving eating disorder treatment in her late teens/early twenties, she began to question how systems of privilege uphold certain versions of recovery that privilege some and exclude others. Her research has since been focused on exploring, through qualitative and arts-based approaches, different experiences of recovery in an effort to enliven change and open new possibilities for living recoveries.

Siobhán Healy-Cullen is a white, Irish, cisgender, heterosexual woman. She is a critical health and social psychologist, and so she uses a social justice lens to understand psychological issues as located in socio-political, historical contexts. She is interested in applying creative and critical research methodologies to explore alternative ways of understanding topics that are often discussed from a clinical lens—such as eating disorders—to learn how to better support recovery experiences. Particularly, she is interested in questioning how power shapes health policy/program development—including eating distress/disorder recoveries—and what this means for intersectional social identities.

Jessica Tappin is new to eating disorder recovery research but is completing her PhD on a topic within critical health psychology. She is a white, cisgender, queer woman. She does not have personal experiences but does have second-hand experiences with eating disorder treatment and similarly to the first author was drawn to this research through considerations of privilege in and complexities of this space (although from an outsider's perspective).

Maree Burns describes herself as a Pākehā, cisgender, heterosexual woman, inconsistently "able-bodied", who has lived experience of dis/ordered eating. Maree's professional activities in the eating disorder space include academic research and publications focusing upon how ideas about gender and health shape (1) how disordered eating is understood, (2) peoples' experiences of eating distress, and (3) options for support and treatment. She worked at the Auckland-based Eating Difficulties Education Network for 10 years and is currently counselling in private practice and in a tertiary setting.

7. Recruitment and Participants

We received ethics approval for this project through Massey University's research ethics board (Northern) in November 2020. Following approval, we set out to recruit both international and Aotearoa New Zealand-based participants. We recruited participants through social media (Twitter, Facebook), email, and word of mouth. A major emphasis of the project was relationship-building; the first author was new to Aotearoa while conducting this research, and a significant aim of the work was to establish relationships in this setting to better understand the specific needs of those with eating disorders and seeking recovery[1] in this context. The project was designed with flexibility built in to foreground the possibility of interactions with participants to shift and change the aims of the project; difference was explicitly welcomed into research processes. After several months of outreach, we assembled an international workshop with four participants based in Canada and the United States. We ran this 3 h workshop in February 2021. In the workshop, we alternated between group discussions about recovery and the research aims and processes, and individual work to create creative outputs (e.g., collages and free writing).

We experienced significant challenges in our recruitment processes for group workshops. Miller (2017) describes recruitment as "unseen work"; recruitment can involve a "fine balance" between seeking people who want to tell difficult stories and being protective of these same people (Gubrium et al. 2014). We found that some prospective participants in Aotearoa were more interested in individual sessions for personal, logistical and/or scheduling reasons and, at times. because they were telling stories they had not talked extensively about in group settings. Thus, following continued outreach in the Aotearoa context, we established that individual sessions would better suit prospective participants. We applied for and received ethics clearance for a change to the processes to enable one-on-one sessions. This change enabled ongoing outreach, and over the following months the first author held one-on-one sessions (online) with eight participants based in Aotearoa[2].

8. Analytical Approach/Processes

Following the workshop and individual sessions, the authors met to discuss next steps. The first author generated summaries of the workshop and individual sessions based on transcripts, which were created with the assistance of Otter.ai software, and sent these to participants for review. These summaries included narrative summaries of the sessions, as well as verbatim quotes and first-glance thematic observations. These thematic observations outlined key points in each session in relation to the question of what the interaction tells us about recovery. Three participants offered small edits to these summaries. Two research assistants (S.H.-C. and J.T.) reviewed the transcripts and noted observations about key moments of difference in each session. A.L. then re-read each session summary, noted further observations on each summary, and generated a "recovery rhizome[3]" outlining various discursive, affective, and material nodes we read in participants' stories and other creative representations. Throughout the analytic process, there was an emphasis on points of difference or divergence. We did not aim to perfectly "connect up" these differences but rather to look at how they move together—and along with our readings of them. The various "traits" within a rhizome are "semiotic chains of every nature [and] are connected to very diverse modes of coding (biological, political, economic, etc.) that bring into play not only different regimes of signs but also states of things of differing status" (Deleuze and Guattari 1987, p. 7). Assembling recovery rhizomes was (and is) an unfinished process. Each return to the data and each engagement with it from our various vantage points caused connections to spark.

This difference-attuned approach is inspired by a Deleuzian theoretical orientation, attending to what recoveries might become, rather than a focus on "what they are". It also foregrounds onto-epistemological entanglement, drawing on Baradian (Barad 2007) insight that "matter and meaning are not separate elements. They are inextricably fused together, and no event, no matter how energetic, can tear them asunder" (p. 3). In what follows, we demonstrate what this approach can offer in analysis of eating distress/eating disorder research. We present methodological innovations in relation to substantive insights from participants around their eating distress/disorder recovering/recovery experiences. Overall, we argue that throwing away the interview guide and engaging specifically with what participants wanted to share—and how they wanted to say/draw/write/design it—generated new insights about recovery and recovery research including *how* that research is conducted. Engaging differently with eating disorder recovery research, as well as with "creative research processes" offers exciting new avenues for this work—and pathways to more inclusive, variable recoveries.

Participant and researcher contributions to the work, and the processes of doing this work, offer up more questions than answers. Below, we discuss three of these questions in detail, namely (i) how participants might re-envision research prompts to generate new understanding, (ii) what it means to be creative in recovery and research, and (iii) how to account for different ways of telling distress and recovery. These questions invite us to consider and account for the importance of differences in recovery tethered to different recovery assemblages. By engaging with differences and questions, we align with Braidotti's (2019) insistence that "instead of new generalizations about an engendered pan-humanity, we need sharper focus on the complex singularities that constitute our respective locations" (p. 53). We understand "complex singularities" as a way to engage with and present data in a way that does not seek to universalize or generalize, but rather to stick with difference, and to welcome disruption to taken-for-granted ways of thinking/doing. For us, these "complex singularities" are made visible through creative research assemblages.

9. How Might Participants Re-Envision Research Prompts to Generate New Understandings?

Given the emphasis of this project on creatively imagining eating disorder recoveries through creative research, prior to beginning sessions with participants, we considered a variety of methods that participants might try out. These included digital collage-making (using online software), drawing, free-writing, found-object stories (i.e., using items in their vicinity to prompt story telling), poetry, photovoice (using photos to tell their recovery journey), or short-form digital storytelling. We also designed a series of prompts which participants could select to explore using these methods. The opening prompt invited participants to consider their journey to the space—a prompt that could be interpreted in relation to their literal journey to the workshop space or to the research, including reflecting on their lived experiences of eating disorders/distress and recovery. Further prompts inviting reflection on recoveries were:

- What makes recovery possible?

- What is missing in talk about recovery?
- How do you feel about the word "recovery"?
- What representations of recovery do you want to see?
- What does recovery mean to you?
- What is needed to support recoveries?

As we discussed core prompts, participants' responses invited a consideration of aspects of the prompts that the researchers had not previously anticipated but that shifted the lens on thinking through recoveries.

For instance, we spent 15 min free-writing about "What makes recovery possible?" in the group workshop. In our debrief, SS (group workshop participant, based in the United States; they pronouns) reflected on how "what makes recovery possible is kind of in opposition to how I feel recovery is not possible". SS chose to write a poem in response to this prompt:

What makes recovery possible?

Community & safety

they say nobody can heal in isolation

they say "when you want to, don't give into temptation"

what is it like to feel held? warm? seen?

I spend so much time worrying about causing harm

that the person who is being harmed is me—

a self-defeating prophecy

what if I am important? favored? free?

It's hard to think of freedom

when I am both captor & captive

when keeping me oppressed is society's prerogative

And how can I think of liberation

when others are suffering?

Do I *deserve* to be sick if I can't fight for those living—

in poverty, fear, abuse, and silence—

sometimes I think AN[4] is the ultimate violence

To imagine a setting of access & care

is all well & good, but we're just not there

Is recovery possible? For some, maybe

But I don't dare think it is possible for me.

The group setting and debrief enabled reflection and analysis of what came up for SS while writing the poem. SS shared that the line that stood out to them in their poem was "it's hard to think of freedom when I'm both captor and captive" and that "the idea of deserving to not be free. It's very pervasive". Their poem illustrates how ideas about what makes recovery *possible* bring up structural and ideological constraints that mean recovery is positioned as *impossible* for some. SS positions anorexia as "the ultimate violence" here and explores the ways in which their activism around eating disorder support entwines with their personal experiences. In fighting for systemic change, their own experiences are sidelined; they are called upon to use their energy to enact systemic change when systems do not themselves enable (via funding, resourcing, etc.) the conditions for more people, particularly people with multiple, intersecting, marginalized identities to recover. Their poem also brings to light the limitations of *imagining* caring and accessible care without the potential for its enactment. While freedom might be configured as a core aspect of recovery, we do not live in a world where freedom (e.g., from poverty, isolation, violence, discrimination, etc.) is equally available and accessible to all. SS later reflected how "community and safety" were necessary—together—for recovery to be possible.

Rhizomes are unpredictable; they branch off in different directions without necessarily following a pattern, but also generate connections across their complex root systems (Masny 2013). Likewise, prior to engagement in the workshop, we did not anticipate how the prompt "what makes recovery possible" might offshoot into a discussion about the potential *im*possibility of recoveries. In practice, conversations leading up to the creative activity in this workshop invited the first author to consider how this question lingers behind her work. This thinking came through in the poem she wrote during the workshop:

I don't know what makes recovery possible

I spend a lot more time thinking about what makes recovery *im*possible

And maybe that's deficit focused.

When I'm doing a project like this

I worry that I will dominate

That my own recovery will take up too much space

And at the same time that it isn't enough.

I think about how and whether I eclipse

Rather than enabling

I think about pain

I think about what I allow myself

And what I don't

How to say the things I want to say

While feeling like when I say things I'm never fully present

In this poem, Andrea (she/her) reflected on the potential dominance of her own perspective within the research space, as well as the potential for a deficit focus in the work. This latter comment relates to the ways in which critical research about eating disorders is often perceived as purely deconstructive rather than hopeful or constructive. Rosi Braidotti (2019) notes the comingling of "potestas and potentia", or the dual negation–affirmation that together enable critical work that presents the possibility of forward motion. Both SS and Andrea's poems illustrate the challenges inherent to doing work that tangles up these two forces—the deconstructive critique and forward, affirmative motion. Furthermore, it illustrates how, on a personal level, this work can lead to questions about one's own role and recovery.

The inseparability of potestas and potentia mirror the inseparability of considering the possibility and impossibility of recovery—and illustrate "the multi-layered structure of power (as both potestas and potentia): it is not a question of either/or, but of 'and . . . and'. Contiguity, however, is not the same as complicity, and qualitative differences can and must be made" (Braidotti 2019, p. 44). Thinking through potestas and potentia as "and . . . and" invites us to consider how seemingly small movements for change may add up. It is unlikely that systems that constrain and delimit recoveries will be transformed overnight. However, it might be possible to make "qualitative differences" by deeply and thoughtfully engaging with creative representations of eating disorder and recovery, by taking such representations seriously—and putting those insights "to work" in the service of supporting shifts in research and clinical praxis.

10. What Does It Mean to Be Creative in Recovery and Research?

In individual sessions, participants engaged in various ways with the invitation for creativity. Crucially, participants' engagement invited the researchers to reconsider the visual and written forms of creativity we had in mind while designing the project. While we may have "plugged in" to the research with a familiar idea of "creativity", engagement with participants sparked rhizomatic reckoning with the de-familiarization of taken-for-granted ways of doing/being creative. Several participants elected to tell stories about their experiences rather than collage/draw/write/digital story them. In discussing creativity, Scout B (individual session participant, based in Aotearoa; they/them) shared that "I think not everyone does creativity in the same way. So, you know, for me coming up with a whole bunch of ideas. That is creativity. But you'd be hard pressed to get me drawing or painting". Rather than drawing or painting, Scout B developed a metaphor around a marble run that was sitting next to them at the time. They described how recovery, for them, was not a singular choice but a series of days moving through life. The systems they were working with did not enable the kind of care that worked for their circumstances. The marble run, then, worked as a metaphor "in terms of the way that you get flung through the system. And once you get to the bottom, there's nothing else, you have to go back to the top". Scout B's story of the recovery marble run evidenced how closed off, universalized, and financially, geographically, and ideologically inaccessible systems generated limited points of entry and engagement.

Diana (individual session participant, based in Aotearoa; she/her) similarly preferred to tell her story verbally, noting that this meant she would be less likely to be "overly perfectionistic" about it, but also that she "look[s] at [her] past as if it was a story". As she noted "I kind of like the goal, like I get perfectionistic, which, I guess, can relate as well to my disordered eating past. But I think like, I just prefer to conceptualize it in story. Because I kind of look at my past as if it was a story". Method and meaning come together in these words—Diana acknowledged how her desire to tell rather than draw/write/collage her experience may be related to her "perfectionistic tendencies". Simultaneously, she invited the possibility that this may not be "problematic" or pathological, but rather a part of her preferred ways of making meaning. Throughout the session, Diana's storytelling invited in perspectives on her recovery that wove together her experiences growing up in North America, surrounded by problematic ideals about bodies—and about womanhood—and her experiences moving to Aotearoa New Zealand and exploring Health at Every Size®[5] communities to support a greater sense of body peace.

Kare (individual session participant, based in Aotearoa; she/her) offered insight into the creative process of storying experiences verbally, reflecting on how "storying my memories, is often quite creative in itself". The creativity of storying memories Kare spoke to carries significant weight when considering how and when to adopt creative methodologies in eating disorder recovery research. That is, rather than only focusing on content participants share *as content* or *objective facts* used to evaluate recoveries, we might spend more time with the ways in which people weave their stories and re-envision "interviews" to invite free-form sharing.

Through storying her memories in a free-form way, Kare, who has European and Māori ancestry, reflected on intergenerational experiences of food and body and the constraints of racism and colonization entwining with norms for womanhood. Echoes of her mother's and grandmothers' experiences clearly shaped Kare's embodied experiences. For instance, she noted that " . . . food scarcity has played a big role in [. . .] intergenerational suffering". She reflected on food scarcity on both sides of her family: her European ancestors' experiences of poverty and rationing in the context of wartime, and her Māori ancestors' experiences of impoverishment and lack of welfare or other government support. Kare described "the kind of the horror of fetishizing small women when this can come from such oppressive circumstances", and described how this fetishization was "carried on through generations and intersected with postfeminist discourses of sexuality and sexualization". Playing out in her experiences of struggle around food and body, "people saw my, my physical appearance as being unattainable, but valorized"—something for which she was framed as a "bad role model". Thinking back on how she did not receive much sympathy around her suspected eating disorder, Kare noted how this kind of (non-empathetic response)

> "has been a theme in a lot of Indigenous women's lives when it comes to whether it's mental health issues, or trauma or things like that, often, it's the woman's

responses that come under scrutiny, rather than the actual circumstances that led them there in the first place".

As non-Indigenous researchers, we propose a *tentative* analysis of the intergenerational interweaving of gender, colonization, and bodies we notice within Kare's story by linking what we noticed to theory-work from Māori scholars. Simmonds (2011) described how "the intersection of being Māori and being a woman posits us in complex and tricky spaces that require careful negotiation" (p. 11). In Kare's story, we might consider how gendered power intersects with colonizing discourses, constraining the possibilities for bodies, and how this might lead to a sense of being "trapped in a space between worlds" (Simmonds 2011, p. 11). Problematizing individual responses rather than focusing on the circumstances that keep people small (physically and metaphorically) distracts from what Kare clearly illustrates is a fundamentally intergenerational story of embodiment. This story is interwoven with the ways in which Māori women's experiences of and access to embodied power and agency has been disrupted (Simmonds 2011) and fragmented (Pihama 2001) through processes of colonization.

These insights came through Kare's stories relatively unprompted; while the first author asked questions about her experiences, she had not anticipated the degree to which Kare's story would return, time and again, to her embodied learning about bodies, food, eating, femininity, and resistance in relation to her ancestors. Working with story represented an opportunity to work through and tease out a recovery rhizome that moved through these various nodes in a non-linear way.

Other participants engaged with visual representations of their recoveries, which likewise added affective resonance and contextual depth to their stories. For instance, Lorraine (individual session participant, based in Aotearoa; she/her) shared "what makes recovery possible" in the form of a drawing with words embedded (Figure 1):

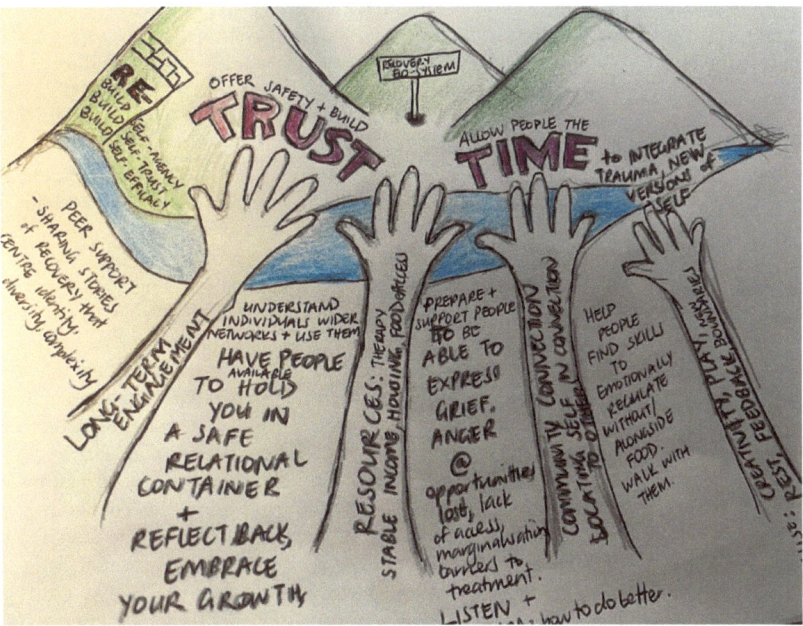

Figure 1. Drawing by participant Lorraine.

Lorraine's drawing shows several mountains bordered by a stream. She described the drawing as demonstrating the "recovery ecosystem", built on twin cores of trust and time. Hands reaching up toward the mountains hold up the ecosystem, and are comprised of long-term engagement, resources, community connection, and creativity. Playing with the idea of "re" in recovery, Lorraine explored rebuilding in recovery: rebuilding self-agency, self-trust, and self-efficacy. In superimposing written thoughts on her recovery ecosystem, Lorraine's drawing can be interpreted on practical and affective levels. On a practical level, the drawing points to the material "stuff" of the recovery ecosystem she imagines—how things such as "therapy stable income, housing [and] food access" are key aspects that prop up recoveries. The drawing also positions the development of trust as central—and evidences how the development of trust takes time—and is rhizomatically linked to the development of the material "stuff" named above. Trust is not a given in eating disorder treatment (Holmes et al. 2021); Lorraine's drawing, and her story, reaffirm how trust might not be easily built when treatments are oriented toward efficiencies and universalities, rather than collaboration and openness. While the insights Lorraine portrayed in her drawing also came through in her verbalized story, wherein she noted, for example, how she needed to "feel safe enough to keep moving through that process [of integrating theoretical knowing and insight about recovery], rather than just like running away screaming", engaging in the creative activity branched into an opportunity to reflect together on what comprises Lorraine's recovery ecosystem.

In summary, these brief reflections on creativity and openness in research encounters signal how our research practices shape who we engage with, how we engage, and what kind of research "outputs" are made possible by different ways of doing. Had we imposed a particular framework for creativity, we may have generated interesting outputs, but these may or may not have resonated with participants' preferred ways of doing and being. This insight might be entangled with aspects of recovery processes themselves—what might be opened up if we moved toward more explicit centering of people's preferred ways of being and doing? Thinking this through means considering the ways in which the voices and preferences of people with living experience are often sidelined within mainstream treatment settings (Holmes et al. 2021). The telling authority of those with eating disorders is often undermined, with the suggestion that "the eating disorder voice" is all-encompassing, rendering the perspectives of people with eating disorders less trustworthy (Holmes 2016; Malson et al. 2004; Saukko 2008).

11. How Do We Account for Different Ways of Telling Distress and Recovery?

Participants' creative engagements offered up new ways of telling "told stories" of eating distress/disorders and recovery. The "complex singularities" (Braidotti 2019, p. 53) of each story invites the question of how to account and make space for different ways of telling distress and recovery. Chun Li's (individual session participant, based in Aotearoa; she/her) story offers an opportunity to engage with questions about what both eating disorders and recovery "are" and "are not".

Chun Li moved to New Zealand from a country in Southeast Asia in her teens; she identifies with the label of "having some problems" around food rather than "eating disorder". Chun Li shared that "this was in [country] in the late 80s and I don't know it wasn't really a thing, you know". Subsequently, Chun Li makes sense of her problems around food as being related to moments of anxiety or depression in her life; she explicitly notes that she is not always aware of the link at the time, but on reflection can often see connections between what she describes as challenges with chewing, swallowing, and keeping down food, and other life stressors. She preferred the terminology of "living with, managing it well" rather than recovery, and likened managing these problems to managing other health problems such as asthma.

Chun Li wrote a short story about her experiences, writing from the perspective of herself as a child. An analysis of that story invites new ways of thinking about eating disorders themselves as well as what it means to "recover". Close to the beginning of her story, Chun Li writes:

> That's what I'm trying to explain. Something is broken. That's why I can't eat. So let me tell you what eating is like for me. It's a daily struggle. After breakfast,

it's a couple of hours before lunch, and I'm already feeling anxious and thinking about lunch. My thoughts go something like, 'It's almost lunchtime. Am I going to be able to eat? Or will I just throw up?' My anxiety about lunch will keep increasing as lunchtime approaches. And now, it's lunchtime. Today, lunch is spaghetti and meatballs. You will see a plate of spaghetti with tomato sauce, a few meatballs and cheese on top. Nothing out of the ordinary. I, on the other hand, will see a mountain of spaghetti, the meatballs are like boulders, and the cheese on top, like snow on a mountain top. This is a mountain that I will have to climb and overcome. If mum puts a big portion on the plate, I will freak out and think that this is a mountain that's too high. I cannot climb it.

The "straightforward" read of this story is that Chun Li was anxious about the food in front of her, which made it difficult to eat. This explanation foregrounds a psychological reading of the situation—the idea that Chun Li's cognitions or misread of the threat of food prevented her from eating. However, Chun Li went on to explicitly position the challenge as a physical, mechanical one, writing "It's as if my muscles don't work properly and my brain can't make the muscles in my throat do the action of swallowing". Throughout her narrative, Chun Li returned to a refrain around voluntary and involuntary actions. Reflecting on her experience, she wrote:

I am trying very hard to be better. I hope that one day, swallowing, eating and drinking, whether they are voluntary or involuntary actions, can one day be enjoyable actions. They don't even have to be enjoyable; I would be fine with achievable actions. I feel I have many more spaghetti mountains and other food mountains to climb before I get there.

Throughout her interview and storytelling, Chun Li engaged in a great deal of self-analysis—again putting the lie to the assumption that people with or in recovery from eating disorders are not trustworthy tellers of their own stories (Holmes 2016; Saukko 2008). On the contrary, the insights Chun Li developed and shared about her experiences—like those of other participants—can be held as their own truths. Within these excerpts, Chun Li's perspectives on her desires and goals, as well as her self-assessment, shine through. Moving through the frame she created around voluntary/involuntary actions, Chun Li wrote about a desire to *achieve* the ability to eat. She edited her own assertion that this needs to be enjoyable, redressing her own recovery aspirations in relation to a perspective in alignment with her current and imagined reality.

Chun Li aligned in some ways with a progress-based perspective on doing better, expressing a desire to "get there" throughout her story. Chun Li emphasized how eating problems were rarely central in her life or top of mind—they materialized in relation to other stressors. The link between exacerbation of challenges with food and stressors is well-documented. However, taking a closer look at the recovery rhizomes Chun Li drew with her words, this might be connected to those stressors, as well as to her biochemistry; in her own words, "Now I know that it's all connected with serotonin". Her *knowing* forms another trait within the recovery rhizome and affectively generates a sense of comfort even in the absence of other pieces of the rhizome (such as the spaghetti mountain) actually moving.

12. Discussion

The stories shared in this article are only a small sample of the rich, complex, and situated stories and creations participants shared. Academic writing could never do justice to the full richness of these stories—and indeed, the full story is not the authors' to share (Limes-Taylor Henderson and Esposito 2019). We selected the excerpts of stories and artistic outputs illustrated here that "glowed" (Maclure 2013) in their difference. Given unlimited space, we could work through many others, and offer these insights as a first step in demonstrating what becomes possible when we revision eating disorder recovery research. Using examples of participants shifting research prompts, doing creativity differently, and telling unanticipated recovery stories, we have illustrated how being flexible in our engagement with creative methods invited new ways of imagining recoveries.

13. The Creative Research Process

Fullagar and Small (2019) explored the value of creative research for offering "different ways of engaging with personal stories as political and affective sites of social change" (p. 123). Similarly, our work invites a reconsideration of taken-for-granted ways of thinking and doing eating disorder, disordered eating, and eating problem "recoveries". Had we not conducted this research in this way, we may have missed affective, material, and relational insights participants shared; indeed, participants' engagement with our work *shifted the research processes themselves* and challenged us to think differently about "doing creative research". Creatively engaging with recoveries is a political act (Fullagar and Small 2019), far from a frivolous exercise. Critically engaging with creative methods can help us "to go beyond taken-for-granted assumptions" (Lupton and Watson 2021, p. 466) to offer something novel and innovative. Eating disorder recovery has been thoroughly explored in academic realms across disciplines and methodologies (see for example Bardone-Cone et al. 2010, 2018; Conti 2018; de Vos et al. 2017; Malson et al. 2011). By working differently, we found ourselves pushed in new directions, working closely and deeply with participants' stories and creations to explore what these creative explorations enable. This represents a step toward prefiguring world making and (re)engaging with recoveries in their differences and pluralities.

We abandoned a desire for sameness across research encounters in this project, a move that could be deemed problematic within a system of knowledge that prizes replicability and universality. In this, we align with those who argue that "if method is pre-given and known in advance, it also suggests that data is an already pre-supposed entity that is waiting to be captured, extracted, and mined" (Springgay and Truman 2018, p. 204). Methods are not neutral, as those working from Kaupapa Māori and other Indigenous methodologies (e.g., Jones and Jenkins 2008) have long shown. In working our creative methods *with* rather than *for* or *on* participants, we opened up to that which we could not have anticipated prior to engaging with them—participants' stories and ways of engaging fundamentally shaped and shifted the research assemblage itself. Our research practices came to matter (Barad 2007) in the divergent, disparate, and different stories—and ways of showing and telling stories—that this research invited. Rather than gloss over the differences in participants' stories and ways of engaging, we center them here (see also Rice et al. 2021).

14. Key Insights

Substantively, participants' stories invite several key insights about eating disorder recoveries. In poetry, participants and researchers in this study puzzled through how the possibility of recovery is entwined with the impossibility of recovery. Various facets of participants' stories crystallized power relations that constrain access to services and align with desired ways of doing recovery and being recovered. Material and systemic factors such as secure food, income, and housing operated within the recoveries participants experienced or wanted to be made possible. These co-mingled with needs to acknowledge how intergenerational body and food experiences shape and shift what people know and feel in their bodies. Participants' stories could be "read" on multiple levels; taking into account histories within treatment praxis and research literature of people with eating disorders as untrustworthy (Holmes 2016; Holmes et al. 2021; Saukko 2008), it becomes particularly important to privilege participants' own articulations of their stories. This is arguably particularly true when a disconnect between dominant "reads" of eating disorders and individual experiences had meant that they did not share their stories with anyone until they participated in this research.

15. Summary

Methodologically, our work invites several provocations for those seeking to dig deeply into the situated, contextualized experiences of people who live in relation to diagnosed or undiagnosed eating disorders and legitimized or delegitimized recoveries.

Firstly, given that many of our participants were undiagnosed and/or had experiences with treatment systems that led to them seeking help and support outside of mainstream systems, this work invites questions about whose recoveries the mainstream academic literatures typically feature. Had we narrowed our selection criteria to those who were diagnosed and/or treated in mainstream systems, we would have missed engaging with those who did not fit this mold. Working closely with those who worked through recoveries alongside, in spite of, or outside of these systems invites new ways of storying and doing recovery. Secondly, remaining open to different ways of engaging with creativity taught us about the value in flexibility of method and how abandoning a desire for sameness invites unanticipated yet impactful differences. Together, our insights on content and method center around a call we issue to those seeking to explore eating recoveries in a richly nuanced way: invite and welcome difference. Doing so opens up opportunities to enable our research—as well as advocacy and treatment—to be driven by collaboration and openness, rather than manualized and universalized approaches.

16. Limitations and Considerations

While this kind of research can open up new ways of engaging with participants and with recoveries themselves, it does not always align with the research agendas, priorities, and practices embedded in neoliberal systems. Both treatment-as-usual and research-as-usual are strongly encouraged—if not enforced—in Western neoliberal systems. A deep dive into the reasons for this is beyond the scope of this paper; briefly, funding systems in private and "public" healthcare systems alike provide for only some forms of treatment, accessible only to those who fit narrow criteria for eating disorders. As several of our participants indicated, even when one does fit those criteria, existing modes of treatment do not always facilitate lasting "recoveries" that align with participants' contexts. In a "managed care" system, evidence-based treatment is upheld as the way to engage with eating disorders (Lester 2019). In its fullest realization, evidence-based practice should include not only research evidence, but also clinical and lived experience (Peterson et al. 2016). As Peterson et al. (2016) note, however, in practice one or more of these "legs" of evidence-based practice may be sidelined. Others have noted the pervasive mistrust of people with eating disorders (e.g., Holmes et al. 2021); this mistrust may lead to the sidelining of lived experience in particular as a "valid form of expertise" in determining treatment approaches and orientations to recovery.

Likewise, in research, there is a strong pull toward delineating what recovery "is" and what it "is not". In transparency, the first author has previously been involved in this kind of work to call a consensus definition of recovery into being. Such a definition—and guidance on how to reach it—has been deemed practically useful for clinical work, as well as to govern inclusion in research studies. There is merit in this view, and we do not wish to ignore the clinical and lived realities facing those working through eating disorders who may find such criteria useful. Indeed, getting on the same page about recovery can be incredibly helpful in facilitating healing (Musolino et al. 2016). And, we cannot ignore the ways in which power flows through attempts to delineate what "recovery is"—nor can we ignore how any normalizing and universalizing definition stands to potentially exclude those who do not fit (Davis 1995).

Even conducting qualitative research in eating disorders is often framed as a sideline consideration or something that will later require quantification in order to "count". Quantitative research can (a) be critical and (b) be conducive to making large-scale decisions about ED treatment and recovery. What may be neglected in discussions of qualitative versus quantitative eating disorder research is that these approaches are fundamentally attempting to do something quite different. In an approach like ours, the priority is on exploring the nuances and needs of people working through relationships with food and body entangled in contexts that constrain opportunities for flourishing. It is not on elaborating a universal approach to either treatment or defining recovery—indeed, it invites resistance to the idea that such a universal approach is the way forward. Altering any aspect of the assemblage shifts the whole assemblage (Deleuze and Guattari 1987).

We anticipate that there will be questions about how such work might make a difference while the broader systems described above continue to exert their universalizing pressures on eating disorder treatment and research. We propose that such an opening presents a crack in the foundations through which to begin to have conversations about the need for both in-the-moment, individual shifts in how recoveries are understood and conceptualized, and broader systemic changes to lead to later, larger, systemic changes. In all of this, we recognize that new is not necessarily better. However, as Gail Weiss (2008) suggests, "If social, political, and material transformation is to have a lasting impact on individuals and society, it must be integrated within ordinary experience" (p. 1). The experiences we have explored throughout this piece offer difference in these ordinary experiences that, in the long run, may help guide (albeit slowly) toward broader systemic change.

Author Contributions: A.L. led the conceptualization of the study and methodological design with feedback from all authors. A.L., M.B. and S.H.-C. were present at the international (online) workshop. A.L. conducted individual sessions. A.L. led analysis, developing summaries and "recovery rhizomes"; S.H.-C. and J.T. worked with transcripts and summaries. M.B. contributed to analysis, providing over-arching feedback and contextual commentary. A.L. led the writing process, with all authors contributing substantive edits on each round. All authors have read and agreed to the published version of the manuscript.

Funding: This research received funding from Massey University through a Marsden Development Support Grant (for A.L.).

Institutional Review Board Statement: This research was approved by the Massey University Ethics Board (Northern), protocol 20/48.

Informed Consent Statement: Informed consent was obtained from all participants involved in the study.

Data Availability Statement: A full dataset is not publicly available as permission for full data set availability was not requested in the informed consent process.

Acknowledgments: We wish to thank all participants for sharing their stories and creativity with us. We learned a great deal from participants—about recovery, about research, and about social justice. We hope that this work represents one step toward honouring differences in recoveries and toward broader systemic changes to support these differences. We also wish to thank Sarah Riley for her consultation on workshop design. Finally, we wish to thank the editors of this special issue—Nadine Changfoot, Carla Rice, and Eliza Chandler, for making space for pieces like ours in the academic peer review landscape.

Conflicts of Interest: The authors declare no conflict of interest.

Notes

[1] It was important for this project to keep recruitment criteria broad to ensure that the study was not restricted to only those with clinical diagnoses. There are significant barriers to eating disorder diagnoses and treatment, particularly for people who do not fit stereotypes about eating disorders (Becker et al. 2010; Cachelin et al. 2001). As such, we invited those whose experiences did not cleanly fit into diagnostic language and/or who had not experienced treatment, as well as those who had been diagnosed and/or treated.

[2] We did not collect demographic information about participants beyond what they shared in their stories, to enable their choice in sharing which social locations they wished to share, in the discussions. We will share those intersections where relevant when analyzing extracts and contributions below, rather than offering a demographic summary.

[3] In constructing the research and analysis plan, we were drawn to rhizomes, as articulated by Deleuze and Guattari (1987) in *A Thousand Plateaus*. Rhizomes are connected, heterogeneous assemblages made up not of ordered points but rather unending and unpredictable "connections between semiotic chains, organizations of power, and circumstances relative to the arts, sciences, and social struggles" (p. 7). Others (e.g., Masny 2013) have explored the potential of rhizoanalysis as "a way to work with transgressive data" (p. 341) that does not propose that the researcher enters into analysis from one particular fixed point. Instead, research is presented as an assemblage and involves the coming together of material and ideological structures including the researcher, the participants, their varied contexts, the processes of analysis, and more (St. Pierre 1997). While we did not follow

4   Anorexia nervosa.
5   Health at Every Size is a framework for thinking about health proposing that "health care must be accessible to people no matter their size, and no matter why they are any given size" (https://asdah.org/health-at-every-size-haes-approach/, accessed on 30 November 2022). It is based around a set of core principles that foreground the importance of looking beyond an individual's size to determine health status, as well as clarifying that health and moral worthiness must be decoupled.

References

Bachner-Melman, Rachel, Ada H. Zohar, and Richard P. Ebstein. 2006. An examination of cognitive versus behavioral components of recovery from anorexia nervosa. *The Journal of Nervous and Mental Disease* 194: 697–703. [CrossRef]
Barad, Karen. 2007. *Meeting the Universe Halfway: Quantum Physics and the Entanglement of Matter and Meaning*. London: Duke University Press.
Bardone-Cone, Anna M., Megan B. Harney, Christine R. Maldonado, Melissa A. Lawson, Paul D. Robinson, Roma Smith, and Aneesh Tosh. 2010. Defining recovery from an eating disorder: Conceptualization, validation, and examination of psychosocial functioning and psychiatric comorbidity. *Behavioural Research and Therapy* 48: 194–202. [CrossRef] [PubMed]
Bardone-Cone, Anna M., Rowan A. Hunt, and Hunna J. Watson. 2018. An overview of conceptualizations of eating disorder recovery, recent findings, and future directions. *Current Psychiatry Reports* 20: 79. [CrossRef] [PubMed]
Becker, Anne E., Adrienne Hadley Arrindell, Alexandra Perloe, Kristen Fay, and Ruth H. Striegel-Moore. 2010. A qualitative study of perceived social barriers to care for eating disorders: Perspectives from ethnically diverse health care consumers. *International Journal of Eating Disorders* 43: 633–47. [CrossRef] [PubMed]
Björk, Tabita, and Gerd Ahlström. 2008. The patient's perception of having recovered from an eating disorder. *Health Care Women International* 29: 926–44.
Björk, Tabita, Karin Wallin, and Gunn Pettersen. 2012. Male experiences of life after recovery from an eating disorder. *Eating Disorders* 20: 460–68.
Braidotti, Rosi. 2013. *The Posthuman*. Oxford: Polity.
Braidotti, Rosi. 2019. A theoretical framework for the critical posthumanities. *Theory, Culture & Society* 36: 31–61.
Burns, Maree Leeann. 2006. Bodies that speak: Examining the dialogues in research interactions. *Qualitative Research in Psychology* 3: 3–18. [CrossRef]
Cachelin, Fary M., Ramona Rebeck, Catherine Veisel, and Ruth H. Striegel-Moore. 2001. Barriers to treatment for eating disorders among ethnically diverse women. *International Journal of Eating Disorders* 30: 269–78. [CrossRef]
Churruca, Kate, Jane M. Ussher, Janette Perz, and Frances Rapport. 2019. 'It's always about the eating disorder': Finding the person through recovery-oriented practice for bulimia. *Culture, Medicine, and Psychiatry* 44: 286–303. [CrossRef]
Conti, Janet E. 2018. Recovering identity from anorexia nervosa: Women's constructions of their experiences of recovery from anorexia nervosa over 10 years. *Journal of Constructivist Psychology* 31: 72–94. [CrossRef]
Couturier, Jennifer, and James Lock. 2006. What is remission in adolescent anorexia nervosa: A review of various conceptualizations and a quantitative analysis. *International Journal of Eating Disorders* 39: 175–83. [CrossRef]
Crath, Rory, Adam Gaubinger, and Cristian Rangel. 2019. Studying the 'sexuality-health-technology nexus': A new materialist visual methodology. *Culture, Health & Sexuality* 21: 1290–308.
Crawford, Robert. 1980. Healthism and the medicalization of everyday life. *International Journal of Health Services* 10: 365–88. [CrossRef]
Crawford, Robert. 2006. Health as a meaningful social practice. *Health: An Interdisciplinary Journal for the Social Study of Health, Illness and Medicine* 10: 401–20. [CrossRef]
D'Abundo, Michelle, and Pamela Chally. 2004. Struggling with recovery: Participant perspectives on battling an eating disorder. *Qualitative Health Research* 14: 1094–106.
Davis, Lennard J. 1995. *Enforcing Normalcy: Disability, Deafness, and the Body*. London: Verso Books.
Dawson, Lisa, Paul Rhodes, and Stephen Touyz. 2014. Doing the impossible: The process of recovery from chronic anorexia nervosa. *Qualitative Health Research* 24: 494–505. [CrossRef]
de Vos, Jan Alexander, Andrea LaMarre, Mirjam Radstaak, Charlotte Ariane Bijkerk, Ernst T. Bohlmeijer, and Gerben J. Westerhof. 2017. Identifying fundamental criteria for eating disorder recovery: A systematic review and qualitative meta-analysis. *Journal of Eating Disorders* 5: 34. [CrossRef] [PubMed]
Deleuze, Gilles, and Félix Guattari. 1987. *A Thousand Plateaus: Capitalism and Schizophrenia*. Minneapolis: University of Minnesota Press.
Friedman, Keren, Ana L. Ramirez, Stuart B. Murray, Leslie K. Anderson, Anne Cusack, Kerri N. Boutelle, and Walter H. Kaye. 2016. A narrative review of outcome studies for residential and partial hospital-based treatment of eating disorders. *European Eating Disorders Review* 24: 263–76. [CrossRef]
Frith, Hannah, and Diana Harcourt. 2007. Using photographs to capture women's experiences of chemotherapy: Reflecting on the method. *Qualitative Health Research* 17: 1340–50. [CrossRef]
Fullagar, Simone, and Iesha Small. 2019. Writing recovery from depression through a creative research assemblage: Mindshackles, digital mental health, and a feminist politics of self-care. In *Digital Dilemma: Transforming Gender Identities and Power Relations in Everyday Life*. Edited by Diana C. Parry, Corey W. Johnson and Simone Fullagar. London: Palgrave Macmillan, pp. 121–41.

Gordon, Kathryn H., Marissa M. Brattole, LaRicka R. Wingate, and Thomas E. Joiner Jr. 2006. The impact of client race on clinician detection of eating disorders. *Behavioural Therapy* 37: 319–25. [CrossRef] [PubMed]

Gray, Ross E., Margaret I. Fitch, Manon LaBrecque, and Marlene Greenberg. 2003. Reactions of health professionals to a research-based theatre production. *Journal of Cancer Education* 18: 223–29. [CrossRef]

Gray, Ross, Chris Sinding, Vrenia Ivonoffski, Margaret Fitch, Ann Hampson, and Marlene Greenberg. 2000. The use of research-based theatre in a project related to metastatic breast cancer. *Health Expectations* 3: 137–44. [CrossRef] [PubMed]

Gubrium, Aline C., Amy L. Hill, and Sarah Flicker. 2014. A situated practice of ethics for participatory visual and digital methods in public health research and practice: A focus on digital storytelling. *American Journal of Public Health* 104: 1606–14. [CrossRef]

Hardin, Pamela K. 2003. Social and cultural considerations in recovery from AN: A critical poststructuralist analysis. *Advances in Nursing Science* 26: 5–16. [CrossRef] [PubMed]

Harwood, Valerie. 2009. Theorizing biopedagogies. In *Biopolitics and the "Obesity Epidemic": Governing Bodies*. Edited by Jan Wright and Valerie Harwood. New York: Routledge, pp. 16–30.

Hay, Phillipa J., and Kenneth Cho. 2013. A qualitative exploration of influences on the process of recovery from personal written accounts of people with anorexia nervosa. *Women Health* 53: 730–40. [CrossRef]

Holmes, Su, Helen Malson, and Joanna Semlyen. 2021. Regulating "untrustworthy patients": Constructions of "trust" and "distrust" in accounts of inpatient treatment for anorexia. *Feminism & Psychology* 31: 41–61. [CrossRef]

Holmes, Su. 2016. "Blindness to the obvious"? Treatment experiences and feminist approaches to eating disorders. *Feminism & Psychology* 26: 464–86.

Holmes, Su. 2018. (Un)twisted: Talking back to media representations of eating disorders. *Journal of Gender Studies* 27: 149–64. [CrossRef]

Hsu, L. K. George, Arthur H. Crisp, and John S. Callender. 1992. Recovery in anorexia nervosa: The patient's perspective. *International Journal of Eating Disorders* 11: 341–50. [CrossRef]

Jenkins, Jana, and Jane Ogden. 2012. Becoming 'whole' again: A qualitative study of women's views of recovering from anorexia nervosa. *European Eating Disorders Review* 20: e23–e31. [CrossRef]

Jette, Shannon, Krishna Bhagat, and David L. Andrew. 2014. Governing the child-citizen: 'Let's Move!' as national biopedagogy. *Sport, Education, and Society* 21: 1109–26. [CrossRef]

Jones, Alison, and Kuni Jenkins. 2008. Rethinking collaboration: Working the indigene-colonizer hyphen. In *Handbook of Critical Indigenous Methodologies*. Edited by Norman K. Denzin, Yvonna S. Lincoln and Linda Tuhiwai Smith. New York: Sage Publications, pp. 471–87.

Krentz, Adrienne, Judy Chew, and Nancy Arthur. 2005. Recovery from Binge Eating Disorder. *Canadian Journal of Counselling* 39: 118–35.

LaMarre, Andrea, and Carla Rice. 2016. Normal eating is counter-cultural: Embodied experiences of eating disorder recovery. *Journal of Community and Applied Social Psychology* 26: 136–49. [CrossRef]

LaMarre, Andrea, and Carla Rice. 2017. Hashtag recovery: #Eating disorder recovery on Instagram. *Social Sciences* 6: 68.

Lamoureux, Mary M. H., and Joan L. Bottorff. 2005. "Becoming the real me": Recovering from anorexia nervosa. *Health Care for Women International* 26: 170–88. [CrossRef]

Lea, Troy, P. Scott Richards, Peter W. Sanders, Jason A. McBride, and G. E. Kawika Allen. 2015. Spiritual pathways to healing and recovery: An intensive single-n study of an eating disorder patient. *Spirituality in Clinical Practice* 2: 191–201. [CrossRef]

Lester, Rebecca J. 2019. *Famished: Eating Disorders and Failed Care in America*. Berkeley: University of California Press.

Levy, Gary, Christine Halse, and Jan Wright. 2016. Down the methodological rabbit hole: Thinking diffractively with resistant data. *Qualitative Research* 16: 183–97. [CrossRef]

Limes-Taylor Henderson, Kelly, and Jennifer Esposito. 2019. Using others in the nicest way possible: On colonial and academic practice(s), and an ethic of humility. *Qualitative Inquiry* 25: 876–89. [CrossRef]

Lock, James, W. Stewart Agras, Daniel Le Grange, Jennifer Couturier, Debra Safer, and Susan W. Bryson. 2013. Do end of treatment assessments predict outcome at follow-up in eating disorders? *International Journal of Eating Disorders* 46: 771–78. [CrossRef]

Lord, Vanessa M., Wendy Reiboldt, Dariella Gonitzke, Emily Parker, and Caitlin Peterson. 2018. Experiences of recovery in binge-eating disorder: A qualitative approach using online message boards. *Eating and Weight Disorders* 23: 95–105. [CrossRef] [PubMed]

Lupton, Deborah, and Ash Watson. 2021. Towards more-than-human digital data studies: Developing research-creation methods. *Qualitative Research* 21: 463–80. [CrossRef]

Maclure, Maggie. 2013. The wonder of data. *Cultural Studies-Critical Methodologies* 13: 228–32. [CrossRef]

Malson, Helen. 1998. *The Thin Woman: Feminism, Post-Structuralism and the Social Psychology of Anorexia Nervosa*. New York: Routledge.

Malson, Helen, D. M. Finn, Janet Treasure, Simon Clarke, and Gail Anderson. 2004. Constructing "the eating disordered patient": A discourse analysis of accounts of treatment experiences. *Journal of Community and Applied Social Psychology* 14: 473–89. [CrossRef]

Malson, Helen, Lin Bailey, Simon Clarke, Janet Treasure, Gail Anderson, and Michael Kohn. 2011. Un/imaginable future selves: A discourse analysis of in-patients' talk about recovery from an "eating disorder". *European Eating Disorders Review* 19: 25–36. [CrossRef] [PubMed]

Manning, Erin, and Brian Massumi. 2014. *Thought in the Act: Passages in the Ecology of Experience*. Minneapolis: University of Minnesota Press.

Masny, Diana. 2013. Rhizoanalytic pathways in qualitative research. *Qualitative Inquiry* 19: 339–48. [CrossRef]

Matoff, Michelle L., and Sabrina A. Matoff. 2001. Eating disorder recovery: Learning from the client's healing Journey. *Women & Therapy* 23: 43–54.

Matusek, Jill Anne, and Roger M. Knudson. 2009. Rethinking recovery from ED: Spiritual and political dimensions. *Qualitative Health Research* 19: 697–707. [CrossRef]

Miller, Tina. 2017. Telling the difficult things: Creating spaces for disclosure, rapport and 'collusion' in qualitative interviews. *Women's Studies International Forum* 61: 81–86. [CrossRef]

Mulderrig, Jane. 2019. The language of 'nudge' in health policy: Pre-empting working class obesity through 'biopedagogy'. *Critical Policy Studies* 13: 101–21. [CrossRef]

Musolino, Connie, Megan Warin, Tracey Wade, and Peter Gilchrist. 2016. Developing shared understandings of recovery and care: A qualitative study of women with eating disorders who resist therapeutic care. *Journal of Eating Disorders* 4: 1–10. [CrossRef] [PubMed]

Patching, Joanna, and Jocalyn Lawler. 2009. Understanding women's experiences of developing an ED and recovery: A life-history approach. *Nursing Inquiry* 16: 10–21. [CrossRef]

Peterson, Carol B., Carolyn Black Becker, Janet Treasure, Roz Shafran, and Rachel Bryant-Waugh. 2016. The three-legged stool of evidence-based practice in eating disorder treatment: Research, clinical, and patient perspectives. *BMC Medicine* 14: 69. [CrossRef] [PubMed]

Pietrzyk, Susan. 2009. Artistic activities and cultural activism as responses to HIV/AIDS in Harare, Zimbabwe. *African Journal of AIDS Research* 8: 481–90. [CrossRef] [PubMed]

Pihama, Leonie. 2001. Tīhei Mauri Ora, Honouring Our Voices. Unpublished Ph.D. thesis, Auckland University, Auckland, New Zealand.

Redenbach, Joanna, and Jocalyn Lawler. 2003. Recovery from disordered eating: What life histories reveal. *Contemporary Nurse* 15: 148–56. [CrossRef]

Renold, Emma. 2018. 'Feel what I feel': Making da(r)ta with teen girls for creative activisms on how sexual violence matters. *Journal of Gender Studies* 27: 37–55. [CrossRef]

Rice, Carla, Eliza Chandler, and Nadine Changfoot. 2016. Imagining otherwise: The ephemeral spaces of envisioning new meanings. In *Mobilizing Metaphor: Art, Culture and Disability Activism in Canada*. Edited by Christine Kelly and Michael Orsini. Vancouver: University of British Columbia Press, pp. 54–75.

Rice, Carla, Eliza Chandler, Jen Rinaldi, Nadine Changfoot, Kirsty Liddiard, Roxanne Mykitiuk, and Ingrid Mündel. 2017. Imagining disability futurities. *Hypatia: A Journal of Feminist Philosophy* 32: 213–29. [CrossRef]

Rice, Carla, Katie Cook, and K. Alysse Bailey. 2021. Difference-attuned witnessing: Risks and potentialities of arts-based research. *Feminism & Psychology* 31: 345–65.

Richmond, Tracy K., G. Alice Woolverton, Kathy Mammel, Rollyn M. Ornstein, Allegra Spalding, Elizabeth R. Woods, and Sara F. Forman. 2020. How do you define recovery? A qualitative study of patients with eating disorders, their parents, and clinicians. *International Journal of Eating Disorders* 53: 1209–18. [CrossRef]

Riley, Sarah, Adrienne Evans, and Alison Mackiewicz. 2016. It's just between girls: Negotiating the postfeminist gaze in women's 'looking talk'. *Feminism & Psychology* 26: 94–113.

Rinaldi, Jen, Andrea LaMarre, and Carla Rice. 2016. Recovering bodies: The production of the recoverable subject in eating disorder treatment regimes. In *Learning Bodies: The Body in Youth and Childhood Studies*. Edited by Julia Coffey, Shelley Budgeon and Helen Cahill. Singapore: Springer Press, pp. 157–70.

Saukko, Paula. 2008. *The Anorexic Self: A Personal, Political Analysis of a Diagnostic Discourse*. New York: SUNY Press.

Saunders, Jessica F., and Asia A. Eaton. 2018. Social comparisons in eating disorder recovery: Using PhotoVoice to capture the sociocultural influences on women's recovery. *International Journal of Eating Disorders* 51: 1361–66. [CrossRef] [PubMed]

Shohet, Merav. 2007. Narrating anorexia: "full" and "struggling" genres of recovery. *Ethos* 35: 344–82. [CrossRef]

Shohet, Merav. 2018. Beyond the clinic? Eluding a medical diagnosis of anorexia through narrative. *Transcultural Psychiatry* 55: 495–515. [CrossRef] [PubMed]

Simmonds, Naomi. 2011. Mana wahine: Decolonising politics. *Women's Studies Journal* 25: 11–25.

Sinha, Sarmila, and Nasir Warfa. 2013. Treatment of eating disorders among ethnic minorities in Western settings: A systematic review. *Psychiatria Danubina* 25 (Suppl. 2): 295–99.

Springgay, Stephanie, and Sarah E. Truman. 2018. On the need for methods beyond proceduralism: Speculative middles,(in) tensions, and response-ability in research. *Qualitative Inquiry* 24: 203–14. [CrossRef]

St. Pierre, Elizabeth Adams. 1997. Methodology in the fold and the irruption of transgressive data. *International Journal of Qualitative Studies in Education* 10: 175–89. [CrossRef]

Steinhausen, Hans-Christoph. 2009. Outcome of eating disorders. *Child and Adolescent Psychiatric Clinics of North America* 18: 225–42. [CrossRef]

Thompson, Becky W. 1994. *A Hunger So Wide and So Deep: American Women Speak Out on Eating Problems*. Minneapolis: University of Minnesota Press.

Viscardis, Katharine, Carla Rice, Victoria Pileggi, Angela Underhill, Eliza Chandler, Nadine Changfoot, Phyllis Montgomery, and Roxanne Mykitiuk. 2019. Difference within and without: Health care providers' engagement with disability arts. *Qualitative Health Research* 29: 1287–98. [CrossRef]

Weiss, Gail. 2008. *Refiguring the Ordinary*. Bloomington: Indiana University Press.
Woods, Susan. 2004. Untreated recovery from eating disorders. *Adolescence* 39: 361–71.

Disclaimer/Publisher's Note: The statements, opinions and data contained in all publications are solely those of the individual author(s) and contributor(s) and not of MDPI and/or the editor(s). MDPI and/or the editor(s) disclaim responsibility for any injury to people or property resulting from any ideas, methods, instructions or products referred to in the content.

MDPI AG
Grosspeteranlage 5
4052 Basel
Switzerland
Tel.: +41 61 683 77 34
www.mdpi.com

Social Sciences Editorial Office
E-mail: socsci@mdpi.com
www.mdpi.com/journal/socsci

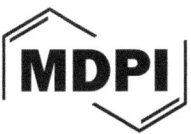

Disclaimer/Publisher's Note: The statements, opinions and data contained in all publications are solely those of the individual author(s) and contributor(s) and not of MDPI and/or the editor(s). MDPI and/or the editor(s) disclaim responsibility for any injury to people or property resulting from any ideas, methods, instructions or products referred to in the content.

www.ingramcontent.com/pod-product-compliance
Lightning Source LLC
LaVergne TN
LVHW072342090526
838202LV00019B/2464

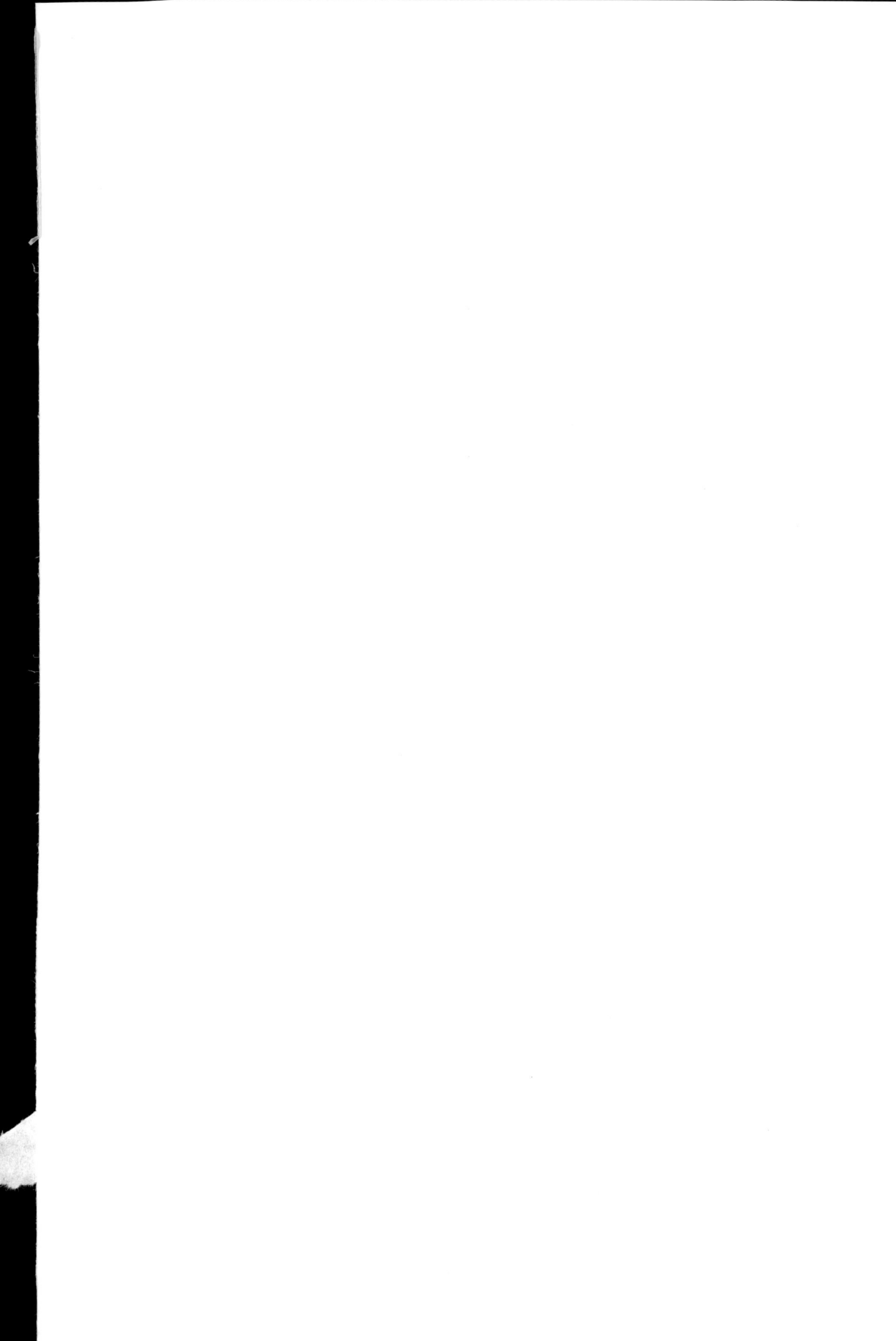